Veins of Devotion

Studies in Medical Anthropology

Edited by Mac Marshall

Veins of Devotion

Blood Donation and Religious Experience in North India

JACOB COPEMAN

RUTGERS UNIVERSITY PRESS

NEW BRUNSWICK, NEW JERSEY, AND LONDON

LIBRARY OF CONGRESS CATALOGING-IN-PUBLICATION DATA

Copeman, Jacob.

Veins of devotion: blood donation and religious experience in north India / Jacob
    Copeman.
p. cm.—(Studies in medical anthropology)
Includes bibliographical references and index.
ISBN 978–0–8135–4448–9 (hardcover: alk. paper)—ISBN 978–0–8135–4449–6
(pbk.: alk. paper)
1. Blood—Collection and preservation—India—Delhi. 2. Blood donors—India—Delhi.
3. Blood—Social aspects—India—Delhi. 4. Blood—Religious aspects. 5. Kinship—India—
Delhi. I. Title.
    RM171.C588 2009
    615.′39095456—dc22   2008016733

A British Cataloging-in-Publication record for this book is
available from the British Library.

Visit our Web site: http://rutgerspress.rutgers.edu

Manufactured in the United States of America

CONTENTS

ACKNOWLEDGMENTS

From the end of 2003 to the beginning of 2005 I lived for fifteen months in an inner-city colony of Delhi. On my arrival in the metropolis, my intention was to pursue a study that would be classically anthropological, insofar as I wished to document holistically the interrelations between voluntary blood donation activity and kinship, politics, economics, and religion. While I did indeed collect data on each of these themes, for reasons of space and coherence this book has ended up focusing primarily on religious aspects of blood donation. It was never my intention to limit the study to Delhi, and I also spent stretches of time in West Bengal, Mumbai, Haryana, Chennai, and even Beijing at an International Red Cross and World Health Organization conference on techniques to promote voluntary blood donation. This is therefore a pan-Indian study of blood donation activity with an ethnographic emphasis on north India, and Delhi in particular.

I interacted with and gathered information on a very large number of different organizations connected with blood donation. Where it seems apt I provide background information on their activities, but allotting an introductory paragraph to each of them would result in constant interruptions to the flow of the argument, so I have included a glossary that provides some details on each of them.

My stay in Delhi was made highly enjoyable through the care and friendship of many. For their warm companionship I am particularly grateful to Neera Bawa, Rachel Berger, Chandan and Gautam Bose, Tim Bray, James Drennan, Rachin Goel, the Gupta family, Satish Kumar Jha, Yunrong Jhang, Sandhya Krishnamurthy, Nishi Mittal, Sudhir Singh, Vijay Singh, and Saroj Thapar.

I am obliged to all those who took time to talk with me and explain things to me. In Delhi I am indebted above all to Neera Bawa and Naresh Kumar Bhatia, who each sacrificed large amounts of their time to provide seemingly limitless fascinating insights. Tim Bray, too, was a very generous guide to the themes I was exploring, as was Kiran Chaudhary. I am also grateful to the following people for sharing with me their time and knowledge: Kavita Chatterjee, Poonam Coshic, S. P. Jindal, Alok Kumar, the late Aneeta Minocha, M. L. Sarin, Bharat Singh, Brigadier Shamsher Singh, Sonu Singh, R. K. Soni, Poonam Srivastava, and

Mahesh Trivedi. I am additionally grateful to everyone at the Red Cross and Rotary blood banks in Delhi, and to all those at the Sant Nirankari Mandal's Social Welfare Vibhag. In Kolkata, Debabrata Ray was an exceptionally kind host, as were others in the Association of Voluntary Blood Donors, West Bengal, including P. M. Banerjee, Ranjit Roy Chaudhury, Sujit Kumar Datta, Subrata Ray, and Prasanta Sankar Sanyal. Also in Kolkata, Saumyendra Nath Brahmachary and the late Father Gerard Beckers were extremely accommodating and helpful. Whilst in Mumbai I received generous assistance from Yogini Patel, B. C. Mehta, and Ameya Naik. I would also like to thank Graeme Woodfield for his insights and encouragement. I am grateful to Prasannanshu and Urvashi Prasannanshu Jain for their warm friendship and extremely helpful practical assistance.

In Cambridge, my greatest debt is to Susan Bayly, who has been a truly committed and inspiring academic guide. The encouragement and guidance of James Laidlaw has also been critical for the coming to fruition of this book, as has the example of his scholarship. Also in the Cambridge Department of Social Anthropology, I have benefited greatly from the support and generosity of Alan Macfarlane and Marilyn Strathern. A conversation with Perveez Mody proved an important and fruitful route into the topic analyzed in this book. I would in addition like to thank Olivier Allard, Alina Bakunina, Rachel Berger, Andrew Brown, Matthew Carey, Mishko Hansen, Tod Hartman, Sarah Hodges, Kriti Kapila, Norbert Peabody, Deepa Reddy, and Rupa Viswanath for kindly commenting on earlier chapter versions. I am particularly grateful to Nathaniel Roberts, Alice Street, and Denis Vidal for many extremely helpful suggestions. Bernhard Krieger kindly helped me with diagrams. Advice from Bob Harwood and encouragement from Erica Bornstein and Jane Springham is also much appreciated.

Jesus College has provided an extremely supportive and congenial environment for the preparation of this book. I am grateful to the Master and Fellows and in particular to Geoff Harcourt, Tim Jenkins, and Nick Ray for their advice and companionship.

I am grateful to the Royal Anthropological Institute of Great Britain and Ireland for permission to reprint here my own material previously published as an article in the *Journal of the Royal Anthropological Institute* ("Violence, Non-Violence, and Blood Donation in India," 2008). The two anonymous reviewers for Rutgers University Press both subsequently revealed their identities to me: Joseph Alter and Lawrence Cohen brought to their reports an extremely stimulating and insightful engagement, from which I have profited greatly.

I am grateful to the Economic and Social Research Council for the two awards which have been my principal financial support. I also thank the Isaac Newton Trust, the Cambridge Department of Social Anthropology's Wyse Fund Committee and Trinity Hall for financial awards. I am indebted to those who gave permission to cite their as yet unpublished works.

The wonderful hospitality of my grandmother, Ann Copeman, deserves special mention. My frequent stays with her in Norfolk provided a superb haven for writing. I would also like to acknowledge the loving care and support given to me during the writing process by my parents, Janet Forsyth and Christopher Copeman, and by my sister, Amy Copeman. It is to my mother, with love and gratitude, that this book is dedicated.

Veins of Devotion

1

Introduction

In 2002 the spiritual head, or guru, of the Beas branch of the Radhasoami movement was given a guided tour of the newly established Rotary blood bank in Delhi. According to the blood bank's director, Dr. N. K. Bhatia, the guru "was extremely happy, he blessed us all, he had some snacks with us, he even took a Coke." Later the guru granted a private audience to a member of the blood bank team. At its conclusion, he presented her with *prashad*, sanctified substance imparted to devotees in token of the guru's divine favor, often consisting of sweets, flowers, and other "leavings." In this instance, the prashad consisted of a small packet of sweets and a piece of paper. On the paper was written: "Every month, one camp." The prashad, in other words, took the form of a promise. The guru would instruct his devotees to organize blood donation events (known as camps, or in Hindi, *shibir*) throughout the year at their different places of worship. Having toured the blood bank, the guru thus offered up his numerous devotees as a new and vital blood donor constituency.

In India as elsewhere, the transfusion and donation of blood are far from being purely technical processes restricted to medics concerned with practical medical matters. Rather, they are procedures that transcend their official purposes, and that, in so doing, shed light on multiple aspects of social life. This book tells the story of the complex intertwinings that have developed over recent years between reform-minded north Indian devotional orders and campaigns to foster voluntary blood donation among the Indian population. Focusing in particular on the situation in Delhi, it documents and interprets the blood donation operations of several high-profile religious movements that organize gargantuan public blood-giving assemblages (camps) involving vast numbers of people, and other heavily publicized campaigns of record-breaking proportions as conspicuous acts of service (*seva*). Blood donation, I shall argue, has become a site not only of frenetic competition between devotional orders

1

but also of intense spiritual creativity. In addition, I explore the persuasive activities of "donor recruiters." These are the blood bank staff and public health officials responsible for increasing the number of voluntary blood donors in India, and whose proselytizing attempts to appeal to all sorts of sentiments of altruism, status seeking, and spirituality in ways that either reflect or cut across existing Indian ideas about virtue, service, kinship, and the nation. This study also situates blood donation within the context of classic themes in the anthropology of giving and exchange, exploring in particular the complex relationship between blood donation, known in Hindi as *rakt-dan*, and Indic *dan* (gift, donation) concepts.

The backdrop to the study is recent legislation initiated by the Indian medical establishment that seeks to stop blood banks from accepting blood on the basis of payment to individual donors and also seeks to end the prevailing ad hoc family-based system of provision. The public policy orthodoxy that informs the legislation asserts that the safety of donated blood is far greater when deriving from voluntary, nonremunerated donors in an anonymous system of procurement.[1] This orthodoxy is supported and maintained by the international arbiters of health policy and funding, the World Health Organization and the International Federation of Red Cross and Red Crescent Societies, both of which subscribe to the findings of influential British policy analyst Richard Titmuss (1970) that voluntary blood donation provides the safest blood for transfusion. Titmuss's study focused on the United Kingdom and the United States, but Indian studies also show that Transfusion Transmissible Infection (TTI) rates are two to three times higher in nonvoluntarily donated blood (Bray 2001; Nanu et al. 1997). Most, though not all, Western countries practice centralized voluntary systems of provision. Blood donation was introduced to India in 1925 when a transfusion center was founded at the School of Tropical Diseases and Medicine in Calcutta, though it was not until 1942 that India's first fully functioning blood bank was established under a government order at Calcutta's All India Institute of Hygiene and Public Health in order to meet the war need (Ray 2003: 32). Since then, the two most common forms of donation have been paid donation and "family replacement" donation—where family members donate to replace the blood withdrawn from the blood bank to treat their ailing relative. India's Supreme Court banned paid donation from 1 January 1998 and directed the government to begin actively encouraging voluntary, nonremunerated blood donation. The government's subsequent National Blood Policy (2002) additionally required the phasing out of replacement donation within five years.[2]

The banning of paid donation, and the phasing out of replacement donation, has required innovative strategies on the part of blood banks, supported by a government body, the National AIDS Control Organization (NACO), to radically increase voluntary blood donation. Despite the assortment of campaigns, however, replacement donation still accounts for more than 50 percent of all donated blood in India. There are striking state-by-state variations: in West Bengal, 90 percent of donations are voluntary. Maharashtra, Gujarat, and Chandigargh also possess healthy voluntary figures. In Delhi, however, less than 19 percent of the total collection comprises voluntary donation.[3]

Though the set of campaigns to foster voluntary donation has faltered, there is one important success story: over recent years religious movements, in particular those led by gurus, have become essential providers of voluntarily donated blood throughout India. In the north of the country, religious movements in the *sant* tradition are most prominent. The Sant Nirankari Mission and the Dera Sacha Sauda devotional orders, the subjects of chapters 4 and 5 respectively, are particularly high-profile contributors. Also in the sant tradition, the Radhasoamis (Beas branch) are prolific collectors in Delhi, as are devotees attached to one of its offshoots, the Sawan Kirpal Ruhani Mission. But religious blood donation activities are also pursued by a wide range of other spiritual organizations: I attended scores of camps organized by Hindu temples, churches, *gurdwaras* (Sikh places of worship), and devotees of Sathya Sai Baba and the Maharashtrian guru Aniruddha Bapu. The devotees of another Maharashtrian guru, Narendra Maharaj, are reported to give blood in large numbers. Devotees of Kerala guru Mata Amritanandamayi also arrange blood donation events (Warrier 2003a: 269). In Mumbai, the Limbdi Ajramar Jains collect huge quantities, and according to Rajasthani blood banking personnel I met at a Kolkata blood donation conference, Jain seva (service) groups in the state collect more blood than any other social service organization. They are reported, for instance, to have exceeded their target of collecting 2,600 units in 2001, the year of Lord Mahavira's 2,600th birth anniversary.[4] I believe that similar activities are to be found in most other parts of India.

Religious organizations are by no means the only contributors to the drive to increase levels of voluntary donation—donation camps are also staged in educational, political, and business settings. The primary focus of this study, however, is on the hitherto unrecognized role of religious organizations in the voluntary donation of blood in India. This is the case for adherents of a very wide range of faiths in India, though is particularly important for movements and devotional networks professing modernist and social reformist aims and values. The study of the enactment of blood donation (*rakt-dan*) by these movements enables me to explore important and widespread new developments in urban religious life through a focus on the interaction between utility and religious thought and practice, and to investigate the ways in which a "Western" biomedical technique has come to be employed by various gurus and sets of devotees for the pursuit of reformist Hindu and Sikh spiritual projects.[5] There is nothing one-sided about the process: blood-giving devotional orders and the project to foster voluntary blood donation evolve together and exchange their properties. Devotees rearticulate blood donation and load it with complex devotional logics in precisely the same process through which the precepts of medical utility are instilled squarely at the heart of these devotional orders' emergent theologies.

Following from this, a key aim of this study is to challenge widespread anthropological characterizations of utility as something diametrically opposed to culture, ethics, and qualitative value. This kind of dichotomy is particularly widespread in the medical anthropology literature on corporeal donation.[6] I shall argue that in the contemporary north Indian devotional and social reformist milieu, this opposition does not hold, and that in a variety of contexts including but not limited to blood donation, utility has been elevated to the stature of virtuousness—hence my term "virtuous utility," discussed in chapter 3, and the concept of "religions of utility," which I employ to refer to what I identify as the phenomenon of utility valorizing devotional orders and spiritual movements.[7] I do not mean by this that these are religions of valueless instrumentality, but that utility has been instilled by them with varying virtuous, richly ethical properties, which make utility precisely irreducible to mere instrumentality.

The term "interoperability," usually used to refer to two or more sets of software able to work harmoniously together, is a helpful epithet for describing the interaction between voluntary blood donation and the devotional orders in question. "Interoperability," states one definition, refers not only to the ability of two or more entities to work in conjunction but also to their ability to contribute usefully to each other's priorities and aims. The concept is particularly helpful, I think, in focusing attention on the practical nature of the operational processes involved when different systems may come to interlock and work through each other. This study argues that voluntary donation and various religious movements are interoperable with, on the one hand, gurus' devotees donating their blood in large quantities, thus contributing decisively to the project of voluntary blood donation, and on the other, the experience of blood donation opening up new devotional possibilities for devotees, while lending tangible force and dynamism to certain of the movements' doctrinal tenets. The collaboration between blood banks and devotional orders is also, of course, marked by numerous tensions and divergent interests, and these are delineated as the study progresses; nonetheless, both entities have come to work through each other in a manner that could be described as "interoperable."[8]

The Sant Tradition

In north India, the three most prominent devotional orders that collaborate with blood banks to organize blood donation camps at their places of worship are the Sant Nirankari Mission (1929), the Radhasoamis (1861), and the Dera Sacha Sauda (1948), each of which, though relatively recent in origin, has arisen out of and draws deeply on the north Indian sant heritage. The Nirankari Mission first began to collect the blood of its devotees in the 1980s, the other movements more recently since 2000.[9] In all of them, though, blood donation is treated now as established convention. Of the three, only the Radhasoami tradition, with its greater number of devotees, has been the object of scholarly study (see Juergensmeyer 1991, 1995; Babb 1986). This movement, though distinct and separate, shares many values and beliefs with the Dera Sacha Sauda and Nirankari Mission. Common to each is *guru-bhakti*—devotion to a living spiritual master, devotee constituencies made up of both Hindus and Sikhs, an emphasis on the recitation of sacred words, a conception of transcendence as being open to all in this birth regardless of caste or gender, a social reformist agenda, and a set of teachings genealogically derived from a family of nonsectarian sants, or saints, which began to emerge in the medieval period.[10] The point about nonsectarianism is important. The sant tradition is not exclusively Hindu or Sikh but venerates the teachings of sants who have been important and influential in each religion. In the devotional contexts explored in chapters 3–6 of this study, distinctions between Hindus and non-Hindus and indeed distinctions of caste and other internal differentiations of "community" are downplayed in favor of shared devotional attachment to a spiritual master.

The fourteenth and fifteenth centuries saw an efflorescence of sant poets such as Kabir, Nanak, Ravi Das, and Nam Dev. Most espoused versions of *bhakti*, defined by Vaudeville (1974: 97) as "a religious attitude which implies a 'participation' in the deity and a love relationship between the individual soul, the *jiva*, and the Supreme Lord, *Bhagavan*, the 'adorable one.'" These sants, often seen as Vaishnavite, though also influenced by Shaivite bhakti, gathered followers and formed communities of mainly low-caste laymen (van der Veer 1988: 91). It has been argued that sant associations underwent "gentrification" in the eighteenth century, with an increase of followers from merchant communities (D. Gold 1992: 33). Though this is borne out to some extent in present-day sant movements, with initiates deriving from a very wide stratum of Indian caste and class groups (see Juergensmeyer 1995), the majority of Nirankari and Dera Sacha Sauda devotees, in my experience at least, remain fairly economically disadvantaged. The implications of this deprivation, as it relates to Nirankari blood donation, are a focus of chapter 4.

Schaller emphasizes the non-Brahmanical tone of much sant poetry. Ravi Das, for example, portrayed Brahmins as proud and hypocritical lovers of empty ritual (Schaller 1995: 106–107). Many sants were themselves from low-status and generally lower-caste backgrounds, and taught that all human births are rare and valuable—not only those of Brahmins (Lorenzen 1995: 18, 24). This kind of social criticism persists in present-day sant movements, which uniformly criticize elaborate ritual, idol worship, and virtuoso displays of asceticism (see chapters 3–5). Devotion, not ritual prowess or caste, so the sants proclaimed, is the determinant of one's worth and ability to attain liberation. Though the all-pervading godhead described in sant poetry is meant to be "without attributes" (*nirguna*), the presiding guru-sants are themselves worshiped. In the case of the Nirankaris, devotees' simultaneous worship of *nirankar* (formless god) and the concrete *form* of the *satguru* appears to allow the Mission to construct itself as superior to idol worshipers (criticized at worship gatherings) while at the same time continuing to worship a living idol.

The Beas (Punjab) branch of the Radhasoami movement is an important provider of voluntarily donated blood in Delhi. Its literature self-consciously employs modern, scientific language—one leader even describing the movement as a "science of the soul" (Juergensmeyer 1991: 51). Some Radhasoami devotees connect their having moved "beyond" idol worship with their enthusiastic approach to blood donation. Several times at Radhasoami donation camps, I heard devotees contrast their own desire to donate blood with people outside the movement who refused to donate on account of "misguided" fears about the physical consequences of donation. Other Indians were idol worshipers, they said, as if that explained their reluctance to donate blood. Belonging to a "scientific" faith, devotees could, in contrast to "benighted" idol worshipers, demonstrate the fact by donating their blood.

Not all sant movements are based around revered living gurus, but the Radhasoami, Nirankari, and Dera Sacha Sauda are, and this has created tensions between them and mainstream Sikhs, for whom the guru is an abstract, trans-historical entity, meant to reside within and not outside the devotee. The final living Sikh guru, Gobind Singh, proclaimed in 1708 that the spiritual energies of the guru had been transferred into the Sikh sacred book, the Adi Granth, thus effectively proscribing the emergence of future human gurus. Juergensmeyer (1991: 85–86) notes that this issue causes Radhasoami-Sikh relations to become fraught from time to time. As chapter 4 illustrates, violent clashes between Nirankaris and mainstream Sikhs over this and other matters played a significant role in the institutionalization of blood donation as an important feature of Nirankari religious life.

Worship among these movements consists largely of devotional singing (*bhajan*), regular gatherings (*satsang*) at which devotees listen to the guru's discourses, and service of the guru (*guru-seva*).[11] The notion of guru-seva is particularly important in this study because devotees' donation of their blood is undertaken as an aspect of this devotional prerequisite. Though gurus say blood donation is *manav-seva* (service of humanity), devotees view it just as much as guru-seva, since it is their gurus who ask them to do it and who, in effect, their donation activities serve to glorify. Juergensmeyer (1991: 127–146) has demonstrated the central role of seva activities in the Radhasoami movement, and this is equally true of the Dera Sacha Sauda and Nirankari Mission (discussed in chapters 3 and 4). Analogous to the making of offerings and sacrifices in a

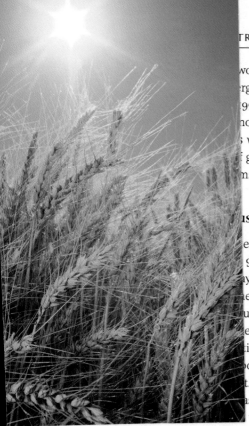

worship and praise and is a critical means of
rgensmeyer 1991: 142). Warrier (2003a), Mayer
996: 9, 140) have additionally highlighted the
nore obviously "Hindu" guru-led institutions
s would suggest, these sant movements form
gurus, and it is in relation to them as much
nselves.

is and Organs

ents based in Rishikesh, and their links with
9) compares gurus with corporate managers
ays, "desire to control subordinates." Gurus,
en" whose attempts to enchant the material
uent consumer-devotees "occult the greed,
eir status as spiritual leaders" (ibid.: 23). In
ical economy of spirituality, McKean draws
ower and domination that any study of guru
t. To be sure, devotees' often unquestioning
s placing them in the gurus' captive power.
the "ideology" of spirituality camouflages,
occults, or masks what McKean calls "exploitative social relations of production
and exchange" ends up, to employ her own term, "camouflaging" any sense of
the devotional specifics that constitute the religious experience of devotees.

McKean contrasts her approach with Babb's supposedly "deferential" attitude toward the three religious movements he explores in *Redemptive Encounters*
(1986). She feels that his professed respect for them blinds him to the movements' political aspects. If McKean had considered Juergensmeyer's study of the
Radhasoami faith, with his admission of holding a sympathetic attitude toward
it (1991: xi), the same criticism would in all likelihood have been leveled.
McKean's argument implies that scholars must make a choice between conducting a naïve engagement that pays heed to devotional specifics and experience, as Babb and Juergensmeyer do in their superbly nuanced and detailed
accounts, and adopting politically aware (and here she means Marxist)
approaches that see the anthropologist's task as one of political unmasking. But
the choice, I think, is an artificial one: the specifics of devotional practice and
experience and those of wider systems of authority need not be in some kind of
analytical zero-sum relationship. My study, which draws liberally on each of the
three aforementioned works, sees no contradiction between exploring and
acknowledging the undoubted power wielded by gurus and recognizing that
motivations for action are rarely if ever "simply political or politico-economic,"
with religion a cover for "thoroughly secular, more or less selfish ambitions"

(Geertz 2000: 178). I thus aim to shed light on both the mechanisms of control through which gurus are able seemingly at whim to establish their devotee bases as blood donor constituencies and the experiential basis on the level of the devotee of being thus mobilized. The point is straightforward: cognizance of the political economy of spiritual systems is imperative—I introduce below the notion of the captive voluntary devotee and conceptualize devotee populations directed by their gurus to donate blood as "donor banks" analogous to the vote banks hailed as mass bodies during Indian election campaigns—but this need not preclude exploration of the values and understandings of those who per-force live as the subjects of these systems.[12]

This book also aims to show that there is far more to the role of gurus in Indian society than "greed, guile and violence" (McKean 1996: 23). Chapters 4 and 6 delineate the important gateway function of gurus in the creation of "Indian moderns." Control over subordinates is a key factor in this but is not in itself sufficient to explain the complex and nuanced facilitative role of gurus in the production of specifically Indian versions of modernity. I argue below that voluntary blood donation in devotional contexts provides critical examples of gurus' wider gateway function—that is, their role as decisive points of access for their devotees into inimitable brands of guru-amended modernity which are irreducible to "Westernization."

The zero-sum analytical treatment of affect and experience on the one hand and political economy on the other is as evident in studies of biological exchange as it is in analyses of devotional movements. The anthropological lit-erature on corporeal transfers had until quite recently been largely character-ized by a logic of debunking and exposé that saw such forms of exchange in somewhat eviscerated terms as reducible to coercion, alienation, and/or mar-ketization. There was rarely any sense in these studies of corporeal donations arising from active, reflective choice on the part of donors. According to such studies, one does not have to be poor to make a corporeal gift, but those who do offer such gifts without being explicitly compelled by debt or as a result of illicit extraction during operations are depicted as being mystified by a predatory ide-ology of extraction masquerading as "gift of life." Such an emphasis on compulsion and false consciousness in discussions of biological exchange has prevented attentiveness to the emergent forms of ethical life grounded in such modes of exchange, as well as their affective bases. Scholars such as Lock (2002, 2007) and Scheper-Hughes (1996, 2004) have been active in highlighting that "the body yields gifts that are deeply problematic" (Simpson 2004: 842), and indeed have established beyond doubt that in numerous sociocultural contexts the body parts of the exploitable poor follow a trajectory upward to the rich. The problem is that such moral commentaries frequently exceed the specificity of the examples discussed, with all biological exchange consequently being cast into the realm of the piratical.

If analyses take as axiomatic that the "gift of life" is merely a "seductive metaphor" (Lock 2002: 207), or begin from a moral position that sees tissue exchange as always already subject to the demands of a rapacious, "gift-wrapped" (Ohnuki-Tierney 1994), and ever more biologically intrusive ideology of late capitalism, then much that is compelling and distinctive about these economies is elided. What, for instance, of ethical self-fashioning? What of possible "marriage[s] of responsibility and faith" (Derrida 1995: 6)? Laidlaw (2002: 324) claims that "by describing the different technologies of the self, one can tell the story of the different ways in which people have purposefully made themselves into certain kinds of person." This, as Laidlaw says, would be subject to existing biopolitical possibilities and in accordance with various constraining norms and regulations. This study attempts to recover a space of the "biospiritual" on this contested anthropological terrain, to give due recognition to the subtle "donation theologies" that have arisen around blood donation, and to show that people can make themselves into certain kinds of distinct person through innovative responses to admonitions to give of themselves.[13] Avoiding analytical moral panic, I seek to show that interpellation by what some have portrayed as a mystifying ideology of "gift of life" does not necessarily strangle the possibilities for ethical self-fashioning as well as theological originality in these contexts. I do not argue that attentiveness to emergent forms of ethicoreligious life should replace the existing focus on political economy but rather that it be insinuated into this focus as a bulwark against existing tendencies toward analytical delimitation.

Cohen (2007) too has noted the panicked language of ardor and elision that pervades many commentaries on biological exchange, a language which seems to suggest that "there is a universal practice of taking organs from the poor." Cohen's (2004: 169) own concept of "bioavailability," a contingency "organized variously around the loving or charitable gift, the commoditized sale, or the authoritarian or piratical forced extraction or seizure," is an important refinement.[14] Though the term seems principally designed for application to populations rendered bioavailable by way of their socioeconomic status—this reflecting Cohen's own ethnographic focus on the recruitment into the organs trade of women in a south Indian "kidney slum" (1999, 2001)—the concept is flexible enough to cover instances of both self-authorized bioavailability and complexly ethicized engagements with medical science concerning tissue supply. For instance, chapter 4 demonstrates that the bioavailability of Sant Nirankari blood donors is on the one hand a kind of "vote bank bioavailability," with recruitment a product of conditioned reflexes to the exhortation of the guru, while at the same time showing that the biospiritual lies at the heart of devotees' bioavailability, with devotee-donors loading their acts of donation with a range of nuanced ideas concerning memorialization, asceticism, and spiritual transformation.

Other exceptions to the reductionism described earlier include Simpson's (2004) sensitive description of different forms of biological exchange in Sri Lanka and sophisticated works by Anagnost (2006) and Shao (2006) on the intricacies and perils of the Chinese blood economy. Also significant is Reddy's (2007) rich study of blood giving for research purposes among Indians in Houston, which portrays the blood sample as a complex form of technoscientific gift, mediated by saints, beloved politicians and other "broker" figures.[15] The mediatory role of the guru is considered at length in the present study: devotee-donors' gifts of blood, I argue below, travel both "to" and "through" the mediating figure of the guru to "humanity." Konrad's (1998, 2005) account of ova donation in Britain is particularly important among these works on biological exchange in providing a powerful critique of anthropological characterizations of anonymity. These, she argues, have tended to discount the imaginative possibilities of "not-knowing." If conventional anthropological treatments have portrayed anonymity as connotative of alienation, passivity, ahistoricity, and asociality, Konrad instead forcefully demonstrates that anonymity in the context of ova donation in Britain can produce "exciting connections between action and relatedness that cannot be reduced to the level of simple misrecognition or oblivious non-identity" (1998: 659).

Anonymity has been recognized as a key aspect of dan categories of Indian gift (A. Gold 1988: 9; Laidlaw 2000: 623; Parry 1994: 75, 80). The most virtuous kind of gift is that made anonymously to strangers. As I noted above, the voluntary gift of blood travels to unknown recipients. Thus, in contrast to the replacement model, the voluntary system is composed of anonymous gift transactions—the blood bank mediating between donors and recipients—and this makes it resemble dan as portrayed in some accounts of the "classical" Indic gift. I return below to the implications of this convergence between classical features of dan and rakt-dan. The point to emphasize here is that, like Konrad's study, this work provides evidence that anonymity need not be synonymous with alienation and passivity but may rather provide a kind of imaginative canvas for novel ideational maneuvers. In particular, this study demonstrates that anonymity is subject to numerous usages and deployments that possess striking spiritual, nationalist, and familial implications. What is particularly important is the way anonymity makes it possible for blood donation to almost mechanically transgress caste and community boundaries, and then for those involved in the donation to construct any number of possible meanings linked to this transgression. Chapter 4 on devotional blood giving examines the importance for the Sant Nirankaris of this mechanical transgression, while chapter 7 explores its nationalist implications.[16]

The anonymity of voluntary blood donation has been criticized in the Chinese case as an alienating contravention of a key tenet of Chinese cultural life, namely, that "gift giving produces reciprocal obligation in the context of building social relationships" (Erwin 2006: 150). Since anonymity between donors and recipients works effectively to block reciprocity (Konrad 2005: xii), it is considered by Erwin (2006: 150) to "contradict . . . the obligations of reciprocity embedded in Chinese kin and *guanxi* relations."[17] This study suggests something rather different; namely, that anonymity can open up new spaces of ideation and relational reckoning—what Konrad (2005: 6) calls "the creativity of non-linkage." I do not mean to suggest that the Indian experience of blood donation is free from disjunction and contrariety. Far from it. But what this study underscores are the ways in which Indian donor recruiters seek to extend existing cultural forms into new territories of signification in order that they may be made to accord with the project of fostering voluntary blood donation. Indeed, a key concern of this study is to explore the specifics of donor recruiters' complex methodology in engaging and operating existing Indian social structures in order to make them supportive of voluntary donation. Often, as I show below in chapter 3, this entails "parasiting" existing giving mechanisms to produce new outcomes that accord with medical utility. Donor recruiters, indeed, are at the vanguard of social change in the subcontinent.

Broken Processes

Returning home after attending a blood donation camp in Noida, south of Delhi, we were stuck in a traffic jam, the car windows wide open due to the torrid heat. A desperate-looking woman approached, holding up what looked like a bloodied rag. She pleaded: *Meri beti ke bacha hone wala hai, isliye ap meri madad karo—beti ka khun baha ja raha hai* ("My daughter is about to give birth to a child, therefore please help me—my daughter's blood is flowing incessantly"). The woman was requesting money in order to be able to pay for the blood required to save her daughter's life.

In most Western countries, such a situation would make no sense. When a transfusion is required, doctors arrange for blood, stored either locally in the hospital, or farther afield in regional storage centers, to be provided for the patient. Doctors thereby draw on the stocks managed by the Red Cross or the country's national blood service which collect blood, usually without payment, from roughly five or six people in every 1,000.[18] Most of these donors give their blood every three months—the officially prescribed time meant to elapse between donations—and are thus "regular, repeat voluntary donors." Worried relatives of the patient are not called on to contribute in any way, and may even be unaware that a transfusion has been called for. In India, on the other hand, where only 2 or 3 people in every 1,000 regularly donate their blood, the families of patients in need of transfusions are required by hospitals to donate their own blood in order to preemptively replace the blood withdrawn from blood banks for their relatives. (Doctors and donor recruiters commonly refer to a

WHO statistic which reports that, though 82 percent of the world's population resides in South Asia, only 13 percent of the world's donated blood is collected there.) In most cases a "processing charge," which ranges from Rs 500 to Rs 1,500 per unit, must also be paid. Government hospitals may waive this fee for the poorest patients, while still demanding replacement donations. Transfusions typically comprise several units of donated blood; six are often required for major surgery. The families of patients must therefore almost always organize donations from not one but several persons. Friends often help out, but the primary obligation of provision lies with the family.

The National AIDS Control Organization (NACO) and National and State Blood Transfusion Councils were established in the 1990s to promote voluntary donation and govern the operations of blood banks, of which there are three main types: government, NGO, and commercial. Government and commercial blood banks tend to be attached to hospitals, whereas NGO blood banks—the two that operated in Delhi at the time of my fieldwork, run respectively by the Indian Red Cross Society and the Rotary Club, have recently been joined by a third, run by the Lions Club—tend to be "stand-alone." Theoretically, one can donate voluntarily at any of these blood banks, though only government and NGO blood banks are allowed to take donor beds to donors, that is, to conduct voluntary blood donation camps at different locations. In Delhi, the Red Cross, Rotary, and Lions blood banks, along with a smattering of government institutions, conduct camps in collaboration with corporate, educational, religious, and political organizations, often at venues convenient to donors (for example, in their places of work or worship). At the time of my fieldwork, only the vanguard Rotary institution collected solely voluntarily donated blood, and did not demand replacement donations from the families of patients; the new Lions blood bank reportedly operates according to similar principles.

"At the city level," write Bray and Prabhakar (2002: 477), "there often appears intense rivalry between and within charitable and independent commercial blood banks and success is usually measured in terms of the number of units donated and hence the number of units transfused—the emphasis is on quantity but not quality." This rivalry extends to the organizing of camps. The Rotary and Red Cross institutions "steal" one another's camps by promising a particular firm, college, or spiritual organization a higher standard of service than the other is able to deliver. One of the reasons that the level of voluntary donation in Delhi has remained static over recent years is the tendency of blood banks to compete to collect from existing locations instead of directing their attention to finding new sources of collection. The proliferation of blood banks in the city—there were forty-one at the time of my fieldwork—has not resulted in more blood donations.[19]

The blood bank, "by mediating between donor and recipient . . . preserve[s] the distance that keeps the different parties separate and separable" (Konrad

2005: 23). It works, says Healy (2006), "to elicit blood donations from donors, to elaborate the meaning of the donation, and to specify the nature of the gift and the obligations that flow from it. This work involves both logistical and cultural effort. The result is a practical system of procurement and distribution, but also a moral order of exchange." The position of the blood banks that solicit voluntary donations, as with intermediaries in other settings (Vidal 2000: 138), is morally ambiguous. This stems from an apparent variance between the aforementioned logistical and cultural imperatives. Having been tasked by the Government of India with fostering disinterested (*nishkam*) voluntary blood donation in place of paid and deal-like replacement donation, blood banks charge recipients varying sums of money for what they receive "for free" from donors. This arouses suspicions among both donors and recipients that find their clearest anthropological expression in Sahlins's (1972: 160) adage that "one man's gift should not be another man's capital." As principal elaborator of the meaning of donation, the blood bank seeks to convert the replacement "deal" into a "selfless" (*niswarth*) offering. The problem, however, is that the very agent of gift purification in respect of donors appears to "degift" (Callon 1998: 36) the gift in respect of recipients; that is, blood banks fail to ensure that what is freely given to them is then made freely available (Reddy 2007: 435).[20]

Further contributing to the blood bank's moral ambiguity is controversy surrounding the Voluntary Blood Donor Card. These are given to voluntary donors, post-donation, and are meant to guarantee free blood, equivalent to the sum of that donated, for the donor and his or her immediate family for the duration of a year. In Mumbai, several blood banks have formed a federation guaranteeing to recognize and honor one another's cards. In Delhi, however, there is no such coordination. Thus, if an individual donates to a particular Delhi blood bank and is later admitted to a hospital affiliated to a different blood bank, they may find that the hospital will refuse to recognize their entitlement to receive the blood they need, even though they have a valid donor card. Therefore, while the cards are meant to be uniform, they are not necessarily treated as such. Such treatment at the hands of blood banks and hospitals understandably creates the feeling among donors that their efforts are not appreciated, and is almost certainly detrimental to efforts to increase voluntary donation.

According to one renowned Indian transfusion specialist, the blood transfusion services "in most of the developing countries in South Asia resemble their highways—chaotic, crowded and swarming with obstacles" (Bharucha 2000: 12). Doctors frequently complain that "the fragmentation grows, grows relentlessly" (Nanu 2004). A recent episode in Delhi, related to me by Dr. Bharat Singh, director of the Delhi State Blood Transfusion Council, epitomizes the problem. Dr. Singh had hoped in 2003 to create a computer system that would network the different blood banks in the city so that the families of patients could log on to the council Web site (http://www.bloodbanksdelhi.com) to view stock levels for particular blood groups at different blood banks. The purpose was to prevent relatives journeying fruitlessly from blood bank to blood bank trying to locate the correct match for a hospitalized family member. The council, however, does not have the power to enforce compliance, and only a handful of government blood banks chose to participate in the scheme. The Red Cross refused to make its stock figures public, since it anticipated the arrival at its blood bank of a deluge of family members eager to obtain blood for their relatives. The Rotary already had its own computer system and declined to coordinate it with the new network.

During my first few weeks in Delhi I thought of the different types of donation and blood bank I saw as resembling something like a structure with "fixed parameters but multiple states or systemic qualities" (Rosin n.d.). However, with several governing authorities, each of them unable to enforce the policies they promote, and competition rather than cooperation characterizing efforts to foster the transition to voluntary donation, in addition to the massive variability in people's experience of donation, the system's parameters are evidently more fluid than fixed, open to manipulation, and frankly difficult to comprehend at any given time. One visiting expert from the American Red Cross described what she saw as a set of "broken processes." This, of course, is not an ideal position from which to initiate coordinated messages designed to persuade a reluctant population to rally to the cause of voluntary donation.

Collaborative Communities

Indian blood donation activity does not offer up an obviously bounded or discrete community. I realized I would have to spend time following and tracking (Marcus 2002: 196) those whose views I sought and whose activities I wished to observe. But that is not to say I did not work with identifiable communities. Of the 1,832 blood banks in India (Ray 2003: 176), 41 were situated in Delhi at the time of my fieldwork. I visited roughly half of them. Though dispersed throughout the city, blood bank professionals meet and exchange recruitment ideas and technical expertise at common forums such as training workshops, conferences on donor motivation, and seminars on quality standards. As a collection of individuals who share a common professional environment, and who also acquire a degree of their identity from that environment, blood bank personnel—medics, technicians, and donor recruiters—may be considered a "community of practice" (Wenger 1998).

The organizational feat of procuring voluntarily donated blood is managed through collaboration between this medical community of practice and other communities of practice such as businesses and educational and religious institutions that conduct blood donation camps. When persons affiliated with different communities of practice coordinate in order to attempt to tackle or resolve a matter of mutual interest, a "community of interest" is formed (Arias and Fischer 2000). The different communities of practice I worked with come together to stage camps at which blood is donated, blood donation being their common concern. I thus studied multiple communities of practice, which, together, form a community of interest concerned with organizing and administering the giving of blood.

The multiplicity and diversity of the actors involved has led to a striking plurality of understandings arising around blood donation. As the concept and activity around which different communities of practice coordinate, blood donation is a "boundary object," an entity that " 'sits in the middle' of a group of actors with divergent viewpoints" (Star 1989: 46). A boundary object "holds different meanings in different social worlds, yet is imbued with enough shared meaning to facilitate its translation across those worlds" (McSherry 2001: 69). Blood donation sits in the middle of various different communities of practice, all of whom imbue the activity with their own contrasting practical, moral, and theological significances: while a doctor may see blood donation as an act of beneficent helpfulness with medical use-value, a Nirankari donor may see it as a means to effect religious conversion (see chapter 4). For a mourner, blood donation may be a way to pay tribute to the soul of the departed, while for a Sikh man with a psychologically disturbed wife it may be a means to remove the inauspiciousness afflicting his family (see chapter 3). The important point for donor recruiters aiming to foster voluntary blood donation is that interpretive alignments between blood donation and disparate other projects and sentiments must be nurtured in order that new donor constituencies emerge: mourner-donors, devotee-donors, and so on. The project to foster voluntary blood donation is necessarily expansive; new constituencies of donors must be sought and enrolled. This is resulting in the rapid proliferation of new relationships and understandings of what it means to donate blood. As I explain below in this chapter and in more detail in chapter 4, all this means that rakt-dan—a dan very much in formation—could never be described as being one dan. Rakt-dan is as heterogeneous as the diverse sets of communities of practice that give and receive it.

The "donor recruiter," states NACO's *National Guidebook on Blood Donor Motivation* (Ray 2003: 50), is a person whose purpose is "to motivate, recruit and retain voluntary blood donors." Most recruiters are employed by individual blood banks to design publicity materials extolling blood donation, organize blood donation camps, educational visits to schools, and events on occasions such as All India Voluntary Blood Donation Day (1 October), or to felicitate regular donors. Their most important task, however, is to pursue strategies that will ultimately result in an increase in voluntary donation. Not all recruiters are in the employment of blood banks: the most impressively innovative and committed donor recruiters in India belong to a voluntary organization based in

Kolkata called the Association of Voluntary Blood Donors, West Bengal (AVBD), of which more in a moment.[21]

Blood donation has become a boundary object through the efforts of the religious, business, educational, and political communities of practice with which blood banks collaborate, but perhaps more important, through the active processes of interpretive entrepreneurship engaged in by donor recruiters. Recruiters are aware that they have to allow blood donation to mean different things to different organizations—that it must of necessity become interwoven with others' narratives and projects in order for collection to be increased.

The proliferation of conceptual alignments and alliances with different communities of practice, however, possesses the danger of the production of "bad meanings"—meanings, that is, that diverge from those deemed acceptable by the medical establishment and policy makers. The AVBD, mentioned above, consequently endeavors to be both a proliferator and a guardian of donation's signification. Founded in 1980 by teachers and ex-students of Calcutta's Jadavpur University, famed for its nationalist origins, its members are professionals and intellectuals who each give a few hours every week to help organize camps, write publicity materials, and engage in other recruitment activities. The AVBD's striking inventiveness and visceral commitment to the cause of voluntary donation has given it a national profile and importance: it organizes national and international seminars and conferences on recruitment techniques, conducts highly effective school visits to promote voluntary donation, and runs diploma courses on donor recruitment and social work; its founder Debabrata Ray is the author of NACO's *National Guidebook on Blood Donor Motivation* (2003). It is no accident that West Bengal is the national leader in voluntary donation, its figure of 95 percent contrasting markedly with Delhi's 20 percent.

I single out the AVBD as an important agent of alignment and alliance in part because of its influence beyond West Bengal, but also because of a specific "signification tool" developed by Ray: the donation calendar. Noting that "different organizations . . . love to organize their blood collection [camps] on a significant day" and that "donor motivators have to be on the lookout for such days and make them popular for blood collection drives," Ray (2003: 263) has prepared a calendar filled with multifarious "days of joys and sorrows, anniversaries [and] historical events" that "may be the days of blood donations."

The calendar presses the boundary object into more and more territories of signification. To take a couple of examples: January 23, the birthday of the "freedom fighter" Netaji Subhas Chandra Bose, is marked as a potential day for camps. Indeed, members of the AVBD told me that followers and admirers of Chandra Bose make an explicit connection between blood donation and the famous request which he made to his countrymen: "Give me your blood and I will give you freedom." March 23 is the day on which in 1931 another "freedom fighter" and nationalist icon, Bhagat Singh, was executed by the British. The

Rashtriya Swayamsevak Sangh (RSS), coordinating body of the Hindu right, stages camps on this day, connecting the blood shed by Indian "martyrs" and that shed by donors. But alignments between blood donation and specific events or social phenomena do not all depend on analogic synergy between blood sacrifice and blood donation (though this is indeed an important analogical relationship that recurs and is analyzed throughout the study); blood donation is often enacted by different constituencies as a mark of their commitment to the values condensed in and by the day in question. The calendar suggests that Gandhian organizations should be encouraged to donate on Quit India Day (August 8), associations of the deaf on World Deaf Day (September 23), the Indian armed forces on Army Day (November 18), Goans on Goa Liberation Day (December 18), Christians on Christmas Day, and so on.

Ray (2003: 266) urges recruiters in different states to prepare calendars based on this model but with local relevance. Armed with the signification tool of a donation calendar—or simply with locally relevant knowledge of notable days—recruiters customize blood donation with "personalized and personalizable referents" (Strathern 1993: 97) to facilitate its appropriation by particular interest groups. In Sirsa, for example, a town in Haryana, an enterprising blood bank asked a gurdwara association if it would consider staging a camp on August 27, the day on which the Guru Granth Sahib was installed in the Golden Temple at Amritsar. It was, and camps are now staged in the gurdwara annually on this date. In Kolkata, the AVBD approached the Muslim community to donate its blood on the birthday of the prophet Muhammad, with similar results.[22]

The problem faced by agents of alignment such as the AVBD and other recruiters is that priming others to make alignments means that recruiters must of necessity loosen their own grip on donation's signification. For an organization that not only wants people to give blood but to give it in the way it wants, this is extremely problematic. At a camp I attended on Rajiv Gandhi's birth anniversary (August 20) in Kolkata, jointly organized by the AVBD and the Congress, large clocks were given to each donor. At the time, local political rivalries were being expressed through the medium of competitive blood donation camps, with different activist groups attempting to out-donate each other. Blood donation had become aligned with political rivalry. The Congress's rewarding of donors with clocks in order to attract more donors, so far as the AVBD was concerned, saddled blood donation with an unacceptable signification. The AVBD campaigns forcefully against the offering of enticements to blood donors and has itself conducted a study that it says "revealed that costly gifts attracted more first time donors, who had a higher prevalence of viral blood transmissible infections" (Ray 2003: 45). The AVBD has accordingly made representations to local political groups and highlighted the issue in Calcutta's newspapers. The AVBD thus attempts, like recruiters in general, to balance the two roles of stabilizer and proliferator of donation's signification.

The Camp as Social Form

Though the heterogeneity of Delhi's urban fabric may be endlessly reiterated by scholars who work on the city (Vidal et al. 2000: 16), there is no escaping the fact that an extremely large proportion of its inhabitants are first- or second-generation migrants from other regions of India. This provides for a wide and exciting array of camp settings: migrants from Kerala stage camps in temples dedicated to Lord Ayyappa; Syrian Christians stage them in their churches; Bengali Hindus donate blood during Durga Puja (the annual Bengali festival in honor of the fierce goddess Durga), and so on.

I worked principally with the Red Cross and Rotary blood banks, Delhi's two most energetic organizers of camps and solicitors of voluntary donors. The Red Cross blood bank is located in the symbolic heart of New Delhi opposite the Indian parliament (Lok Sabha). The Rotary blood bank lies in an industrial area to the south of the city. The Red Cross conducts camps almost daily, the Rotary sometimes holds two per day in different locations. As NACO's *National Guidebook on Blood Donor Motivation* (Ray 2003: 107) puts it, blood donation camps are premised on the idea that blood banks should take donor couches "as close as possible to the donors on their convenient date and time rather than expecting the donors to come to the blood bank. The closer the bed to the potential donor, the stronger is the likelihood of success." The blood donor sessions held at United States university campuses and corporate offices are equivalents of the Indian "camp." While one can walk in to donate at blood banks and hospitals in the United States and in India, it is largely true that "All over the world, most blood from voluntary blood donors is collected from outdoor camps in rural and urban areas" (ibid).

Despite the forcible sterilization camps conducted during Indira Gandhi's Emergency (see Tarlo 2003), "camps" in India are seen mainly positively, especially by the less well off, as opportunities for free medical treatment, which can include basic surgical operations such as the removal of cataracts. The Rotary and Lions Clubs are particularly prolific providers of treatment, as are the devotional and guru-led movements introduced above. The staging of free treatment camps is also a populist political instrument, especially during election times or on the death or birth anniversaries of past and present political leaders. Residents' associations in wealthy Delhi suburbs stage more commercially oriented camps in the form of "health *melas*" (festivals) where basic treatments are provided at subsidized rates, various new medical products and treatments are advertised, and famous doctors, familiar to residents from daytime television chat shows, lecture on healthy lifestyles. It appears likely that the recent striking expansion of religious and corporate charity, which frequently takes the form of services and treatments provided at camps, has partly been in response to the government's liberalization policies of the 1990s, with the state, having abandoned its commitment to socialist principles, no longer able to represent itself as the benefactor of the masses (McKean 1996: 11). This is an important point to which I return later.

What is distinctive about blood donation camps is that those who attend become donor-providers as opposed to recipient-patients. The widespread expectation that camps are a medium for giving out to a needy population can lead to confusion at blood donation camps which seemingly turn such a dynamic of give-and-take on its head. Although many blood donation camps are staged in private spaces such as office, worship, and college buildings, they are also frequently conducted outdoors on the roadside or in car parks under colorful marriage tents. Such tents are markers of camps in general and are not specific to the blood donation camp. Hence, when a blood donation camp is staged in a less well-off area it is not uncommon for passersby to cross its threshold in the full expectation of fulfilling the role of recipient (of free medicines, health checkups, etc.) only to be asked to register as a donor. Because of widespread fears about the physical consequences of giving blood, a quick exit usually follows. (These fears are considered below.) The confusion caused by a camp form that reverses the usual source of beneficence is exacerbated in the style of donation camp which is advertised as a health checkup camp in a ploy to ensure a ready supply of persons for blood donation—again, such camps are most common in poorer locales and usually organized by the smaller blood banks. Having gratefully received the checkup (which is in fact nothing other than the blood donor screening process), the "recipient" is asked to turn voluntary donor and give his or her blood as a means of repaying a debt which has to all intents and purposes been imposed upon them.

Blood donation camps are unamenable to categorization according to the classic delineation of state—the legal and formal apparatuses of governance through which interests are negotiated—versus civil society—the more chaotic space of interaction between state and population as mediated by political parties and other more informal networks. As collaborative endeavors between state or NGO medical institutions and a mixed assortment of associations and *samitis* (societies) of primarily religious, corporate, educational, and political provenance, some of which enlist the camp as a medium for their agonistic relations with one another, what on one level are state ventures of medical provision are at the same time wholly entangled with the divergent priorities and imperatives of an array of informal networks and competitive-minded groupings.

How does a blood donation camp function? Before being declared eligible to donate, prospective donors undergo "donor screening." They first answer a donor questionnaire on their medical histories, before being weighed and having their blood pressure and hemoglobin levels measured. If qualified to donate, donors take a blood bag to a table on which they are bled; 350 ml of blood is usually extracted, taking about ten minutes, and as many as ten or fifteen donors will donate at one time on adjoining tables. After donating, donors are provided with a *frooti* soft drink, a banana, a voluntary donor card, and often a cup of tea. Some blood banks also offer donors tokens of appreciation such as a wallet or a coffee mug.[23]

The camp structure enabled me to move fluidly between doctors, recruiters, donors, and representatives of the institutions with which the blood bank had collaborated to organize the camp. This latter participant often provides a photographer so that its virtuous deeds can go recorded, perhaps in the next day's newspaper or on its Web site. Garlanded politicians inaugurated a large number of the camps I attended; some even donated their blood in highly visible acts of seva for their constituents (see Mayer 1981 on politicians and seva, and chapter 3 on involvement with blood donation as a political virtue). Photographic inscription is vital for both the politician and the camp organizer. At one camp, the local MLA (member of the Legislative Assembly) arrived hours late to "open" the camp just as it was drawing to a close. There were no donors left, so the politician stood next to a blood bank technician feigning donation in order to secure the necessary photographic inscription.[24]

The blood donation camp is an extremely variable social form. Those conducted in corporate offices can be dull and routine, with quiet, orderly employees queuing to donate. One of the most striking features of voluntary donation in India, however, is the gargantuan scale of the camps staged by certain devotional orders. These can resemble large devotional convocations like the great melas at which sadhus and pilgrims congregate. But in this case it is a "modern" biomedical treatment procedure that is the occasion for gathering, with "this-worldly" service activity sanctified by the electrifying presence of gurus or other holy figures. As chapter 5 shows, these devotional orders compete to attain the Guinness world record for most donations made in a single day. Indeed, record-breaking blood donation camps have become a key indicator in what I call the national league of virtuous beneficence. These kinds of camp are great spectacles of devotional fervor and donor excess. Chapter 5 explores the various religious implications of this "obsessional theater" (Barthes 1959: 163) of spectacular camps, while chapter 7 focuses on a further key aspect of Indian blood donation camps: the ways in which they have come to be seen as situational enactments of the Nehruvian post-Independence ideology of "national integration."

The gender composition of camps is quite even, except when they are staged at professional/corporate and political locations, when gender disparities among donors reflect those of the surrounding environment. As I note below in chapter 7, however, for reformist campaigners the value of blood donation camps in Allahabad lies precisely in their not reflecting the gender inequalities of the wider locale in which they are situated. The camps of one blood donor association in the city are said to have "acquired the status of a social movement where boys and girls mingled freely."[25] A very different situation, however, pertains at Radhasoami and Dera Sacha Sauda camps, where men and woman tend to queue to donate in separate lines (I did not witness such a separation at Sant Nirankari camps).

That a fairly equal number of men and women attempt to give blood does not result in an equal level of accepted donations, since a large number of females are disqualified due to inadequate hemoglobin levels. Many aver that this is the result of a north Indian situation in which women tend to eat only the leftovers of the food consumed by the male members of the household, their poor diet being reflected in the low hemoglobin levels that disqualify them (see chapter 4 on diet and blood donation). Menstruation also acts as a bar to donation, in India as elsewhere. Moreover, though women contribute a far lower quantity of blood than men, it is reported that 60 percent of donated blood is transfused into females (Ray 2003: 105). This can result in highly moralized narratives such as the following which, far from focusing attention on the reasons for their disqualification, instead rebukes women for their parasitical reliance on men: "in [the] case of blood transfusion, [the] women of our country are dependent on their men-folk . . . women should not forget that they require quite a large quantity of blood in treatment of various surgical cases and particularly at childbirth. So they have an obligation to donate back" (Ray 2003: 106). The narrative focus here on dependency and moral debt obviates the critical issue of physical disqualification, an issue which devolves from far wider questions concerning gender asymmetries. It seems likely, after all, that the reasons many women are ineligible to donate are connected to the reasons why they require more transfusions than men; that is, just as anemia necessitates transfusion so does it thwart donation.

So the multiple camp contexts discussed in this study tend not to be marked by gender disparities in terms of *attempts* made to give, and the views and sensibilities of women of many different ages and backgrounds are as central to the following arguments as those of men. This study also considers gendered ideologies of blood donor recruitment, a focus of chapter 2 being depictions of the generic "mother," who is viewed somewhat ambivalently as both an obstacle to voluntary blood donation and as the ideal model for blood donors to follow as providers of pristine care. In addition, chapter 2 explores the gendered imaginings of donors who see their donated blood as a force of familial continuity which, in "saving" a male transfusion recipient with a dependent family, is considered to "save" the family as well—not only in the present but reproductively speaking also in enabling a generational continuity that, were it not for donated blood, would be precluded.

Blood/Substance

Weiner (1995: 5) reports the response of an Australian aboriginal artist who, when asked about the significance of his bark paintings, declared: "There are too many meanings. Later on, when you know more, you'll know which ones to choose and which ones to discard." Blood has myriad meanings and connotations in India. I focus here only on "meanings" that I take to have specific situational relevance to practices of blood donation in India.

Blood (in Sanskrit: *rakt*; in Hindi: *khun*) is seen by many South Asians as a repository of strength; its loss understood as weakening (Starr 1998: 186). Equivalence between semen and blood is a prominent theme in South Asia generally (Alter 1994, 1999; Parry 1994: 214; Juergensmeyer 1991: 132). Fear of impotence, linked to issues of strength, has been depicted as a critical reason for people's unwillingness to donate blood in India (Vicziany 2001). Parry's (1994: 202) Banaras informants held that a man should ideally drink milk after sexual intercourse "to replace what he has just discharged." I was told several times by doctors in Delhi that some donors in north India similarly seek to replenish their extracted blood by drinking milk. This, added to Parry's data, again points to an important association between blood and semen loss that would appear to negatively affect men's willingness to give blood.

Blood has additionally been described by anthropologists as a particularly defiling substance in South Asia. "Throughout India," notes S. Bayly (1989: 127), "bodily secretions, especially blood, semen, saliva and human wastes, are thought of as being charged with a form of power and energy which may be both menacing and protective." If the belief that, along with food (Appadurai 1981; Dumont 1966) and cloth (C. Bayly 1986), "detached parts of the body . . . can be conduits of spiritual and personal qualities" were to coincide with deeply held investments in certain differentiations, as it does for example in the ideology of the caste system, then practices of blood donation and transfusion might imply "moral entanglement" of the highest degree (Laidlaw 2000: 629). Vicziany, however, argues forcefully in reference to colonial medicine in India that these ideas "vanished in the twentieth-century quest for longevity," that revulsion toward these substances has been overcome, indeed, that "there are no cultural obstacles to the development of world class blood banks in contemporary India" (2001: 393). Vicziany is largely correct that "purity and pollution" issues are not significant barriers to blood collection. At the same time, however, traditional beliefs in the transforming power of blood (S. Bayly 1989: 264) in India should not so easily be dismissed.

Donors do on occasion construct themselves as agents of purification. In chapter 4, I document Nirankari devotees' view that the blood they donate, imbued with their spiritually purifying love (*pyar*), will remove the faults of recipients, instilling them with grace. For many devotees, therefore, the blood they donate is indeed charged with power and energy. Moreover, I show just below that there is also an emphasis in recruitment lectures and materials on blood donation as a means to "take care of thyself" (Rabinow 1994: xxv)—one should donate to purify one's body, to expel one's aged "senile cells," in the words of one doctor. For some, blood donation is a chance to purify their bodies, for others it is an opportunity to purify or positively affect others in a manner that transcends the gift's official purpose. All this signals that purity concerns are distinctly present in the Indian blood donation scenario, but not in ways that necessarily hinder collection. This study is therefore supportive of Alter's (2004: 176) claim that although Marriott and others may have performed a useful service in deemphasizing the dichotomy of purity and pollution as the determining principle of South Asian life, "purity as such has tremendous power and persuasive force as a cultural ideal in modern India."

Rather than concerns relating to purity and pollution, it is the perception that blood donation is a dramatically unhealthy, even life-threatening activity that discourages many from donating. The "prick" of donation is particularly terrifying. As one donor told me: "When I got vaccinated and my skin was pierced I felt it was bursting my body and everything inside would spill out. It will never stop. Syringes, needles—pain, such a pain." Many donors find the vision of their blood leaving their bodies and coursing into bags highly disturbing. Doctors in one government blood bank cover blood bags, while they fill, with a green cloth: "otherwise they shout, 'This amount of blood you have taken doctor!'" It is well known that relatives play a prominent role in the treatment of their sick family members in various Indian medical contexts (see Minocha 1996: 41; Halliburton 2002: 1127). Several doctors informed me that when there are too many family members crowding a particular ward, they say: "Okay, we need [you to donate] two units." This technique is apparently extremely effective in quickly dispersing inconvenient crowds.[26]

Apart from impotence and infertility ("I can't donate. I'm getting married next month!"), I heard a litany of other grounds for declining to donate, which ranged from fear of resulting blindness to unamenable weather conditions—some hold that the summer heat dries up their blood. The most important reason, however, is the widespread understanding of blood loss as leading to permanent volumetric deficit. This is frequently expressed in the formulation: "If I donate blood I will need a transfusion, so why should I give?" The Hindi phrase *khun ki kami* (less blood) is also often employed. In an effort to counter this "misconception," donor recruiters compare blood donation to having one's hair or nails cut: blood, they say, like these other detachable substances, reforms and returns. The biomedical term for the recuperative power of blood is *hematopoiesis*. As I note below in chapter 4, Nirankari devotees, having donated, give their guru credit for the replenishment of their blood. This shows that they do not necessarily take seriously recruiters' claims about the recuperation of donated blood; rather, they see their devotional relationship with their guru as ensuring a replenishment that would not otherwise transpire.

The socioeconomic basis of some of these apprehensions is clear. At a camp in a busy commercial district in the center of Delhi, I joined a blood bank team in attempting to recruit passersby. Manual laborers often expressed their reluctance by connecting their profession with what they saw as their deficient blood quantum: "I'm a laborer, I have no blood." Similarly in a study of a Delhi slum, respondents said that "they already felt weak and that they did not have 'even a drop of blood in their bodies'" (Singh et al. 2002). While the poor do see themselves as having proportionately less blood, *khun ki kami* was a refrain I heard in a multitude of settings, by no means all of which were populated by the poor.[27]

The central point is that it is not anxieties about pollution but anxieties about strength depletion which deter large numbers of prospective donors. Some recruiters attempt to overcome this objection through their promotion of a definition of blood donation as a practice of purgative self-purification. In devising a strategy to counter the pervasive view of donation as weakening through the employment of purity concepts which, as I show below, bear a striking resemblance to those delineated by Marriott (1989), recruiters attempt to resignify blood donation from being a practice that induces weakness to one that promotes strength.

Recruiters throughout India have attempted to counteract the perception that blood donation is an activity that leads to permanent volumetric deficit through an emphasis on blood's capacity to regenerate, producing slogans such as: "Saving the life of a needy person without causing slightest harm to donor is the beauty of blood donation," and the following, drawn from sayings attributed to the Buddha: "Thousands of candles can be lighted [*sic*] from a single candle, and the life of the candle will not be shortened."[28] Similarly, in Kolkata lines from Tagore's *Gitanjali* are employed to explain to donors the "endless" quality of their blood:

> THOU hast made me endless, such is thy pleasure.
> This frail vessel thou emptiest again and again,
> and fillest it ever with fresh life. (1)

This approach, however, which focuses on the unharmful or health-neutral effects of donating blood, is increasingly being supplemented by a set of claims and slogans that go a step further in calling attention to the health-enhancing properties of blood donation. This strategy is reflected in slogans such as the one that advertises blood donation as "The only transaction where the giver is the gainer!"[29]

The attempt to connect blood donation positively with prospective donors' concern with their own physical good health is pursued in a very particular manner that constructs an affinity between blood giving and established ayurvedic and yogic principles of purgation. Recruiters suggest that blood donation purifies donors' blood through the removal of their aging blood cells. This principle of purification appears to correspond with Marriott's (1989: 30) conception of purity as a three-dimensional concept for South Asians, involving "movement towards unmixing, matching and unmarking of coded substances" (Rosin 2000: 383). This can be illustrated with a citation from a Delhi-based doctor who was speaking at an event called Rakta Kranti (Blood Revolution), staged before a set of Delhi schoolchildren to try and raise their enthusiasm about donation:

> I started donating blood in 1972. All my blood is young. The red cells are younger in me and with better functioning. If you have a younger red cell mass in your body you have much better hemoglobin, because the senile cells go out. With the new cells, the red cell function (one's oxygen carrying capacities) increases. A regular donor, after five years, gets 30 percent more oxygen capacity. This is at the experimental stage but it is just common sense. . . . Regular donors don't get hypertension or heart attacks, so if all our population starts donating blood, heart attacks can even be removed from India! It is a gift of nature that you can give and you don't lose anything—your blood will be fresher like water in a well.

What is notable here is the emphasis on the removal of "senile cells" leading to the formation of "younger" red cells. He continued: "You give old blood and what you get back is fresh blood. When RBCs [red blood cells] are given you receive much younger age cells and better capacity to function." Through this "somatically introverted logic" (Alter 2004: 182),[30] blood donation is shorn of the sense it carries of being a transaction with another (the transfusion recipient), becoming instead a transaction with and within oneself: the donor will "get back" fresh blood, "receive" younger cells in a hematopoietic exchange, with blood donation coming to appear more like bloodletting than an act of beneficent helpfulness. It would seem that the doctor's purgative logic is related to certain ayurvedic principles, which, as Langford (2002: 265) notes, often center on "evacuative therapies" such as purgation, emetics, and bloodletting for the removal of excess *dosa*. I suggest that this doctor's enlistment of an indigenous purgative idiom in order to encourage Indians to become voluntary blood donors demonstrates at the same time the enlistment of blood donation into the Indian armamentarium of purification.[31]

Marriott's conception of the different trajectories involved in Hindu processes of purification is echoed in recruiters' depiction of blood donation as a movement toward unmixing and matching. Following the purging of the donor's "senile cells"—what in fact would be a mixed crop of cells of different ages—the bone marrow is stimulated to produce new cells at a quicker than usual rate so that what results is indeed a higher concentration of matched (i.e., self-similar), less mixed-up cells.[32] With the mean age of cells thus reduced, their effectiveness as oxygen carrying agents increases. As Dr. Alok Singh from a government blood bank informed me: "Now you are twenty-five. Another person is fifty years old. Suppose both of you are asked to do the same physical work. Who can do more work? The answer is the younger person, because the younger one is more energetic. Similarly, the new red cells have more oxygen-carrying capacity. After donation you will feel stronger because old cells are replaced by new cells." The pervasive view of blood donation as weakening is thus turned on its head in a manner which can be compared with *soma*, the elixir of immortality, which, in foundational ayurvedic texts such as the *Sushruta Samhita* (circa 200 B.C.E.), is understood to "produce immortality by 'killing off' the body prone to aging, disease and death and replacing it with a flawless reproduction" (Alter 2004: 192). Recruiters' marketing of blood donation is structurally similar, with the blood donor expunging his dead, dying, or "senile" cells, thereby stimulating the bone marrow to reproduce a fresh concentration of vigorous, youthful cells in replacement of those removed. "A pure body," states Alter (2004: 176–177), "is, in a very literal sense, a powerful and supremely strong body." As Dr. Alok Singh said, the "purified" concentration of younger cells is more energetic and powerful. The inner logic of the recruitment strategy is therefore one of profound (Hindu-filtered) revaluation: from weakness, via purification, to strength.

The idea of donation as a technique of purification is remarkably widespread among donors and was spoken of enthusiastically by many of my donor informants in Delhi. A security guard giving blood at a camp staged in a Delhi hotel said: "Blood donation purifies the body—we do the camp here twice a year so that we [the hotel staff] can purify our bodies twice a year. To be healthy you have to eat well, do exercise and give blood. *Rakt-dan, jivan-dan* [Give blood, give life] is the [Red Cross] slogan. But it should be *Rakt-dan, shuddhikaran karo* [Give blood, get purified]. All the old cells are extinguished." I met Akash, a student, at a camp held at a Delhi University college: "I have donated many times. It is for my own good, nothing else. All the impurities go. I read somewhere that if you don't donate cells die and take a long time to leave the circulation—so I do it for myself."

Evidence from Delhi suggests that biomedical blood donation may be in the throws of being added to the Indian armamentarium of purification techniques as found in branches of yoga and ayurveda. The mobilization of purity concepts in the swadeshi campaigns of the early twentieth century (see Tarlo 1996: 91), which involved redefinition of purity (C. Bayly 1986: 312), Mahatma Gandhi's concern to purge the body of its "toxins, waste, and unnatural substances" (Alter 2004: 267), his follower Raojibhai Manibhai Patel's adoption of auto-urine therapy, and now depictions of a purgative blood donation reveal the interesting and enterprising ways in which Hindu Indians continually contrive to amend and expand their armamentarium of purification. My examination here of an innovative strategy to counter a pervasive view of blood donation as weakening has thus highlighted the growing importance of purity concepts in the solicitation of donation, exploring how blood donation has been maneuvered into conceptual alignment with indigenous purgative praxis.

What I have been describing also underscores the complex and paradoxical nature of blood donation's relationship with dan (gift, donation) concepts.[33] Dan is paradigmatically asymmetrical and disinterested. According to both ancient Hindu law (Parry 1986: 461) and virtually every person with whom I discussed the matter during fieldwork, dan is a gift for which no return can be countenanced. Since blood donation was first practiced in north India, however, rakt-dan has been the euphemistic administrative label for all the varieties of blood donation: paid, replacement, and voluntary alike. For many voluntary donors and donor recruiters, the use of dan to denote paid and replacement donation was and is a disgraceful misapplication of a revered term and concept. However, the recent focus on the promotion of voluntary blood donation, necessitated by the 1998 legal ruling that forbade payment, has made the use of the term *rakt-dan* seem less reprehensible to doctors and recruiters. This is because in the new voluntary system, donors are meant to receive no payment and also to remain unaware of the recipients of their donations. Voluntary donation thus promises to provide the asymmetry and anonymity held to characterize many classical notions of dan. For doctors, the conceptual convergence between disinterested dan and voluntary donation is of practical importance: voluntary blood donation must conform precisely to the highest ideal of disinterested dan since disinterested giving is seen to ensure the safety of donated blood.[34]

And yet, as I have demonstrated, some recruiters portray rakt-dan as a gift that purifies its giver, and as such it resonates with accounts of dan that have depicted its expiatory and cleansing qualities (Parry 1986; Raheja 1988). Ann Gold's (1988: 292) remarks on giving in rural Rajasthan as a process of emptying and refining are particularly pertinent here. The recruitment strategy I have been describing therefore appears to diverge from the disinterest meant to characterize idealized conceptions of dan, for it reflects a view among recruiters, to paraphrase Adam Smith (1976: 27), that it is not from the benevolence of prospective donors that they can expect to receive their blood but rather from this population's regard to its own interest in self-purification: donors should donate to receive the "return" of purified blood. This, of course, underlines the fact that dan is not one thing. Just as rakt-dan appeared to many donors and doctors to be becoming asymmetrical, and thus like the revered nonreciprocal version of dan, recruiters have begun to employ other understandings of dan as a mode of emptying and refinement as a solicitation technique through which donation comes to be a means to "take care of thyself."

In fact, rakt-dan takes us straight to the paradox at the heart of classical forms of Indian gift; namely, that such gifts are conceptualized as being at once pure and purifying. As Parry (1989: 75) has noted, a gift capable of purifying its giver appears "to subvert its own ethic of disinterested generosity." Similarly, the purifying gift of blood through which "senile cells" are removed makes it a gift with a built-in return (purer blood). Thus the "classical" sense in which dan constitutes "its own counter-prestation" (Parry 1980: 105) is also a key structuring element of this "biomedical dan." Not only does recruiters' message about donation subvert doctors' orthodox depiction, it does so in a manner directly comparable to the way in which the ethic of disinterested generosity is breached in the Banaras case, that is, through purification of the donor. Once again, the ideology of the gift's purity is compromised by virtue of the fact that it is also purificatory.

Rakt-dan should be thought of as a dan in formation. Different parties imbue it with various differing conceptions associated with assorted forms of dan and in so doing reveal that all conceptual definitions and activity attached to dan are internally differentiated and dynamic, not static—that is, "in formation." In other words, the diversity that inheres within rakt-dan enables us to see the diversity of dan in general. This recognition informs the discussions of chapters 3 and 4, which return to the complex relationship between blood donation and dan concepts.

From Replacement to Voluntary Donation

As I mentioned above, family replacement donation is now being phased out in favor of an anonymous voluntary system. Although the practice of replacement donation is not unique to India, its practice is marked by particular features in the subcontinent, one of which is that its family basis can make it appear "natural" to some Indian doctors and donors, thereby weakening their resolve to promote the voluntary mode. Such persons often disapprove of what they see as the "parasitical" features of a voluntary system in which the role of the family in a relative's illness decreases. According to some doctors and donors this is a reprehensible abdication—they protest that this removes provision from its properly moral (familial) domain. Cohen (2001: 18) has recently pointed to Indian assumptions about the need to reestablish "the familial order of giving eroded by selfish, western modernity." In a seeming paradox, some doctors I worked with equate voluntary blood donation with selfishness because it will ultimately result in relatives being able to acquire blood without themselves donating. "Selfless" (*niswarth*) voluntary donation, in enabling relatives to acquire blood merely by paying a processing charge, thus removes blood donation from the domain of intrafamilial ethics, and thus breeds a "selfish" (*swarth purn*) dependency on others' altruism. Healy (2006) sums up the paradox well: "Altruism is parasitic on self-interest . . . because altruists need at least one self-interested person to be altruistic towards."

This institutional transition which is underway from "specific" replacement to "abstract" voluntary donation would thus appear to eliminate the familial and personal elements associated with replacement blood donation. However, much of this study concerns the processes through which those factors characteristic of the replacement mode that are apparently repressed in its successor form resurface in transfigured ways in the voluntary system. That is, much of this study is concerned with intricate and paradoxical processes of the reinstallation of the personal and the familial in a donation environment apparently hostile to them.

This study thus focuses on the complex interrelations between the formal conceptual logic underpinning functioning systems, and the more subjective experiential logic that donors bring to the activity of blood donation. What I particularly have in mind here is something for which I use the term "directional intentionality," by which I mean the ideas that donors have of the routes traveled by the blood they give. This requires emphasis: the whole business of soliciting and organizing blood donation, both in the West and in India, is ordered around large-scale processes of publicizing and solicitation addressed to potential donors. Within India, organizations like the Red Cross and its many Indian counterparts, which have come to include large proselytizing Hindu and other devotional networks as well as political parties and ostensibly secular medical charities, all have one thing in common. They seek to engage the imagination of potential donors, encouraging them not just to envisage their blood as being productive but also as undergoing a productive kind of physical movement through time and space from virtuous donors to particular kinds of recipient-beneficiaries. And the crux here is that whereas in the still predominant replacement system several donors are asked to give to a specific person (usually a relative), donors in the nascent voluntary system are required to give as an act of high-minded citizenship rather than familial obligation, their recipient being an anonymous "any" rather than a specified known individual.

I regard this issue of donors' imagined conception of the journey taken by their blood and the direction in which this travel takes place as crucial to the understanding of this form of gift exchange. When people embrace so-called voluntary donation, what they are being asked to do as donors is to imagine their blood traveling in the way that the technology of blood processing operates on the blood they donate. Much donated blood is centrifuged; this is a laboratory process that separates component elements of blood by rotating it at high speed, thereby creating centrifugal forces that move the substances being treated in an outward direction. Anonymously donated blood is also to be imagined as traveling in an external or outward direction: away from the donor to unnamed recipients whose identities cannot be specified or known. The direction of travel is precisely the reverse in the replacement system, in which a circle of donors, usually family members, all focus their donation inwardly, that is, centripetally, on the needs of a specified, known individual recipient (see figure 1.1).[35] I thus refer to the underlying principle of donation in the replacement system as "centripetal" in direction, and to that of the voluntary system, now being promoted, as "centrifugal."

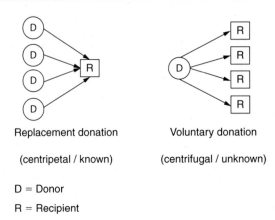

Replacement donation   Voluntary donation

(centripetal / known)   (centrifugal / unknown)

D = Donor

R = Recipient

FIGURE 1.1. Formal Intended Structure of Blood Donation Reform.

The variant of donation in reference to which I am using the term centrifugal and which is characterized by so-called voluntary giving to unknown and unnamed recipients has another important aspect: its multiplicity. This is manifested in several ways. First, the committed donor repeats his or her donation every three months, and therefore gives for multiple recipients. And second, the anonymity of voluntary donation creates a kind of blank page that in a sense primes donors to engage in imaginative acts of enumeration in regard to possible future beneficiaries. I use the term "m/any" as shorthand to describe those aspects of the voluntary system in which donors think of themselves as giving both to an unnamed "any" and at the same time to a pluralized or multiple "many."

Though the principal stated reason for the promotion of voluntary donation is the requirement to improve the safety of donated blood, its anonymity connects it to the kind of giving that is widely favored in a host of other contexts both within and beyond India in which philanthropic action is considered to be both modern and moral only when directed untraceably to anyone in need. This kind of philanthropy promotes "idealized solidarity reigning in abstract humankind" and fosters bonds between "abstract subjects" (Godelier 1999: 5). The switch from a replacement to a voluntary mode of donation appears to instill blood donation activity with the anonymity and generality characteristic of this modernist philanthropic principle.[36] However, just as Oxfam and other international aid organizations personalize their exhortatory posters with pictures of needy-looking children, the present study focuses on particular processes of repersonalization in Indian blood donation settings, even as efforts are redoubled to foster depersonalized voluntary donation. The specifically Indian implications of this point can be elucidated in reference to a set of arguments put forward by Ramanujan.

The presence of organized campaigns to promote voluntary donation—an abstract and decontextualized mode of giving in comparison with the family-based specificity of the replacement mode—appears to reflect Ramanujan's observation that modernization in India can be seen as a movement from the context-sensitive toward the context-free. Ramanujan makes the further important point, however, that in India the context-free is liable to become just another context (1989: 55, 57).[37] This is vitally relevant to the Indian experience of voluntary blood donation: the desired centrifugal trajectory of blood donation (from being given to someone in replacement, to anyone in voluntary donation) is very often actively facilitated by centripetal foci. Donation camps are frequently organized in honor of specific persons. For example, a camp I attended at a Delhi insurance company was arranged by the father of a thalassemic child. A severe form of anemia, thalassemia requires a transfusion every three or four weeks in order to bolster hemoglobin levels. I soon learned that the donors at the camp, moved by the plight of their colleague's child, were, emotionally speaking, giving for the child—despite the fact that their blood would actually be transfused to "anyone." Camps are similarly staged on gurus' and politicians' birth or death anniversaries. The honored figure, whether live or dead, thereby becomes the emotional focus of the camp; a specific object is relied upon to facilitate the abstracted gift. The movement to the context-free is thus installed within and structured by an array of highly specific memorial and celebratory contexts.

Centripetal giving for specific persons thus interlocks in vital facilitative ways with abstract (centrifugal) giving, and results in the repersonalizing of the de-personalized gift. In chapters 4–6, I show that gurus are particularly important repersonalizing agents. Whereas figure 1.1 portrays the formal conceptual logic in directional terms of the transition to a voluntary system, figure 1.2 depicts the prevalent subjective structure of this transition, which takes the form of an interlocking of different directional intentionalities, with donors at once donating specifically to the guru and abstractly to anyone. The gift, in other words, travels both to and through the guru to "humanity." The "to" and "through" model possesses a broad applicability—as was noted above, Oxfam and other international aid organizations also engage in various processes of personalization as a means of securing donations to help "lives uncontextualized and unknowable" (Reddy forthcoming). I show below, however, that the pivotal role in India of devotional cynosures as facilitator-catalysts of philanthropy has its own particular implications.

There are further important differences between the replacement and voluntary systems. Replacement donation is in essence a "forcible deal" (Tarlo 2003), for doctors lead family members to believe that if they do not arrange necessary replacement donations, the treatment required by their relative may be withheld. As one recruiter informed me, this led to a situation in which

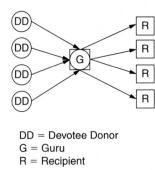

DD = Devotee Donor
G = Guru
R = Recipient

FIGURE 1.2. Subjective Structure of Transition (or, a schematic rendering of how the intended reform is brought to fruition in practice, depicting the "to" and "through" model of interlocking directional intentionalities, with guru in role of simultaneous donor and recipient). For illustrative purposes the diagram depicts the triadic donor-guru-recipient relationship, but the model has wider applicability, with other facilitative figures such as politicians substituting for the role of the guru as represented here.

replacement donors were frequently treated by blood bank staff as "two-legged cows that you milk." In the less agonistic voluntary system, the tables are turned, with donations—at least in theory—arising from self-will (the equivalent Hindi term, *svechha se*, is commonly employed by recruiters) rather than from force of circumstance; consequently, in the voluntary system blood banks are more dependent on donors than donors on blood banks. Doctors and recruiters are thus acutely aware that far better donor care is required, that voluntary donors must be accorded greater courtesy and respect, and thereby encouraged to return to donate again.

Whereas replacement donation is a one-time, singular event, undertaken in emotionally extreme circumstances, the voluntary campaign "aims at [the] creation of a culture of donation ... the culture of helping somebody."[38] Voluntary donation requires that lifesaving becomes a lifestyle. In contrast to one-time replacement donation, voluntary blood donation—ideally performed every three months—involves "the continual reinscription of one's role as [a] donor" (Erwin 2006: 150). Like Kierkagaardian repetition, the committed voluntary blood donor repeats forward "by a creative act of sustaining a commitment from day to day. The 're-' of Kierkagaardian repetition means to keep coming back in the future to the self which one sets out to be.... It is an ethicoreligious act of faithfulness, of constituting and creating a moral self" (Caputo 1987: 58).

There also arises the issue of class. The relationship between voluntary blood donation and class is complex. As in the United States, where paid donors were thought of as social "undesirables" who sell their blood for cash to buy drugs and alcohol, so too in India, where the selling of blood is widely thought to be a practice of the very poor, and their blood to be a menace to those receiving it. Recruiters stigmatize paid donors as drug-addicted rickshaw drivers who place others at risk. As the Indian Red Cross Web site puts it: "Whenever [paid donors] run short of money for drink, drugs or gambling they sell their blood. They care little for their health and suffer from various ailments and disabilities. They are often carriers of blood borne diseases like malaria, hepatitis, syphilis and AIDS. It matters little to them whether the recipient suffers or dies because of poor quality of blood."[39] Class is an equally important feature of the replacement system. The well-off are just as likely as the poor to be asked to donate for ailing family members, but it is common knowledge that those with sufficient means very often employ their servants or professional donors to donate in their stead.

In contrast, and in Delhi at least, recruiters concerned with promoting voluntary donation actively solicit the "cleaner" blood of the comparatively well-off. Indeed the urban middle classes are now widely thought of as ideal blood donors, and recruiters stage donation camps in such places as shopping malls and the premises of multinational corporations. As the honorary director of a Delhi blood bank, a retired policeman, put it me: "We go out in the van to middle-class areas so as to get safe, healthy donors. No slum dweller's or poor person's blood is allowed."

Yet, as was noted above, the devotees of the mass devotional movements which are now so prominent in blood donation activities are mostly people of very modest means: if not the very poor, that is, the so-called slum dwellers whom recruiters so disparage, then definitely not from the upper-level commercial and professional middle-class backgrounds of most metropolitan donor recruiters. So what is happening is more complex than a simple movement from lower-class to middle-class donors. Even as moves are afoot to secure "well-off blood," a countervailing trend is gathering apace which sees the underprivileged adherents of a range of devotional orders provide an increasing proportion of voluntarily donated blood. The shift from replacement to voluntary donation thus possesses key distinguishing features connected to class as well as to atmosphere, ethics, and the directional orientation of the giver.

As I explained earlier, Delhi collects fewer voluntary donations than the national average. In addition to apprehensions about the physical consequences of blood donation, doctors see particular features of Delhi's urban culture as an obstruction to increasing voluntary donation. One doctor, now practicing in Mumbai, but who had previously run a blood bank in Delhi, says of the city: "It is a political place and they are all at war. You are related to this minister and only then do you get an appointment. You are related to a politician and they call the blood bank and say, he is my relative, give him the blood.[40] Mumbai is less political and more philanthropic." For one Delhi doctor, the situation provokes shame: "In West Bengal there is 90 percent voluntary donation, 80 percent in Maharashtra. In Delhi it is less than 20 percent. In the national capital we cannot have this situation." Another, the director of a large government blood bank, told a seminar for the promotion of voluntary donation: "Blood donation is a special culture. But the culture in Delhi is to manage blood, not to give it." Yet another exasperated doctor disparaged Delhi as a "callous, easygoing city. It's like: 'I need blood [for my relative]. Oh, I know a doctor so I'll get it arranged. I have a business, I have no time. She'll arrange it for me.' That's the culture of Delhi—you know someone, or you know someone who knows someone, and it will get arranged. I just bought a ticket for a concert next week. . . . I told my friend and she said, 'You stupid! I would have arranged passes for you.' It's the same with blood banks."

According to these complaints, Delhi's low voluntary collection figures are a direct reflection of a regional culture which they see as being politicized in pathological ways. Vidal et al. have called attention to the all-too-prevalent "impoverished image" of Delhi as "a hall of mirrors," always "reflecting the power of the moment." These authors consider that though such an image "may be colonial in origin . . . it is not without contemporary relevance. For it is this idea that continues to inspire many of Delhi's bureaucrats and politicians even today" (2000: 17). This is a vital point. The fact that doctors and donor recruiters see Delhi as a city of politics and arrangement, antithetical to notions of neighborliness and philanthropic activity, means they are disposed to treat it as if it were so and thus to help constitute the stereotype as a living reality.[41] More important, their subscribing to this prevalent image of the city absolves them from responsibility for the bleak blood donation situation. As I noted above, the lack of cooperation and coordination between blood banks led one visiting expert to describe what she saw as a set of broken processes. Delhi's political culture may be at fault, but it surfaces among blood banks at least as much as among the city's resident prospective donors from whom blood bank personnel rhetorically attempt to separate themselves.

As was seen above, some Delhi recruiters, seemingly in line with such stereotypes, seek to depict blood donation as an almost yogic practice of purgation, and thus as a health-giving activity not merely for recipients but for donors as well. Chapter 2, which explores interrelations between religious merit, technology, and ideas about the family, documents further novel ways in which recruiters portray blood donation as a self-interested activity. Further, while the transition to voluntary donation would appear to remove the familial focus that characterizes replacement donation, chapter 2 demonstrates how ideas about the family have come to be reinstalled within the voluntary system.

Chapter 3 considers the relationship between blood donation and Hindu social and religious reform movements. I emphasize the role of blood donation in the constitution of reformist "religions of utility," showing how the giving dynamics that conventionally proceed upon the occasions of mortuary rituals, death anniversaries, and even marriages are rechanneled into "useful" blood donation rather than other "useless" forms of giving (such as food for the deceased). Chapters 4 and 5 deepen the exploration, begun in chapter 3, of the interoperable relationship between projects to foster voluntary blood donation and north Indian devotional orders. Just as chapter 2 documents the "refamilialization" of blood donation, these chapters show how the figure of the guru repersonalizes what at first glance seems like a depersonalized voluntary system. Chapter 4 focuses on the origins of devotional blood donation and considers Nirankari devotees' emphasis on the transformative qualities of their donated blood for transfusion recipients. It also demonstrates how some devotees treat blood donation as an ascetic ordeal.

Based principally on a case study of the Dera Sacha Sauda, chapter 5 shows how world-record–breaking blood donation camps have in recent years become a means for spiritual organizations to attain prominence in a highly competitive national league of virtuous beneficence. Chapter 5 also explores the constitutive role of these camps in what I identify as an emergent zone of religious spectacles, while additionally highlighting the work they do in the formation of a new order of the miraculous. Another important emergent trend—blood donation as a means of enacting protest—is also investigated.

Chapter 6 examines the rich and multifarious "donation theologies" developed by different gurus and the movements they head. It also elucidates the gateway function of gurus in Indian society, documenting in particular the special ways in which they operate on and transform the array of modernist practices they facilitate. A further issue explored in chapter 6 is that of the complex relationship between blood donation and issues of violence and nonviolence. Evidence is presented demonstrating why blood donation might be viewed as *the* exemplary practice of nonviolent behavior in modern India. And yet at the same time, I argue, blood donation possesses structural features which directly enable specific forms of violent engagement, but from a distance.

Turning next to nationalist interpretations of blood donation activity, chapter 7 examines how Indians read Nehruvian-style integrative messages into the practical procedures through which blood is donated and distributed. Chapter 8 then delineates and connects together the several forms of ascetic and sacrificial logic that surface in Indian enactments of blood donation, arguing that they can help explain several important features of the wider (international) corporeal donation ecumene. Specifically, I elucidate concepts of "donation asceticism" and "corporeal trusteeship," both of which I hope to show possess explanatory purchase beyond the Indian scenario.

The eclectic, wide-ranging nature of my many rich conversations with Debabrata Ray, founder of the AVBD and author of the *National Guidebook on*

Blood Donor Motivation (2003), prompted him to reflect, "The more you think about blood donation, the more you can think of many things." This book, a study of Indian people's multiple and diverse experiences of blood donation, will, I hope, show how right he was.

I thus present a study of religious, conceptual, and institutional change through the unique lens of a set of medical practices whose breadth of social implications has so far remained unrecognized.

2

Generative Generosity

This chapter concerns the re-production of donated blood in the blood bank through a technological procedure called blood component therapy and explores connections that have developed between this technology and some Indians' ideas about the reproduction of families and the calculability of spiritual credit. It demonstrates that familial narratives are not restricted to the intense dramas of replacement donation but, perhaps paradoxically, are also highly significant in the voluntary context, that is, in situations where donors are not donating for immediate family purposes.

In demonstrating how kinship reckoning, spiritual merit, and technology come together in powerful and unexpected ways in the process of soliciting and organizing blood donation, this chapter joins works by scholars such as Bharadwaj (2003, 2007, 2008) and Cohen (1999, 2001, 2004) in documenting the configuration of new biosocialities in the subcontinent. It reflects further on the interlocking set of widening movements I described in chapter 1, arguing that the condition of the resurfacing of "the family" in voluntary donation is its reconceptualization according to a broader template—this being in line with and in part a consequence of the "centrifuge" of directional intentionalities required by the institutional transition to an anonymous voluntary blood donation system in which blood is donated for m/any.

The Procedure

Blood component therapy is a technology designed to enhance the efficiency of distribution and accuracy of prescription of donated blood. A centrifuge machine spins whole donated blood, thereby separating it according to the relative gravity of its constituent components. These are principally red cells, platelets, and plasma.[1] The divisions of blood component therapy are held by doctors and donors alike to multiply the substance because this permits the treatment of at least three people from one donated unit of blood. In the medical view, component separation produces both quantitative and qualitative benefits: more patients can be treated from a single donated unit; and not only that, blood division also allows patients to be treated for the specific ailment from which they are suffering. For medic-proponents of component therapy, therefore, the transfusion of a whole unit of blood, now reperceived as three components as opposed to a single unit, would not only represent the quantitative waste of two units but it would also provide patients with components that are qualitatively unnecessary for their specific condition. The re-production of blood therefore introduces a new particularism into transfusion therapy.

The counterpart to this qualitative particularism, however, is a new imprecision in regard to the numerical relationship between blood providers and transfusion recipients. This imprecision, I explain below, provides donors with new imaginative possibilities in conceptualizing the pathways of their gifts. The scenario recalls Konrad's study of ova donation in Britain, which documents the efforts of fertility experts to "re-source" ova through multiplication techniques in the laboratory as a countervailing action to what the profession views as their progressive "loss" by women. Noting that the gift "does not travel in just one direction," Konrad explains that exteriorized ova are divided into dispersive sets of three which are then sent along "alternative ova pathways" (Konrad 2005: 183, 175). These pathways are "contingent" because the quantity of extractable ova cannot be predetermined, and hence, "the would-be donor can never be set as a pre-fixed or stable formula in relation to the would-be recipient" (ibid.: 176). The statement is equally valid in regard to the Indian blood donation situation. I consider below certain spiritual and familial effects of the relational destabilization consequent upon the advent of component therapy.

In their important work *Tissue Economies*, Waldby and Mitchell rightly note that whereas some tissues such as solid organs are not amenable to "complex technical ordering," and thus tend to be transplanted in their "native" states, other sorts of tissue such as blood are "open to the micro-technical manipulation of productivity." Indeed, a large portion of medical biotechnology is "devoted to this amplification or modification of the biological capacities of tissue fragments" (Waldby and Mitchell 2006: 32). Blood component separation is, of course, a prime example of a technology of augmentation designed to make cells more prolific. What Waldby and Mitchell emphasize is that "surplus in vitro vitality may eventually be transformed into surplus commercial profits, as well as in vivo therapies. In this way, the productivity of tissues intersects with the productivity of markets" (ibid.: 33). The point is compelling but in the present case too narrow; as we shall see, the productivity of tissues may intersect with, and indeed augment, not only the productivity of markets but the productivity of other phenomena too such as spiritual merit and genealogies.

Developed in the United States in the 1950s (Copeman 2005: 471), the tech-nology of component therapy had become widespread in developed countries by the late 1960s. The technology requires a linked set of three blood bags (called triple bags) for the components to subsequently be separated into. Indian blood banks, however, only began to move beyond crude glass bottles and introduce PVC collection bags in the early 1980s. It has been estimated that 25 percent of donated blood in the country is now separated into components.[2] In Delhi the percentage is much higher. Blood banks that do not possess this technology invariably plan to acquire it as soon as sufficient funds become available to them. Blood separation technology may be said to be a "default descriptor" (Corsín Jiménez 2005: 167) of modernity and sophistication in Indian blood banking circles, its availability advertising "the hypermodernity of a clinic" (Cohen 2004: 170). According to medico-marketing campaigns, those who persist in prescribing whole blood are blinkered and benighted. I once heard a proselytizer of "componentization" refer to a colleague who prescribes whole blood as a "thief" (*chor* in Hindi). The prescription of whole blood "steals" use-value.[3] Advertisements which inform the public that "One blood donation of yours can save three lives, not just one" point to the inadequacy of the singular. Saving only one life is insufficient, derisory.

In a discussion of different forms of counting and their relation to concepts of ownership, Strathern (2005b: 161) writes of contrasting types of multiplicity: the "multiple origins" of Euro-American commercial creations are multiple by virtue of "the way persons are added to one another's enterprises." For Melanesians, conversely, "multiplicity comes from the way persons divide themselves from one another." Both of these types of multiplicity surface in the blood-banking scenario: transfusion is effectively an aggregate term—rather than the transfer of a single unit, a transfusion should be multiply composed through addition.[4] Donations, on the other hand, are made multiple through division—the additions of transfusion being made up of divided donations. The "singular" transfusion derives from multiple origins; the "singular" donation is propelled toward multiple destinations.

This chapter explores the intersection of several forms of multiplication. The reproductive powers of donated blood in terms of familial "life-saving" are examined in relation to the divisional reproduction of the substance itself by blood banks via the use of centrifuge technology. Blood component therapy is a technique that re-produces blood outside of bodies in order that it may be inserted into more than one body—and, further, these will be bodies for which it will now be qualitatively appropriate. Many Indian donors I encountered hold donated blood itself to be reproductive in the standard "kinship" sense of pro-ducing offspring. This view derives from the objective fact that donated blood is capable of facilitating the familial reproduction of "saved" persons. I thus define "primary recipients" as those into whom donated blood is transfused, and "secondary recipients" as the primary recipient's dependents and/or descendents. The sum of these two arguments is that blood both is re-produced and reproduces; and that it is because blood is itself re-produced technologically that it can reproduce more in a familial sense.

Following from this, slogans of solicitation—and quite a few donors as well—seek to give donors and the blood they donate "credit" for the future reproductive activity of those who are "saved." Discussing song transactions in Melanesia, Strathern (n.d.) explains that those who obtain a song become its source just as much as those who previously held the song (that is, it has multiple origins). Thus, she writes, "other people's generative power can be appropriated for oneself"; potency is an appropriatable phenomenon. One could similarly say that attaining "fruits" or any other kind of credit for the primary recipient's ability to produce future descendents both enables and appropriates those persons' generative power.

There is also an Indian precedent for this kind of taking on of responsibility for the actions of others. Members of the modernizing order of Shvetambar Terapanth Jains teach that if a person were to intervene to save the life of a rat being chased by a cat, that person would take on all the sins the "saved" rat goes on to commit (Laidlaw 1995: 164). Though I never heard the suggestion that a blood donor takes on the sins of those that he or she "saves," some donors and recruiters suggest that those who give their blood can take on the credit for recipients' future reproductive activity. Clearly, transfusions can be life-saving; in those situations in which they cannot be mustered for want of donations, patients can die—sometimes without having produced offspring. Those persons who would not have been born were it not for a transfusion received by their pre-reproductive parents are a good example of what I call the secondary recipients of blood donation. As in the Terapanth case, there is much more to blood donation than saving one life—what can result are exponential spiritual effects. This chapter shows that donors are being encouraged to imagine a kind of open-ended continual numerical growth in regard to the recipients of their donations, and that this connects with Indian ideas about units of time, space, and spirituality.

The Multiplication of Blessings

Blood bag manufacturer Terumo Penpol has produced a poster that asks, "How many patients can benefit? Since your blood is going to be separated into components, you can save more lives every time you donate blood." Like an investment or share that yields great fruits despite being divorced from the actions of the investor in the present, or a supermarket that advertises its prices as enabling customers to make more of their money, the value of donation is stressed to donors as consumers of a technology that enhances not only blood banks' but also donors' effectiveness in life saving. This effectiveness, quantifiable in terms of the number of destinations, can possess, I hope to demonstrate, a correlative spiritual feedback, quantifiable in terms of the number of obtainable blessings (*ashirvad*) or fruits (*phal*).[5]

The frankest purveyor of this kind of association was a donor I met at a Sathya Sai Baba donation camp in Chennai. The devotee in question, who had played an organizational role in the camp, explained to me that the choice of blood bank had been influenced by its use of component therapy. He painted a picture to me of blood donation as a supremely efficient means of both helping numerous others and acquiring blessings: "Four persons will be treated from my one unit. The name of the blood bank is Jeevan—this means life. Four persons will get life and I will get blessings from four persons." I asked what these blessings would mean for him, and he replied: "Maybe I will live longer, be successful, maybe my son gets a good job." Several others I spoke with made the same connection. "There is no time to earn *punya* [spiritual merit] anymore," said a government employee at a camp in the center of Delhi, "but they bring the camp here [that is, conveniently close to his place of work], and they say the blood will be divided (*taksim kara jayega*) so three people will be helped (*isliye tin logõ ki madad karega*), so the gift's benefit is more for me also." This recalls the statement reported to have been made by the notorious Poona-based guru Bhagwan Rajneesh to a magazine correspondent: "My followers have no time. So I give them instant salvation" (Fuller 1992: 180). The division of donated blood does not offer donors instant salvation, but its appeal may lie partly in its condensation of virtuousness. Or put another way, it is not difficult to see why a concentrated form of merit acquisition might appear attractive to those with busy professional lives, who are concerned that there does not seem enough time in modern, "globalizing" India to perform adequate amounts of meritorious actions.[6] In a more secular idiom, the condensation of merit afforded by blood donation is exactly what makes it attractive to university students participating in the National Service Scheme (NSS). With a Gandhian heritage and the motto "Not Me, But You," the program stipulates that student volunteers complete 120 hours of community work over the course of each of two years. The certificate awarded upon successful completion is known to be looked upon favorably by some employers and universities for graduate admissions.[7] In some institutions, such as the Indian Institute of Technology (IIT) in Delhi, a single blood donation counts for as much as ten hours, making blood donation a highly speedy and efficient means of reaching the requirement of 120 hours. So in secular contexts, too, blood donation possesses efficacy as a concentrated form of merit acquisition.[8]

The division of the gift thus creates the efficient donation not only for blood banks but also for donors who attain three or four blessings, fruits, or merits from singular donations. Punya (merit) in India paradigmatically results from the giving of generous gifts (Laidlaw 1995: 27). The technology of component separation makes a generous gift more generous, the technological multiplication of substance viewed by some donors at least as multiplying their attainment of punya.

There are obvious precedents in India for this multiplication of meritorious feedback—oftentimes, the same act, performed in different spatio-temporal circumstances, produces different magnitudes of spiritually advantageous effects. At certain times or in certain spaces there occurs a special economy of worship, or as Michaels (2004: 288) puts it, "identifications can be dilated or compressed. Thus, in Benares there is the Pancakrosi Temple with 108 reliefs, which represent the [108] shrines of the procession [that circles the city]; there, walking around Kashi—an ancient name of Benares—can be performed in one place: with a walk around the temple, which brings as much religious merit as the five-day procession [around the city]." If there is agency evinced here by pilgrims, it is that of performing alignment—one aligns oneself with compressed identifications in order to attain a compressed set of credits. The point is that one does not necessarily have to "do" more to "get" more. Hinduism's "calculative repertoire" extends to the giving of *dan* (gifts, donation).[9] A male schoolteacher told me that, "especially in *kaliyug* [the present dissolute age], dan gives great blessings (*dan, maha kalyan*). It says this in all the religious books. And in holy places like in *mela* or by the Ganga, your charity is multiplied by thousands. If you give Rs.1, you have given Rs.1000. Just as prayers are multiplied by thousands if you pray between three and five [in the morning], similarly your charity is multiplied at an eclipse." Or as one Sikh donor put it to me on the occasion of the Punjabi Lohri festival, on this day his *thoda-dan* (that is, his "small" donation of blood) becomes *maha-dan* (a great or big donation).[10] Spatio-temporal alignments can thus produce multiplications. This is not a feature only of Hinduism's calculative repertoire. For Muslims, too, a prayer in Mecca is said to be worth 100,000 elsewhere. But the multiplication of benefits through specific kinds of alignment is particularly pronounced in Hinduism—multiplied spiritual returns accumulate not necessarily through the giving of more but through the correct alignments of the giving practices themselves.[11]

I suggest that the proliferation of advertisements for component separation in the subcontinent has the effect of priming a connection between the novel arithmetic of component separation and Hinduism's existing calculative repertoire. It is not difficult to see why this might be appealing to (principally Hindu) blood donors. India is not the only country where the advantages of component therapy are depicted in advertisements for donation. In one of several examples I have found from the United States, the Detroit Red Cross, publicizing a forthcoming camp, reminds donors that "A single blood donation can benefit as many as four different patients."[12] It seems likely, however, that the intensity of the Indian focus on these techniques is unique. The examples I have already given of donors who have made just such a connection suggest that the subtext of such advertisements has either been effective or will be so. A Mumbai doctor told me that his blood bank advertises the technology precisely to prime an association between it and correlative multiplied feedback: "We tell them about component therapy because, it's like, give a little and get a big result" (again, *thoda-dan* becomes *maha-dan*). The Rotary blood bank in Delhi provides every donor with a mug adorned with a picture of four sunflowers symbolizing the four lives they claim are saved. The same picture is reproduced on a poster with the slogan, "Save four lives—not just one."

On October 1, 2004, All India Voluntary Blood Donation Day, the Delhi State AIDS Control Society placed a notice in several newspapers that read, "Remember, just one unit of your donated blood can save as many as three lives." One Mumbai donor recruiter delivers lectures to students in the city:

> I tell them a story. I tell them your blood will be split into three components. The red cells will go to a thalassemic child, the platelets will go to a cancer patient, and the plasma to a third person. There will be at least three beneficiaries of your one act of lying in a bed. I compare it to a film situation in which the hero is dangling from a rope, battling the bad guys to save the heroine. I say, you can save three heroines by lying flat on a bed!

Dr. Kumar, from the Association of Voluntary Blood Donors, Tamil Nadu, told me how he explains the procedures to donors: "*Rasam* is a food of liquid tamarind and *dal*. If you keep it for some time the upper portion is liquid. And this is like plasma which is on the upper side. The down side of the *rasam* is thicker, like red cells. Then they understand and I tell them this: it is such an advantage—you save so many more lives now with component separation!" The "advantage" is that just as certain times and spaces produce an economy of worship, the gift of blood possesses an analogous efficiency in terms of the attainment of "spiritual" remuneration or feedback. It is just such a connection, I suspect, that is primed by the proliferation of component therapy publicity.

Existing Calculations

Konrad (2005: 41) distinguishes between "reproductive gifts" (such as ova, sperm, and embryos) and other corporeal donations that do not engender new life but "help sustain an existing life" (she mentions hearts, kidneys, and corneas). This is, of course, a valid distinction, with donated blood seeming to fall unambiguously into the latter category of sustenance rather than reproduction, but I argue here that blood donation is held by many Indian donors not merely to sustain but to engender new life; for example, in saving the life of someone yet to produce offspring.

It should be emphasized that a concern with the quantification of effects of blood donation was well established even before the advent of component therapy. I therefore do not claim that component therapy has resulted in a set of unprecedented multiplications. Rather, component therapy, as it were, adds a new multiplication to an already existing set of multiplications. This is pertinently illustrated by the recruitment tactics of two donor motivators from Vellore: "We used to say that your one donation will not only save one, but a whole family also. Now we say your donation will save not only one but three, and not only three people, but three families also." Blood both is re-produced and reproduces—in the sense of facilitating reproduction—and, as I noted above, it is because blood is itself re-produced that it can reproduce more.

Recruiters are keen to attribute to donors an effectiveness that goes beyond helping merely the transfusion recipient—to do this, as the example of the Vellore recruiters indicates, they engage in a rhetorical projective maximization of donation's effects that emphasizes the present and future kinship implications of donation. In so doing, they formulate new categories of primary and secondary recipients, and construct the family as a kind of infinity of eternal reproduction that is safeguarded and maintained by donated blood.

First, there is the emotive idea of saving kinship relationships. A very prominent recruitment poster depicts a child alongside the text, "My mummy is back home because you donated blood." Additionally, the idea of saving one upon whom others are dependent—and hence saving them as well—is particularly powerful, and is reflected in the common rhyming slogan, *Ap ke rakt ka ek ansh bacha sakta hai kisi ka vansh*, that is, "A part (*ansh*) of your blood can save somebody's generation/family line (*vansh*)." "Give blood save *vansh*," says another slogan. These are highly gendered expressions, for one's *vansh* can be passed on only through the male line. If your blood saves a providing male at a certain point of time, the assumption is, his whole family will be saved, not only in the present but generatively speaking also. According to such slogans, donated blood acts as a kind of progenitor. Far from there being merely one recipient, both dependents and descendents are factored into a substantially enlarged category of "recipient." The slogan thus emphasizes the familial reproductive power of blood. The familial aspect is stressed in addition by donors. For instance, in a discussion with a student donor I was told, "A drop from me can be a life for someone. A drop from me may be life for a full family. Who knows? The patient who survives may be the earning breadwinner of the family." Other donors I spoke with alluded to the possibility or the hope that their gift would save a person—male or female—who was yet to produce children. Such imaginings depict donated blood as a profound force of genealogical continuity.

In saving family relationships, dependents and descendents in addition to primary recipients, donated blood is defined as a substance imbued with "temporal potentiality" (D. Gold 1987: 48), an indispensable force of conservatism.

Like the ova donated by the British donors studied by Konrad (2005: 124), which she sees circulating as "'other' time," full of generational potential, donated blood is viewed as reproductive in its capacity to produce infinitely ramifying generational effects. Examples of the focus on the gift's magnitude abound—for instance, a slogan used by a Delhi motivator reads, *Thoda sa rakt-dan bachata jivan mahan*, that is, "A little donation of blood saves many lives." A poem read at a motivational gathering of school students by a trainee doctor contains the lines: "Just sit and think for a while. / Your donated blood may save millions of smiles." A slogan at a government blood bank in Delhi encourages fantasies of enumeration: *Ek ikai rakt-dan bacha sakta hai kitnõ ke pran*, that is, "One unit of blood can save how many lives!?"

The kinship effects of donated blood—the saving of present relationships, of reproductive potential, and of all those whose births would otherwise have been foreclosed—are potentially so great as to defy the specificity of number. One can "count" them in a projective, hypothetical manner, whilst accepting that they are beyond counting—such may be their magnitude. Numbers have been described as acting to establish certainty and to help resolve situations of doubt and mistrust (Poovey 1998), but this can only happen when they are constrained as "stable objects" (Zaloom 2003: 259). Obviously, blood donation has become a gift of adjusted magnitude by virtue of being "newly multipliable" (Konrad 2005: 15). The numbers associated with it have ceased to be stable objects and this has helped in the formation of this new arithmetic of component therapy.

The enumeration of possible future effects is by definition a practice lacking specificity. Donation's "uncountable" effects share the quality of numeric abstraction with a spiritualized rhetoric of solicitation which emphasizes that blessings and merit will be "multiplied by a thousand." Another poem delivered in front of an audience of schoolchildren contained the lines, "Come sisters, come brothers, all come forward. / You will win the credit of hundreds of thousands of merits" (*Bahanõ ao, bhayiõ ao, sab age ao / Tum karoge lakhon lakh punya*). At another public presentation in front of prospective donors, one donor recruiter declared, "When you give blood you get the fruits (*phal*). I will quote from the epics to prove this to you. A devotee was sitting at the feet of god and he said 'I am hungry for you Oh Lord. Give me such courage (*himmat*) that I can do work to benefit (*bhala*) others, since when I benefit others it will benefit me.' I say concentrate on god, organize a camp, give blood, and earn the greatest good deed (*accha karm*) multiplied by a thousand (*hazar guna*)."

The important point is that this propensity toward spiritual inflation and hyperbolic numbers comes to share imaginative terrain and intersect with donors' and recruiters' projective inflation of future secondary recipients (that is, dependents and descendents of primary recipients). In a debate before schoolchildren on the merits of blood donation, one lady declared that "the blood you give goes to the blood bank, and when, to whom, and where this blood goes, you never know. And how many blessings that person *and his family* have given you, you never know. They will come to you and give you inner strength (*atma-shakti*). At that time the blessings are unknown to you, you are spending your life peacefully" (my emphasis). The reference to receiving blessings from both primary recipient and from this person's family members (the gift's secondary recipients) is significant, suggesting that it is certainly not far-fetched to propose a correlation or "secret sympathy" between projective quantification of humanitarian effects and the quantity of reverberating spiritual effects.

Familial Ambivalence

There are further family implications of these strategies of solicitation. In chapter I I discussed the centrifugal forces brought to bear on the form of donation (the fostering of outward giving for anyone rather than inward giving to a specified someone), and this chapter has focused on the centrifugal technological operation performed on donated blood. The two centrifugal modes are connected: centrifuge technology facilitates the centrifuge of economic forms, for a gift split into multiple parts can hardly be directed toward a specific person. The family too is part of this interlocking set of widening movements.

The phasing out of family-based donation in favor of voluntary donation for an unspecified anyone might appear to be a process involving the removal of the family from its central role in the organization of blood donation in India. This would be consistent with the modernist practices of philanthropic activity outlined in chapter I which eschew known in favor of unknown recipients. We have seen, however, how kinship ideas are reinstalled within the domain of voluntary donation. And yet, it is not an identical set of familial ideas that has resurfaced. The emergent Indian ideology of voluntary donation conceptualizes the family in centrifugal terms: it is anyone's family rather than one's own family which benefits. Donor recruitment activity is, of course, only one instance of what is a larger phenomenon of "family widening," with social reformers actively attempting to expand "care" beyond the immediate family, not by denying the integrity of family bonds of care but by extending their reach to include m/any. To take a famous example: Mahatma Gandhi (1949: 222) sought a centrifugation of the Indian family comparable to that of donor recruiters in declaring to his brother that he would no longer provide his family with his future earnings, which would instead be directed toward community projects. When his brother criticized him for neglecting his duty toward his family, Gandhi retorted that "the meaning of 'family' had but to be slightly widened and the wisdom of my step would become clear." The poet Tagore, too, wrote of "ever-widening thought and action" (1912: no. 35).

What I wish to draw attention to here is how recruiters depict the figure of the "mother" in strikingly ambiguous ways as both impediment and exemplar in their quest to widen the directional intentionalities of blood donors. I was frequently told by blood bank staff and donors that altruistic or disinterested (*nishkam*) behavior is only ever really evinced by mothers in reference to their children. But disinterested service (*nishkam seva*) is exactly what recruiters say they require of donors. The relation between voluntary donor and transfusion recipient thus needs to mirror that between mothers and their children. This is reflected in the slogan: "Blood donation is like a mother's love moving from the healthy to the ailing."[13] Blood donor Satish Gupta offered a typical example of the many idealized projections of motherhood I heard: "A mother serves and nourishes her son, and the son doesn't pay her anything. The voluntary blood donor should be like the mother."

Another striking example is found on the Indian blood donation Web site http://www.bloodgivers.com. In a section designed to illustrate the "joy of giving," an arresting short story is available with the title "Mother—The Selfless Giver." It relates the birth of a baby born without ears: "Time proved that the baby's hearing was perfect. It was only his appearance that was marred." Bullied at school, a solution is found: " 'You are going to the hospital, son. Mother and I have someone who will donate the ears you need. But it's a secret' said father." The operation was a "brilliant success." Later in the boy's life, the identity of the mysterious donor is revealed: "He stood with his father over his mother's casket. Slowly, tenderly, the father stretched forth a hand and raised the thick, reddish-brown hair to reveal . . . that his mother had no outer ears." The father comments to his son, "Real giving lies not in what is given and known, but in what is given but not known."[14] Again, attention is drawn to the selfless giving of the mother as exemplar and archetype for the voluntary blood donor whose gift will never be acknowledged by recipients.

The generic Indian mother, however, is a figure of profound ambivalence: she is both archetype and obstacle in the pursuit of voluntary blood donation. She evinces pristine altruism, but it is centripetal altruism. Directed only at her (principally male) children, her altruism actually restricts the giving actions of her children because her fears for her children's health cause her actively to prevent their giving for others. As a recruiter from Chandigargh told me, "we target the mothers because it is the mothers who put the fear of giving blood into the child—the misconceptions must be removed from the mothers first of all." In my discussions with students at college donation camps, I frequently heard those unwilling to donate say it was their mothers who had forbidden them to give blood. In 2003, one Delhi blood bank team wrote and performed a play designed to encourage donation. Shown on state television on All India Voluntary Blood Donation Day (1 October), it dramatized the plight of a woman with a stomach tumor. For the necessary operation, four units of blood were required. Brought by her son Kushi Ram from their ancestral village in Bihar to Delhi for treatment, Kushi initially refuses to donate to replace the blood she requires. It is significant that the patient in need is a mother: the figure seen by recruiters to inhibit their children's donations becomes precisely the person that would benefit from the donation she prevents. The mother, it seems, is getting her comeuppance.

As I have noted, the mother's narrowly familistic form of altruism is viewed by many recruiters as stifling the expansion of the altruistic impulse beyond the familial domain. At the play's denouement, when Kushi Ram has finally seen the light and makes his donation, he declares he will return to his village and become a blood donation proselytizer. Thus, while expansion of altruism beyond the sphere of kinship does eventually occur, it has to begin first within its "natural" familial abode. As I explained above, it is the mother who principally bears the weight of this classification. Altruism starts within the family (in replacement), but then it must be brought outside in new circulations of altruism. What recruiters concerned with promoting voluntary donation seek to do is not to deny the naturalness of the family as the consummate site of altruistic feeling and action, but to widen people's notion of family. What can be called civic duty in India is in effect a function of the extent to which the family can be understood as having been centrifuged.[15] Voluntary donation for anyone's family members, by virtue of recruiters' solicitation strategies, is thus less a break from the family replacement basis of donation than that system's abstraction and generalization.

Mazzarella (2003: 139) notes that Asian "kin-mindedness" has been seen by both colonial and postcolonial commentators as detrimental to the formation of Western-style "bourgeois civic culture." The interesting point about recruiters' deployment of familial ideas and narratives as a method of obtaining voluntary donations for anyone is that the family is understood not to be a hindrance to civic duty but its condition and starting point. Indeed, "kin-mindedness" has come to facilitate an example of the kind of social form it had previously been seen to obstruct.

Conclusion

Lest this study be seen as another example of the supposedly cliché-ridden scholarly accounts of India's "essentially familial self" criticized by Cohen (1998: 105), I emphasize that donor recruitment strategies in other countries also make personalizing appeals based on the saving of family relationships (see Copeman 2005: 474). What is unique in the Indian context, I think, is the development of novel conceptual interrelations between kinship reckoning, spiritual merit, and technology. Moreover, it is significant that the centrifuge of the economic form of donation and consequently of donors' directional intentionalities forms the basis of an interlocking set of widening movements. This chapter has dealt with family widenings (a theme developed further in chapter 7), while chapter 4 explores a spiritual variant of the phenomenon of widening movements enabled by voluntary blood donation, with Nirankari devotees employing its anonymous structures in order to centrifuge (widen out) their spiritually transformative love to m/any.

Projective multiplications were already operational before the coming of the new arithmetic of component therapy. The incorporation of the technology into Hinduism's calculative repertoire, however, underlines the adaptability of Hinduism's apparatuses of return, pointing once again to the religion's faculty of " 'translat[ing]' one group of basic meanings into [an]other" (Wagner 1981: 9). I have tried to show the ways in which the arithmetic of component therapy has begun to be enrolled into an already existing and polyvalent concern with quantification and spiritual efficiency. Recruiters' energetic publicization of the gift's division draws attention to the gift's quantifiable effectiveness; an effectiveness which, I have attempted to demonstrate, is potentially convertible into increased magnitudes of spiritual return. The consistently kin-based and generation-based language employed by donors and recruiters in their representation of the virtues of blood donation is, I have argued, intimately connected to these notions of return. Blood component separation acts as a kind of technological supplement to auspiciousness.

I do not claim that enhanced spiritual return necessarily motivates a majority of donors. I do hope to have demonstrated, however, the possibility of translation between the gift's multiplicity and its reverberating "credits." It is of course significant that the division of blood multiplies a saleable product, three or four prices emerging from where there had been only one; but I do not think that this suggests the instrumental usage of a spiritualized rhetoric of solicitation. Publicity centering on component therapy indeed enables the blood bank to attain more divisible blood, and therefore more "prices," but, as I explained earlier, the therapeutic benefits of the technology are understood by doctors to be as much qualitative as quantitative, so it would be overly cynical to propose naked instrumentalism as primary stimulus behind the publicity. Instead, interests are accommodated in a way which is of mutual profit: the division of the gift, for donors, makes their generosity more generous; for doctors, it makes their profits more profitable. The profane and the sacred nourish each other, demonstrating "the power of the gift to move between the two realms of the ostensibly 'sacred' and the ostensibly 'secular'" (Coleman 2004: 432).

This chapter has shown that the technological multiplication of use-values may simultaneously multiply donors' attainment of blessings or *punya*—merit and utility can be understood as part of the same calculation. The next chapter deepens this study's exploration of merit and utility. I turn now to an exploration of the relationship between projects to foster voluntary blood donation and the social and spiritual reformist valorization of social utility.

3

The Reform of the Gift

Modern Hinduism, it has been argued, is a fractured world consisting of "a curious medley of ancient monuments and half-formed new structures" (Madan 1987: 15). This chapter explores in detail the nature of this medley, arguing that one set of highly significant, and yet markedly undertheorized, "half-formed new structures" are those existing rituals, occasions, and in particular giving mechanisms, that have been or are in the process of being "made social"—that is, rechanneled or redeployed "intelligently" (Roberts 2006: 88) and reflectively according to a teleology of social production. Conventional modes of giving—money to temples, food to the dead, the staging of feasts, and so on—come to be viewed as wasteful and asocial in the light of the emergent imperative to give that which will be useful (*upyogi*) for an "in-need" society (*samaj*).

Though I describe this imperative as emergent, the obligation to give to what counts as "society," rather than, say, to temples, has been recorded for pre-Independence India by Haynes (1987) and Watt (2005). This chapter seeks to show that calls for "useful" giving, such as those documented by these two historians, have reached a new pitch and level of diffusion in contemporary India. My concern is to document the pivotal role of blood donation in this larger social trend, and to provide conceptual tools in order to be able to apprehend more precisely the forms and religious implications of these changes. My term "in need" draws on Corsín Jiménez's (2007) depiction of allocational models of utility and well-being in which society is "in place"—drawn into models and schema—by virtue of invocations of a "utility" that stands for it. Similarly, an "in-need" society is drawn into place in rituals and giving mechanisms through conscious provision for it.[1]

In a recent essay on how invocations of "society" in the United Kingdom can throw a cloak of virtue or respectability over a host of disparate causes or projects, Strathern asks: "What will count as 'society'?" In stating that society is that for which entities bracketed off from it (such as science) need to show they do "useful things" (2005a: 476), Strathern provides an answer that is pertinent to my discussion. Deaths, marriages, anniversaries, birthdays, even suicides—as I show below—may be spoken of and understood by donors and event-organizers as opportunities for providing society with "useful things." Such occasions usually involve different sorts of offerings, for example, money to the bride the night before her wedding. Giving blood instead of, or as well as, this money would be (and is, as I demonstrate below) a principal way of bringing in utility and therefore society—"society" having being bracketed off from religious, economic, and family life largely as a result of the widespread acceptance among modernizing Hindu activists of European cultural assumptions about the "bifurcation of the social realm" (Sen 2003: 16). This bifurcation has given rise to a situation in which society is summoned in diverse contexts as an entity to which useful things should be contributed. Enactments of "utility" thus ensure the presence of "in-need" society. Though the Hindu reformist milieu has always been internally differentiated and characterized by competing aims and methods, the shared imperative to make society present in all occasions, ritual or otherwise, is one of the important filaments that crosscuts and unites the many movements and associations that form it.

Of course, blood is not the only useful thing that can be given to society: pledging bodies for dissection and organs for transplantation, or giving wheelchairs to hospitals, where previously a religious organization might have offered a feast for its followers, or gifts might have been given by mourners to Brahmins in order to transfer to them the pollution produced by a death, would also count as instances of "making social." It is in the arena of blood donation, however, that one finds some of the most vivid and arresting examples of this rechanneling of existing giving dynamics.

The emerging giving structures documented here are related to and yet distinct from existing scholarly characterizations. Those structures reported in the most important anthropological writings on gifts in India (principally Laidlaw 1995, 2000; Parry 1986, 1994; Raheja 1988) are by no means mere "ancient monuments," but in certain, mainly public, settings there is mounting evidence that they are in the process of critical thought and reformulation, in part through active initiatives involving groups and individuals who profess reformist spiritual and social aims. As shorthand, I refer to the forms of gift explored by the abovementioned anthropologists—all of whom have produced ethnographies of the gift from within comparatively traditional settings—and the important differences between these forms notwithstanding, as "classical dan." I present evidence of the infusion into classical dan categories of what I call "virtuous utility," with modernizing adherents of medical or social utility seeking to convert what they view as nonproductive or wasteful dan into productive dan—that is, gifts that are useful for society.

Virtuous Utility

Utility, says MacIntyre (1981: 62), is a "pseudo-concept available for a variety of ideological uses"—it is nothing more, he says, than a "conceptual fiction."[2] Utility is undoubtedly a problematic concept and requires clarification. It is principally understood, both inside and outside anthropology, according to the quantitative delineations of classical economists, for whom, says Bataille, utility is on the one hand "limited to acquisition (in practice, to production) and to the conservation of goods; on the other, it is limited to reproduction and to the conservation of human life." This implies that all social activity, "in order to be valid, must be reducible to the fundamental necessities of production and conservation" (Bataille 1985: 116, 117). For Mauss, utilitarianism was equally reductionist—synonymous with "the brutish pursuit of individual ends"—and he famously proposed "the gift" as an alternative. Reciprocal gifts, in contrast to "icy, utilitarian calculation," would institute and sustain enduring social relations (1990: 98). The important differentiation here is that for Mauss gifts did indeed have utility in establishing relations and social solidarity but were not utilitarian. Gifts for Mauss were useful in a sense that classical utility could not recognize. Parry (1986) has demonstrated the limited applicability of Mauss's *The Gift* to Indian categories of dan. Spirit (sin, impurity, inauspiciousness, and so on) is indeed present in Indian gifts, argues Parry, but paradoxically in light of the prevailing interpretations of Mauss's essay, the norm of reciprocity is denied (Parry 1986: 463).

Processes of "making social" in which gifts of blood, eyes, or bodies are made unilaterally by donors thus do not represent the progressive ebbing away and replacement of Maussian reciprocal gifts—Indian dan was not reciprocal in the first place.[3] Instead, this chapter provides examples of the "exaptation" of the gift, exaptation being the "process of co-opting one structure to do a different job from that for which it was originally adapted" (Ingold 1997: 119). Exaptation, here, neither departs from nor moves toward a version of Maussian utility—rather, the exaptation of the gift is in the direction of production and conservation, and hence of classical utility. Importantly, however, exaptation is mostly enacted only in a partial manner (that is, the structure's ability to serve its original purpose is largely maintained, even reinforced, as the structure is adapted to serve another purpose). The partial nature of this exaptation is significant because the reform of giving practices is characterized both by conceptual retentions and by departures that consolidate those retentions through being dependent on them. Reformed gifts, or gifts "made social," tend not to efface existing giving structures, but rather to enroll and become parasitical upon them. The "parasiting" of one calculative agency by another, says Callon (1998: 45–46), involves the imposition of the interloper agency's calculative rules and the consequent forcing of the "host agency to engage in its own calculation." In the cases documented in this chapter, existing giving structures become the host agencies for the particular calculations of medical or social utility.

According to Bataille's portrayal of utility as a creed that recognizes social validity only in actions reducible to production and conservation, adherents of utility would view actions of "disutility" as wasteful and in need of reform. This of course recalls Weber's claims about the rationalizing effects of industrial modernity, and related transformations in giving activities from "wasteful" to "useful," or efforts in the direction thereof, have been studied ethnographically in several contexts. Yang, for instance, who also draws on Bataille, notes that the burning of money at funerals and other displays of "ritual excess" in Wenzhou, southeast China, are viewed by Chinese Communist reformers as wasteful and stupid. The irony here is that such "illegitimate" and extravagant consumption of wealth can only take place because the region is so prosperous and thus fully cognizant of the economic rationality it so strikingly suspends on these occasions. Thus, Yang concludes, "the opposition between ritual and religion, on the one hand, and economic development, on the other, does not hold in rural Wenzhou" (Yang 2000: 479–480).

Whereas Yang documents attempts by the Chinese state and its officials to prohibit excessive expenditure, Haynes considers attempts made by the British authorities in nineteenth-century Surat to reform comparable varieties of expenditure in a "socially productive" direction: officials urged the city's wealthy elite to adopt an attitude of philanthropy, "hoping to divert some of the money spent on religious festivals, offerings to deities, and marriage ceremonies into channels they regarded as more 'productive.'" Colonial officials argued, "Far better it is to lay out your riches on such lasting objects [as school buildings and suchlike] than to waste them on fireworks, in music and other extravagances." It was by no means only colonial officials, however, who exhorted the Indian elites to reform their giving practices. The Gandhian National Education Society in particular portrayed itself as a "sacred focus for charitable donations, one that was more deserving than Vaishnavite or Jain festivals and temples" (Haynes 1987: 350, 356).

Haynes concludes his study of Surat philanthropists' gift giving with the observation that there occurred a "negotiated accommodation to the value system of the rulers rather than an abandonment of traditional preoccupations" (1987: 353). Secular giving was now pursued in tandem with religious offerings but in different transactions. For the most part, the wealthy elite partitioned its giving into separate spheres, continuing to offer resources to festivals and temples while also making "modern" charitable donations to "society" (for example, to schools and hospitals).

In the cases of "making social" I document below, however, a kind of volitional conjunction or "fusion force" (Kapferer 1997: 261) is developed whereby both secular and religious giving commitments are sustained simultaneously within the same giving actions. Philanthropic gifts of utility come to be enacted in "sacred" settings for purposes that are as much spiritual as secular. In his study of the renovation of giving practices in colonial India, Watt finds comparable instances in which "new" giving is justified in relation to older charitable concepts. When, for example, in the early years of the twentieth century Brijendra Nath Roy and others sought to raise funds for the founding of Benaras Hindu University, the revered concept of *vidya-dan* (the gift of learning) was mobilized in order "to sanction the transformation of traditional charitable institutions to suit modern educational needs" (Watt 2005: 71). Though Watt is careful to say that "the shift toward social service . . . was inflected by indigenous traditions of giving" (ibid.: 88), the story is still largely one of replacement, hence his chapter title: "From Dana to Associational Philanthropy." In the face of Western ideological influence, the Indian giving mentality is ultimately revealed by Watt to be "something like a glass, which when it becomes full, begins to shed its old content as the new is poured in" (Macfarlane 1997: 23). In exploring blood donation's role in making existing giving mechanisms "social," I aim to show, conversely, that even when groups professing reformist aims actively seek to replace established practices of giving, what actually results are complex accommodations between different aspirations and imperatives.

Watt additionally invokes Parry's (1986) argument that regions dominated by "world religions" such as Hinduism and Christianity are the most susceptible to conceptions of the free gift for the reason that such religions restrict reciprocity to the realm of salvation and "unseen fruits" in the next life. Watt (2005: 70) adds to this the insight that although in the early twentieth century, "many Indians did indeed hope to acquire *punya* (and thus improve their *karma*) through acts of giving . . . this is precisely what social activists wished to change." Rewards would henceforth be detached from "spirit," recompense now coming in the form of this-worldly social improvement. Indeed, Arya Samaj leader Lala Lajpat Rai (1865–1928) thought Hindus' quest for spiritual reward should be replaced with an emphasis on social service: "The brahmanical emphasis on 'self-realization' he condemned as mere selfishness" (Sen 2003: 14).[4]

The mutual exclusiveness of service-oriented giving and spiritual reward may well have been the desired objective of modernizing social movements— their goal a kind of radicalizing of the free gift through which it becomes drained not only of this-worldly but also other-worldly recompense—and both Watt and Lajpat Rai portray acts of social utility as being exterior to spiritually remunerative virtue. In the examples I document below, however, the targeting of practical utility emphatically does not preclude the attainment of spiritual aims; in fact, the fulfillment of practical goals becomes the very condition of their achievement. Simpson's observation that body commoditization debates are cast largely as a struggle between intrinsic value and utility is certainly germane as regards wider debates on the theme of corporeal donations for medical purposes (2004: 841). The interesting thing about the contexts that this chapter explores, however, is that utility has been assigned a virtuous or pious aspect and is regarded by many of the donors and medics I met as itself something like an intrinsic value. This is apparent, for instance, in the phrase, often repeated by both doctors and donors, that "Donating blood once is better than giving to a temple a hundred times."

This leads to a further key aspect of the reformed gift—the question of its recipients. In the examples I explore below, blood donation comes to possess superior virtue compared to temple giving in part because it presupposes a need that cannot be guaranteed in the case of temple priests, who are often viewed with suspicion as grasping intermediaries.[5] The superiority of blood donation also obtains from the fact that it more safely secures the benefits of giving (dan ka labh) to the donor. It can at times seem as though the individual spiritual goals attainable through giving can now only be secured by way of an expansive (or centrifugal) movement that, as it were, makes the gift social. Such a logic appears to invert the idea that "moral obligations to others can be satisfied [best] . . . by first satisfying obligations to the self" (Wolfe 1989: 33). Indeed, the logic of "making social" seems to indicate that only through adding to "in-need" society can self-oriented spiritual aims be satisfied. In the discussion in earlier chapters, blood donation was "made selfish" through recruiters' emphasis on donation as an act of physical purification and a means of acquiring maximal quantities of merit, whereas in the present discussion it is "made social." However, these seemingly contrasting approaches are in fact the two sides of the same coin, with both seeking commensuration between apparently incompatible requirements as the means to obtain donations. Mandeville's celebrated observation in his Fable of the Bees—that Publick Benefit derives from Private Vice—also embodies a commensuration of self-love and the overall welfare of society, where a privileging of the former supposedly has epiphenomenal benefits for the latter.[6] A large measure of self-love's value was this socially beneficial overflow. This chapter documents the same commensuration but from the opposite angle, where part of the value of the making social of "host agency" ritual and giving forms lies in the way this process better enables the attainment of spiritual merit.

Making Social as Reformist Activity

The "making social" of structures of giving is a process of reform. The word "reform" could be viewed as problematic in that it may imply relative stasis prior to recent moves to update established transfer practices. The term "reform," however, is appropriate here since it invokes a much-studied, avowedly reformist milieu of social and religious activity from which transformations in giving practices cannot be dissociated. Indeed, the reform of giving is indivisible from the reform of Indian religion which has also, in many contexts, been made social.

In a comparative study of trends in Vietnamese and Indian religious reform, S. Bayly (2004a: 117) notes that reformist thinkers sought to purify and rationalize religiosity: "The characteristic model for these reformers was and still is a religion of doctrinal coherence whose prevailing mood or disposition was one of reason, sobriety, and selfless service." This disposition has had an impact not only on giving practices but also on a series of interlocking social phenomena which have all been subject to reformist redefinition: the concepts of *seva* (selfless service), *sannyas* (renunciation) and *dan* have all undergone or are undergoing similar centrifugal movements from being targeted toward specific people's material or spiritual statuses to mass social uplift and society in general.

To take renunciation: definitions of Indian religiosity as being "the cradle of those religious ethics which have abnegated the world, theoretically, practically, and to the greatest extent" (Weber 1958: 323) rightly remain integral to understandings of Indian renunciation. However, certain innovative forms of asceticism that do not entail withdrawal from society have been receiving increasing scholarly attention (see Copeman 2006; Alter 1992a; Khare 1984; Warrier 2003a). Swami Vivekananda, founder of the Ramakrishna Mission in 1897, is often credited with initiating a redefinition of asceticism as the truest template for socially oriented seva (Warrier 2003a: 255).[7] Beckerlegge (2003: 59) notes that "Vivekananda's use of the *sannyasin* [renouncer] as a deliverer of organised service to humanity has frequently been acknowledged as an astute retention of a powerful Hindu symbol." In a discussion of the increasing entwinement of asceticism and seva, Mayer (1981: 170) declares that "renunciation of selfishness through social service has taken the place of the traditional form of renunciation as leading to spiritual merit." Though I do not agree that "spiritual merit" has been expunged from the realm of asceticism, Mayer rightly argues that the "selfless" orientation of the truest seva has become indivisible from contemporary definitions of renunciation. As I illustrate below, the Dera Sacha Sauda devotional movement provides a particularly striking example of the "making social" of renunciation.

Seva is a polyvalent term enacted and enunciated as a claim to virtue in a variety of settings: children do the seva of their parents in old age (Cohen 1998; see also Gandhi 1949: 24), devotees do the seva of a particular deity or guru, and politicians are ideally supposed to do the seva of their constituents (Mayer 1981: 158–159). Like philanthropic giving and asceticism, however, seva is increasingly directed toward service of "humanity" (*manav seva*) or nation rather than merely parents, gurus, or deities. As stated, the historians Haynes (1987) and Watt (2005) have both undertaken interesting and important studies of changing Indian giving dynamics in pre-Independence India. In anthropology, however, though the reform of asceticism and the correlative redefinition of seva have been touched upon, the reform of the gift has received negligible attention thus far.[8]

Gurus, Death, and Blood Donation: A Winning Combination

As was noted in chapter 1, the Dera Sacha Sauda is a devotional order in the sant tradition which undertakes large-scale social welfare projects. I undertook a month's ethnographic research in one of its ashrams in the city of Sirsa, Haryana state, in 2004. One of the ways in which the movement proclaims its reformist credentials is through its professed disdain for conventional asceticism. The guru's public declarations are often directed toward the demystification of the figure of the sadhu:

> We met a man who said you will find god in forests. We said, just think! If you find god in forests then all the wild animals living there must have found god way back, but have they?! Somebody said to us, wear clothes of a particular color [i.e., saffron] and you will find god. Think! If you can meet god by changing the color of your clothes then there is nothing to do! Change the color of your clothes; god will come to your home. And when you want to make god leave, just change your dress to different color clothes.[9]

The Dera Sacha Sauda at once retains and reformulates classical concepts of asceticism in housing roughly 350 "sadhus" and 100 "sadhvis" at its Sirsa ashrams. Dedicated to the giving of seva (service) to the guru and to "humanity," these renouncers claim to work eighteen-hour days tilling the fields, writing and publishing the organization's newspaper, *Sacha Kahoon*, serving at the Sacha Sauda petrol pump or restaurant, or engaged in other labors. They wear plain, non-saffron clothes, many sadhus donning cockney-style flat caps. There seems very little visually to link them with classical representations and definitions of the sadhu. They have, however, left their families to live in the ashram—an archetypal Indian ascetic requirement—and further, the claim to work eighteen-hour days appears to be a kind of practical analogue of the feats of endurance associated with classical renouncers. Indeed "practical sadhus" would be an appropriate term for these renouncers whose activities correspond to Swami Vivekananda's call for a "Practical Vedanta," which "propagates an ethical and social application of the *advaita vedanta*" (Hellman 1996: 241) and which stresses the supremacy of action as worship. One extremely important way in which their behavior diverges from (and implicitly critiques) that of classical renouncers is in their not accepting alms. The guru strongly criticizes the giving of money to temple priests, and his organization professes never to accept donations. In one discourse the guru contrasts useless offerings

of money to God with superior offerings of utility such as medicine and blood
for human beings:

> Nobody reached God with money. We can give this to you in writing. Yes!
> Donate, but where it is needed. . . . If somebody is dying from a disease,
> then it's your duty to help him. Donate blood and money; bring medi-
> cines for him. . . . This body will vanish to soil so donate your eyes for
> somebody. It is really a great donation and God must bless you for this. So
> brother! Saints never stop you from donations but they ask you to do so
> *at the right place, for the right person* [my emphasis; see above, note 5].
> Donate with your own hands. Don't bring anybody in between. O! You
> give a donation of money and say it is given to God. Does God sign
> on that?[10]

Since Dera Sacha Sauda sadhus and sadhvis were firmly at the fore in donating blood at a donation camp staged by the movement in October 2004, the
occasion forcefully demonstrated the interlocking nature of reformist redefinitions of giving and asceticism, for each was manifested simultaneously and
interdependently in this singular event.

Articles published in regional newspapers by journalists covering the camp
recount the guru's address at the inauguration in which he reportedly declared
that the decision to hold the camp was taken at the *pagri* ceremony of his father,
Sadar Magghar Singh. It was staged in order to "contribute towards the service
of mankind rather than having a public feast."[11] In another article on this "great
yagna [fire-offering ritual] of blood donation," the guru is quoted as claiming
that manav seva (service of humanity) such as blood donation is "of greater significance than organizing any type of feast." The reflective replacing of customary feasts and rites with blood donation in "the service of mankind" may be
termed "substitutive ennoblement." Another article puts this clearly: "A rare
example was witnessed on the occasion of the homage paying function (*shrad-
dhanjali samaroh*) of the father of the present *gaddinashin* of the Sacha Sauda,
Sirsa . . . a massive blood donation camp was organized on the occasion of this
homage paying ceremony instead of indulging in the numerous rites and rituals
which usually follow the death of elders in order to create a reputation for
oneself."[12]

In addition to making statements similar to those cited above from the
local media, devotees in Sirsa told me explicitly that they thought of themselves
as performing rakt-dan in replacement of *pind-dan*: the giving of food to the
deceased. As Banwari Lal, editor of *Sacha Kahoon*, told me: "Guru Ji said our aim
is to serve society (*samaj*). So [when his father died], instead of pind-dan, which
is actually just a waste (*bekar*) of money, we did rakt-dan, which is a great donation (*rakt-dan maha-dan hai*). In pind-dan a cow is given to a Brahmin, but this is
not useful (*upyogi*)."[13] My guide in Sirsa, Dr. Soni, also describes the instigating of

blood donation as the substitutive ennoblement of conventional mortuary ceremonies: "Instead of pind-dan and other orthodox customs, Guru Ji did a blood donation camp and gave free houses to the poor and widows. Pind-dan is for the peace of the soul of the departed. But it's not true! Old people say give pind-dan, give a cow to a Brahmin. But the pandits are rich. If you give money to the rich, how will anybody be benefited?" Part of the virtue of blood donation, according to this view, is that it possesses built-in means testing—a person doesn't receive a transfusion, Dr. Soni surmises, if they do not need one: the transfusion recipient is needy and therefore worthy.

Extensions of Death and Marriage

Soon after my visit to Sirsa I met with the donor recruiter Vinay Shetty in Mumbai. I mentioned to him the extraordinary scale of the Sirsa camps, and he laughed: "Religious leaders and death is a fantastic combination! It really hits you. Indira dies and Rajiv wins the elections. You have a death and everyone is more sympathetic to you. Death, gurus, and blood donation is a winning combination!" He has a point. The first blood donation camps conducted by the Sant Nirankari Mission took place on the death anniversary of its former guru, Gurbachan Singh, who was assassinated in 1980 (see chapter 4); the Dera Sacha Sauda's first world record–breaking donation camp was conducted on the death anniversary of its preceding guru; the Youth Congress holds camps on the death anniversaries of Indira, Rajiv, and Sanjay Gandhi, respectively.

Deaths and death anniversaries precipitate giving practices that spiritual movements and medical institutions seek to "parasite" in order to reconfigure their calculative goals in accordance with the aims of medical utility. Devotional orders and political parties are not unique in attempting to "make social" events staged in the immediate aftermath of deaths. The Shiv Shakti blood bank, located in Sirsa (but not connected to the Sacha Sauda), takes active steps for the initiation of (reformist) rakt-dan in the "spaces" of classical dan. It uses its literature and expertise to campaign for both eye and blood donation, and its medics regularly travel to Haryana's more remote rural areas to educate villagers about donation and to encourage the staging of camps. A blood bank director named Dr. Arora whom I met in Sirsa at a blood donation camp conducted at a marriage function (discussed below), recalls holding roughly ten blood collection camps at the *uthala* and *rasam pagri* ceremonies of persons who had donated their eyes or bodies on either the fourth or the thirteenth days after a death: "We get a good response—usually 25–30 units. It is an emotion by which they pay tribute to the departed soul (*jane wale*). It is a prayer to god, an offering to the god that the soul will rest in peace. By doing something good, they want something in return—peace for the departed soul." Uthala is the "getting up" ceremony when mourners are no longer expected to sit patiently on the floor; rasam pagri is the passing of the deceased male's turban to the new head of the family. The blood bank's founder, Dr. Banerwal, explains: "When people have the funeral gathering, a turban (*pagri*) is put on the elder son to show he is now responsible for the family, and we have convinced people that after wearing that pagri, the first thing to do is to donate blood. This is the noblest (*sab se nek*) way to begin your regime."[14] Banerwal continues: "I went to mourn the death of a friend and I said to his children, if your father can donate his eyes, why can't you donate blood on rasam pagri? At first they said no but they called me up two or three days later and asked me to address the mourners." The alliance between reformist Hinduism's focus on practical action over existing formal procedures and campaigns to solicit blood donation was again clearly present in Banerwal's appeal to the mourners: "We have come here to pray for the peace of his soul and it doesn't come through words but through action."

In the "active" focus of rakt-dan lies its reformist superiority. In his address to mourners, Banerwal succeeded in making social the occasion of rasam pagri by stressing the virtues of utility. The soul of the departed person, he asserted, would find peace through offering the productive dan of rakt-dan, the strong suggestion being that this soul's "peace" is most safely secured through the giving of a dan made social.[15]

Miyazaki has recently written of extensions in gift-giving practices in reference to Fiji. He describes different "terrains" of extension (Miyazaki 2005: 279) which may be glossed here as "indigenous" and "analytical": indigenous Fijian gift-giving appeared, in one historical moment—though in fact ultimately failed—to provide a template for future relations between native Fijians and the state; indigenous gift-giving appeared to possess "extensible potential." Another terrain of extension is that of anthropological analysis: through extending the insights gained through his analysis of gift giving in numerous contexts, Mauss (1990), as discussed above, formulated a diagnostic tool for certain problems characteristic of Western society. Following from this, it is evident that Banerwal, in "parasiting" existing giving practices in order to collect blood from mourners, rendered rasam pagri "extensible-to-utility."

Raheja (1988: 148–156) provides a detailed description of the funerary gifts given on the deaths of male householders in Pahansu village, Uttar Pradesh. She explains that on the day of death, four balls of dough are placed in the corners of the stretcher carrying the deceased. They are later removed to a space outside the boundary of the village in order that the body's inauspiciousness (*nasubh*) be removed from the vicinity of mourners. On the third day, milk, honey, and flour are offered to the wandering ghosts (*prets*) of the locality. More offerings of yoghurt and sugar are made in the house to the deceased's pret to sever connections with it and to transfer its inauspiciousness. On the thirteenth day, offerings are now given to human recipients. By this time the pret has become an ancestral deity and is no longer a potentially malevolent force. Thirteen measures of certain types of uncooked foods (*karva cun*) are transferred from the wife-giving side of the deceased's family to the wife-taking affines who then symbolically offer them to the deceased before finally they are (reluctantly) accepted by the family Brahman. In Pahansu, the thirteenth day is also the day on which the pagri is tied onto the eldest son of the deceased man. His mother's brother gives him money and the turban. The mother's brother later places "the cloth of widowhood" onto the head of his sister, which she must wear for several months in order that its inauspiciousness remain contained in her person. The cloth is finally disposed of in the Yamuna River or given to a sweeper at Haridwar. A final prestation on the thirteenth day is called "the coins of the hand washing" and involves women mourners washing their hands and offering coins into a vessel provided by the barber's wife. This, again, is done to transfer donors' inauspiciousness to the recipient (the barber's wife).

Though I did not witness any mortuary rituals in the villages surrounding Sirsa in Haryana, and though the details provided by the blood bank doctors are far from comprehensive, the information I gathered does suggest that certain of the prestations described by Raheja were indeed conducted at the mortuary ceremonies in which blood was donated. Drs. Arora and Banerwal specifically mentioned gifts made to the pret (ghost of the deceased) and to a Brahmin. Rakt-dan performed in such settings thus appears to represent the reformist "ennoblement" rather than simply a replacement of existing dan transfers. And yet, while much is seemingly retained of the "traditional" mortuary rites, even as a reformist departure is undertaken, the blood bank, with its emphasis on the importance of rakt-dan as a theology of action and a socially conscious method of ensuring the peace of the deceased, is clearly a significant agent of Hindu reform.

Raheja's description of Pahansu mortuary gifts additionally raises the issue of inauspicious or impure transfer. In reference to the mortuary rituals under consideration, the matter of impure transfer cannot be authoritatively resolved given the paucity of data, but there are clues. Säävälä (2001: 314) has recently argued—though in a different context—that the removal of inauspiciousness by one party need not necessitate its transfer to another. Similarly in Pahansu, the four balls of dough, placed in fields surrounding the village, simply propel the dead body's inauspiciousness outside the bounds of the village. The accounts provided by Dr. Arora and Dr. Banerwal appear to suggest that, in certain Haryana villages, rakt-dan may also remove inauspiciousness or sin. It would be going too far, however, to suggest that these qualities become located within delineable others. Rather than being propelled toward transfusion recipients, it may be the case that inauspiciousness is instead minimally impelled away from the vicinity of mourners, just as the balls of dough in Pahansu remove without necessarily transferring inauspiciousness.

A further purpose of rakt-dan in this setting, according to Banerwal, is its symbolic role in the immediate institution by the successor pagri recipient of a "noble regime"—a further indicator of the propensity of reform-minded Hindus to see utility as a virtue. Finally, to the extent that rakt-dan is aimed at the pret (for its peace or its sustenance, see Parry 1994: 196), the mutating form of the deceased assumes a role similar to that of the Nirankari guru as an agent of multiple refraction. Chapter 4 details how Nirankari devotees' blood donations are given both *to* the guru and *through* the guru to "humanity." Similarly, securing the peace and sustenance of the pret may be the principal aim of the mourners, but, as in the Nirankari example, the recipient turns facilitator, converting a centripetal aim (securing the soul's peace) into centrifugal (socialized) effects. Exaptation—the coopting of existing giving structures to effect new outcomes— thus signals not the prior gift's effacement but the newly formed gift's duality: rakt-dan, as a mortuary gift extended-to-utility, comes to serve several different purposes at once.

I provide examples elsewhere (Copeman forthcoming) of execution and euthanasia as actions extensible-to-utility. I also heard of a case in Delhi where a student killed himself because he failed his exams, having left a suicide note expressing the wish to have his eyes donated for medical use. I came across numerous further instances of Delhi blood donor recruiters seeking to exploit the "extensible potential" of death-related giving procedures. A medical student at the All India Institute of Medical Sciences (AIIMS) exhorted an audience of schoolchildren to "choose one important day of your life like your birthday (*janam din*) or *shraddh*," when rites for the dead are performed, on which to give blood. "Give blood on shraddh in memory of your dead elders (*bhuzurg*). Choose the day of shraddh, the day to honor and respect your elders, so that from their souls (*atma*) will come blessings (*ashirvad*) for you." Once again, it appears that the impulse to "make social" through "useful" giving to m/any as opposed to "useless" giving to specific dead elders becomes the condition for the fulfillment of the self-oriented component of offerings (here, the wish to attain blessings).

A notable feature of the blood donation-mortuary rituals I heard about in Haryana is that they were conducted by mourners partly in tribute to the deceased's donation of his or her eyes. This phenomenon of donations being made in tribute to donations made by others was also a feature of a marriage ceremony I attended in Sirsa in which the well-educated couple's friends and family were encouraged to give blood. The bride's brother had died a year before of muscular dystrophy. Before dying, according to his cousin Sandeep, he had said: "Please donate my eyes and they will go on seeing after my death." Thus, said Sandeep, "Social service is in the family's blood right now." I describe such modes of dying elsewhere (Copeman forthcoming)—in which dying persons pledge parts of their bodies—as "consecrations" of misfortune indicative of an emerging Indian aesthetics of dying that foregrounds utility, this being consistent with what has been described as the widespread Hindu ideal of playing an active part in one's own death (Madan 1987: 11).

Inspired by her brother's example, the bride Yukti's blood donation initiative was endorsed by her parents, who stated on the wedding invitations: "Blood donation is a great donation (*rakt-dan, maha-dan*). Please take part enthusiastically (*barhcharh kar*). This only (*yahi*) will be the true blessing (*sacha ashirvad*) for the *kanya* [daughter/virgin]." There is the suggestion, once again, that "true blessings" accrue only from offerings of virtuous utility. The occasion was *ladies sangit* (ladies' music), a function that precedes the wedding proper, in this instance involving the bride's female relatives performing a broad range of songs on stage, from classical *bhajans* (devotional songs) to contemporary Bollywood hits. In the adjoining room of the *dharmashala* (pilgrim lodge) at which the event was held, beds were laid out for blood donation, and it was indeed a remarkable sight to witness the guests and family members donating in their finery. This donation of blood was performed explicitly in place of the small offerings of money which I was told would usually be given to the bride on ladies sangit. I gained the impression, however, that gifts were to be given to the couple as usual at the wedding proper. Blood donation in this marriage context was thus part substitutive ennoblement of a prior gift-form, and part ennobling addition. It was the innovative Shiv Shakti blood bank, described earlier, which bled invitees, and the blood bank's founder, Dr. Banerwal, who declared on stage, microphone in hand: "People give gifts and blessings to the bride in marriage, and sometimes it reaches a million rupees. But what people are giving today is the gift of life (*jivan-dan*) which is priceless (*anmol*)."

The reflective nature of this "parasiting" of marriage offerings should be emphasized—the bride and her family were well aware of the novelty of the event, inviting journalists and television crews to cover the "first ever blood donation marriage."[16] This appears consonant with Cohn's (1987: 229) argument about cultural objectification, whereby the "Western educated class of Indians" began in the twentieth century to "stand back and look at themselves," making their own culture into a "thing." Once culture has been turned into a conscious object, states Cohn (ibid.: 250), it can be used for "political, cultural and religious battles." One such battle, perhaps, is the "making social" of existing offerings, with classical giving structures being objectified in order to be subjected to ennobling reform. Having drawn this parallel, however, it should be emphasized that I do not subscribe to Cohn's claim that all this amounts to "Westernization," since, as I hope has been made clear, in many cases reformist giving practices are highly dependent upon and actually reinforce the giving structures they "parasite." What results is not Westernization but complex accommodations between differing imperatives.

Differing Instances and Intensities

The set of processes I term "making social," it should be clear, are taking place on multiple different levels. Moreover, it is by no means only classical dan offerings that are subject to this dynamic. In February 2004, Delhi University was the venue for the Society for Unexpected Goals and Means (SUGAM) to induct Valentine's Day into the realm of the reformed gift. The society was formed in north Delhi by a handful of local traders and businesspeople for the express purpose of refurbishing the narrow and exclusive romantic exchanges they hold to be characteristic of Valentine's Day into expansively reformulated, "inclusive" gifts of love. It capitalizes on the emotional content of valentine gifts, declaring that celebrants must expand and despecify the circle of valentine beneficiaries and thereby discover the "true" meaning of the occasion. Blood donors each received a red rose, provided symbolically by future recipients. A poster adorning the donating area declared: "All humanity, my Valentine. Selfless love—The poor and destitute—The downtrodden—Accident victims—The suffering—The old and infirm—Indian values—Spiritual values—My India, my Valentine. True love, my Valentine. Give blood for Valentine." Student donors I spoke with appeared to subscribe to SUGAM's message. As one male student told me: "Love is for everyone, not just for a girl or boy. It is also for the poor and for my mother. Today I gave for the poor and for my mother. My mother is my valentine."

SUGAM's nationalist reformulation of Valentine's Day invites a contrast with the Shiv Sena's stance on this "Western" festival. The Shiv Sena political party was begun as a vehicle to promote the interests of the Marathi-speaking population of Maharashtra, but in the 1980s turned to "rabid Hindu communal rhetoric" (Hansen 1999: 162). The party epitomizes the politics of violence and has engaged in numerous anti-Muslim pogroms. Hansen describes the Sena's public spectacles of violence as "the very generative and performative core of its being" (2001: 65). The SUGAM donation camp I attended was at one point interrupted by a Shiv Sena demonstration against the festival which passed close by. The Shiv Sena has declared that "Western culture is injected into people's mindset by these celebrations" and that this represents "cultural corruption of the youth."[17] The irony is that the party advocates the organizing of blood donation camps instead of Valentine's Day celebrations so that youngsters can "express their love for the motherland."[18] SUGAM's blood donation camp certainly included the nation as beneficiary, and maybe even encouraged youngsters to "express their love for the motherland," but not as an alternative to Valentine's Day. Rather, the narrow anti-valentine nationalism of the Shiv Sena contrasts sharply with the integrative reformism of the NGO for which "utility" reaches out to absorb "alien" practices into the canon of virtue.

The diversity of the levels and locations subjected to processes of "making social" is indeed striking. The phenomenon is evident, for example, in Bollywood films in which, according to Vanita (2002: 155), problematic "love" relationships come to be sanctioned and recognized as virtuous by the romantic protagonists' families and friends if they can be "demonstrated to be socially

useful and out-reaching rather than inward-turning." I have been arguing, however, that what is not happening is the unilateral conversion of practices, occasions, or giving structures to a state of virtuous utility. The picture that emerges
is more multifaceted. The following example should make this clear. In 2004 the
Rotary blood bank conducted a donation camp at a huge congregation of 12,000
people in Delhi who had gathered to learn a form of yoga under the tutelage of
Swami Ramdev.[19] Yoga techniques—for Swami Ramdev and his followers at
least—are oriented to the physical fitness of the practitioner: Swami Ramdev
claims that the breathing exercises he prescribes purify the blood, ward off cancer, and make one live longer.[20] In his pre-camp address in front of Ramdev's
devotees, blood bank director Dr. Bhatia related blood donation to devotees'
concern to improve their physical fitness: "Blood donation is another way to
prevent you from falling sick—your whole health will become better."[21]

I suggested earlier that the two seemingly opposite tendencies in donor
solicitation—conceptually rendering blood donation "social" on the one hand
and "selfish" on the other—are two sides of the same coin. From one angle, the
example of the yoga camp appears to invert the claim that Publick Benefit
derives from Private Vice, since a yoga event is "made social" through its integration of an archetypal practice of virtuous utility. As a self-oriented practice,
yoga, like a Bollywood love relationship, comes to secure its own piety and worthiness through the inclusion of an "in-need" society to which its practitioners
contribute. In other words, the starting point of the process of commensuration
was apparently Publick Benefit, whereby adding to "society" served to make virtuous a self-oriented activity (Private Vice)—an analogous but inverse commensuration to that proposed by Mandeville. However, in the same instant that the
yoga gathering was "made social," the blood bank director portrayed blood
donation as a self-oriented activity in his depiction of it as a method "to prevent
you from falling sick." Each practice took on a quality of the other, donation
being "made selfish," yoga being "made social." The blood donation yoga camp
thus operated simultaneously according to the two "opposite" modes of commensuration, with each of its two main operational aspects functioning in
reverse but complementary ways.

Enigmatic Utility

The focus turns now to the ways in which utility may defeat itself when it is executed with hyperbolic intensity, its pursuit somewhat paradoxically producing
effects of disutility and waste. With its "practical sadhus" and voluminous medical contributions to an "in-need" society, the Dera Sacha Sauda enacts what in
chapter 1 I called a "religion of utility." Yet doctors who seek to foster the "doctrinal" variety of regular, consistent, and moderate blood donation activity view
the movement as being hopelessly compromised by disutility and destruction,

since the quantities it collects far exceed immediate requirements, thus leading to expiry and waste.

In Sirsa I visited Dr. Aditya Arora, an eye specialist in a Sacha Sauda–run hospital. Long lines of pilgrims crowded the hospital corridors, their pilgrimage doubling as an opportunity to obtain free treatment. Large television screens relayed the guru's oration before a gathering of his devotees, which was then being delivered in the nearby ashram. Arora described to me a forthcoming Sacha Sauda "mega eye camp" in which he claimed 1,000 cataract operations would be completed in three days: "This eye camp will also [in addition to the movement's blood donation feats] be a world record." Arora was well aware of other doctors' criticisms of the waste resulting from Sacha Sauda blood donation camps and of the lack of patient/donor care they see as characterizing these contexts of mass treatment and collection: "The way we treat patients may not be approved of in the so-called civilized world, but we have a problem to solve with limited resources. The standards of care at our blood donation camps are on the lower side, but if you look at the functional side, we are treating so many people."

The movement's philosophy of mass treatment is epitomized by Arora's own frighteningly speedy method of screening pilgrim-patients: "It's a cost benefit screening analysis—in 45 seconds I do a screening for three eye diseases. It is so we can get rid of them and treat more. Similarly at blood camps there is an emphasis on saving time so there might be a 10–20 ml discrepancy in the amount collected. It hardly matters if a little less is collected." Therefore, due to the temporal constraints of the camp, blood bank teams may compromise on the inner quantity of individual units, thus producing quicker bleeding times and, consequently, optimization of the overall quantity of units collected. In other words, under-collection on the micro level leads to more abundant macro-level collection. Arora's argument is consonant with the Dera Sacha Sauda's philosophy of mass treatment. It would not be overly cynical, however, to suggest that the desire to achieve world records is the primary incentive for under-collection on the level of individual units. The criteria for the Guinness world record is explicit in stating that the record must take place within twelve hours. Even for this religion of utility, utility is ultimately subordinated to the desire for recognition through records—"demonstrable utility" (Ssorin-Chaikov and Sosnina 2004) takes precedence over the actually utilizable.

The hyperbolic intensity of the movement's mass provisioning exercises—its embracing of utility to the point of its erasure—suggests the culturally productive nature of uselessness for the Dera Sacha Sauda, with wastage and tales of voluminous extraction creating "material reports" of the guru's extraordinary capacities of mobilization (Ssorin-Chaikov and Sosnina 2004). The under-collection of blood in singular blood bags results from the rush to achieve world records within the stipulated amount of time. With medical utility thus subjugated to quantity, the organization's covert ambivalence toward utility becomes clear, its excessive collection appearing, to paraphrase Bhabha (1984), to be both within the rules of utility and against them.

Further examples of an "inappropriately" enthusiastic attitude to utility are to be found in the several cases reported in Indian newspapers in which people have sought euthanasia for the purpose of donating their organs. In one case in 2004, Venkatesh, a twenty-five-year-old hospital patient, was facing imminent death from the degenerative condition known as Duchenne's disease, a rare form of muscular dystrophy. He had written a note explicitly stating that it was not a "mercy killing" that he sought, but a killing that would enable his organs to be extracted for the benefit of others before the disease wasted them further, making them unusable—what was being proposed was euthanasia for the purposes of postmortem organ donation. Venkatesh's mother, who fought the legal battle, ultimately unsuccessful, to have euthanasia performed on her son, declared that up to six persons could benefit from her son's extractable organs.[22] In 2000 it was further reported that two applications were made by retired schoolteachers to the High Court of Kerala seeking euthanasia. Both deployed the possibility of transplantation as aim and justification for the procedure: "69-year-old Mukundan Pillai . . . prayed he was contented and believed his mission in life had been fulfilled. He wanted the Court to issue directions to the State to start 'Mahaprasthana Kendra' (Voluntary Death Clinic) so as to facilitate death and donation/transplantation of bodily organs."[23]

There is a well-established genre of philosophical writing (and some legal and medical writing besides) that explores the implications of the familiar Benthamite utilitarian credo, "the greatest good for the greatest number," for questions of transplantation (Bailey 1997: 92; Hogan and Lairet 2007: 17; Bergman 2006: 247). In a literalist application, the credo would appear (for the "act utilitarian" at least) to license the killing of a person so that their heart, lungs, liver, kidneys, and other useable tissues could be used to save the lives of several others. Such inquiries are always hypothetical, the cases being presented as thought experiments. But Venkatesh's case is a literal one. What his case and others demonstrate is that far from being a mere hypothetical abstraction, utility is increasingly aligned with the virtuous in an array of Indian contexts, to the extent that some people clearly seem to wish to die to facilitate it. Venkatesh's mother's emphasis on the six possible beneficiaries of her son's death mirrors the emphasis on quantification in the Benthamite thought experiments; only her emphasis is not in the least hypothetical but strikingly current and actual.

Lock (2002) has provided a comprehensive overview of debates on "brain death" as a modern redefinition of the cessation of life. She treats the concept skeptically as oriented toward the particular demands of rapacious medical establishments all too willing to define bodies as ripe for harvesting. Venkatesh's situation was rather different and, in terms of Lock's account, far graver, given that he was still fully conscious—it was a "heartbeat death" for which his mother was campaigning: "There is no possibility of brain deaths for patients of this type. This wish of my son is due to the fact that infection starts before his death and his organs will not be useful if sepsis starts."[24] In seeking to make a fatal disease that happened to him into something that he did, Venkatesh's legal fight in a sense "overtook" the injunctions of medical utility, the state, and its legal system, none of which could keep up with his envisioning of utility's hyperevolution.[25]

The hyperbolic tenor of some Indians' commitment to utility may be suggestive of their simultaneous "deification and defilement" (Lal 2002) of its maxims. Cohen (1999: 161) might well view these examples as further evidence of a burgeoning "donation madness."[26] In the case of the Dera Sacha Sauda, its extravagant events of utility maximization actually reveal the enigmatic nature of the movement's commitment to utility. Such events show how "demonstrable utility" may be deployed as a kind of virtuous capital in Indian public life— the Dera Sacha Sauda, as it were, performs utility. The cases of Venkatesh and others seeking euthanasia for the donation of their organs do, however, say something significant about the preeminent positioning of utility within an emerging Indian aesthetics of dying. What is clear, I think, is that the intensity of some Indians' embrace of utility pushes its logic to its limits and therefore enables us to see it afresh, not as the detached concept against which ethics and virtues are inevitably composed and defined, but as itself an instantiation of virtue and intrinsic value and therefore not merely an abstraction divorced from context.

Religions of Utility

One notable way in which utility becomes "virtuous utility," of course, is through its divinization. Each religious group that collects blood—and there are many—places a different theological emphasis on it. What these "donation theologies" have in common, however, is their valorizing of social utility. Calling these groups "religions of utility" therefore draws attention to this commonality while recognizing that their individual theological emphases are likely to differ.

As the examples above have demonstrated, blood donation is not the only method of "making social." It is, however, one of the principal means, and its study creates a privileged vantage point from which to observe the wider processes of which it partakes. It is clear, I hope, that blood donation on the one hand, and Hindu projects of reform on the other, are interdependent projects— donor recruiters' frequent declarations to the effect that giving blood once is better than giving to a temple one hundred times is co-extensive with, and reinforcing of, the reformist message of action as worship. As I show below in chapter 4, a further aspect of the interoperable relationship between these spiritual movements and projects to foster voluntary blood donation derives from the latter's anonymity. The anonymity of donation means that donors donate for anyone rather than someone, and it is this practical feature of donation activity that the Sant Nirankari Mission conceptually aligns with its own professed universalism. Perhaps most important of all for these movements, however, is blood donation's status as an unambiguous practice of social utility. It is thus from the veins of the devotees of avowedly reformist religious movements that an increasingly large proportion of voluntarily donated blood in India originates.

I have noted that blood donation has been instituted in several ritual settings as the substitutive ennoblement of classical dan. In this reformist medical milieu, there is a case for going further and viewing blood banks as the substitutive ennoblement of temples. The blood bank attains the status of a sacred setting through its reputation as a consummate arena of utility. Prime Minister Jawaharlal Nehru famously declared of the new dams under construction in 1950s India that "these days the biggest temple and mosque and gurdwara is the place where man works for the good of mankind" (Khilnani 1997: 61). The frequent assignation I found of temple status to blood banks probably borrows from Nehru's paradigmatic comments, which are themselves phrased in a richly reformist idiom, suggestive both in terms of economic and religious transition. Calling a dam a temple because a dam "works for the good of mankind" suggests a conception of temples already congruent with Swami Vivekananda and others' promulgation of action and service as worship. Although Nehru's comments are often interpreted as emblematic of modern India's political orthodoxy of secularism and secularization, they may equally be viewed as exemplifying an opposite formulation: modernity's divinization, with the dam—symbol of social utility—being elevated to the status of a temple rather than the temple being relegated to that of a dam.

The Sirsa-based Shiv Shakti blood bank, introduced above, houses a framed photograph of Nehru himself donating blood in 1942. Four years later, in 1946, *Time* magazine reported that "Jawaharlal Nehru, 56, drew a rebuke from followers for donating to a blood bank. His health, they protested, is 'national wealth, which should be preserved.' He should really 'abstain from such destructive sacrifices.' "[27] "Sacrifice for the nation," notes Parry (n.d.), "had been a leitmotif of the Independence struggle, the 'freedom fighters' offering their lives as *bali dan* [a term usually used in reference to animal sacrifice] that India might shake off the imperialist yoke." Songs from this era are often played at blood donation camps in Delhi as rousing calls to donate. Nehru probably felt that he *was* sacrificing for the nation, but his followers viewed his donation as unpatriotic in their presumption of its harmful effects on his health. Nehru's donation, they thought—because of his political indispensability—was a sacrifice *of* rather than *for* the nation. Such protests against the giving of blood would in the present day be unthinkable, blood donation having become a key mode of articulating ethical and patriotic citizenship. Nowadays, gurus and politicians vie to organize donation camps, and politicians disclose on their CVs the number of blood camps they have arranged and number of times they have personally donated—all these being attempts to enclose for themselves a share of the available "national capital." The Association of Voluntary Blood Donors of West Bengal has designed a recruitment poster containing a photograph of Nehru's grandson, Rajiv Gandhi, donating blood, with the slogan: "A nation is great when its leaders are great." The Indian Parliament (Lok Sabha) Web site contains "Biographical Sketches" of Indian Members of Parliament. The entry for Dr. Vallabhai Kathiria, BJP MP for Rajkot, lays emphasis on his "medical patriotism": "as a surgeon, operated over 7500 patients and diagnosed and cured over 1,00,000 patients . . . donated blood 104 times; organized over 500 general diagnostic camps and 350 blood donation camps; imprisoned during Emergency; introduced the mobile hospital concept, especially mobile dispensary service in rural areas . . . instrumental in organizing . . . Blood Donation Camp in which 5174 blood donors donated their blood at a time following the unprecedented earthquake in Gujarat in 2001, undertook untiring work of rescue, relief and rehabilitation of affected people . . . professing faith in 'Nothing but the hard work succeeds' and nurturing vision of 'The glorious, the great and the divine India' of 21st Century."[28] Blood donation has clearly joined having been imprisoned among the litany of nationalist virtues. Nehru, having been both a prisoner and a blood donor, was ahead of his time.

To return to the matter of sacrifice: despite the efforts of recruiters to convince their fellow countrymen that giving blood is not an unhealthy activity, the association with sacrifice persists both in the rousing patriotic songs played at camps, which exhort the public to shed their blood (that is, sacrifice their lives) for the country, and in the minds of the many Indians who hold the view that if they were to give blood they would subsequently require a transfusion. While many recruiters seek to dislodge such conceptions and indeed try to emphasize the health-enhancing properties of donation, others actually use sacrifice as the basis of their appeal to donors, thus contributing to the circulation of inconsistent messages about donation. Additionally, it is possible that the fact that classical dan is "officially" a surrogate for both asceticism and sacrifice in the Age of Kali (Parry 1994: 190), and therefore suggestive of both, underscores the widely made association between blood donation and sacrifice.

Parry (n.d.) has illustrated the remarkable ways in which customary forms of local sacrifice in Chhattisgargh came to overlap in workers' understandings with Nehruvian "sacrifice for the nation" upon the building of the Bhilai steel plant in 1950s India. Nehruvian sacrifice was "reformist" insofar as it was certainly not traditional blood sacrifices that it advocated. Instead, it referred to the efforts required to secure Independence and then to bring India into the new socialist modernity—going to prison, renouncing one's property in favor of the poor or new construction projects, or indeed providing industrial labor for those projects were all modes of nationalist sacrifice. However, the furnaces of the steel plant in Bhilai had to get their power from somewhere, and for many in the outlying areas, it seemed obvious that human sacrifices for the goddess Kali were their vital source of energy. The steel plant, like the dam, was an emblem of a modernist social utility for which sacrifices were necessary.

The blurring of the "two different discourses" of Nehruvian and Kali sacrifice holds a lesson for the present analysis. For reformist activists, blood sacrifice is "a barbarity inconsistent with Hinduism's central tenet of non-violence" (Fuller 1992: 101). Shedding one's blood for the nation, on the other hand, is highly approved of. Indian soldiers who died in the 1999 India-Pakistan Kargil conflict are now remembered annually through blood donation camps staged in their honor; the same is true for the policemen who were killed defending the Indian Parliament building (Lok Sabha) when it was attacked by militants in 2002.[29] For donor recruiter Dr. Ajay Bagga from Hoshiarpur, Punjab state, it is "the memory of the bullet-ridden, blood-soaked body of his father [a political leader in the Punjab Pradesh Janata Party, who was assassinated by militants in 1984] which propelled him towards the blood donation movement."[30] The commemoration of bloodshed for the nation through acts of blood donation shares at least partial structural affinity with the immuring of the bodies of workers who died in the construction of the Bhilai site: these victims, the sacrificial remainder, represent the "regenerative element that is the seed of new life and a guarantee of continuity" (Parry n.d.). In remembering blood sacrifice through blood donation, the formula is spelled out literally—the deaths of the soldiers and policemen are regenerative in precipitating blood donations that will plant "the seed of new life and a guarantee of continuity." The microevent of a donation camp is both expressive and constitutive of the soldier's role more generally—his bloodshed ensures the continuity of the nation. Blood donation, in these contexts, embodies the extensibility of blood sacrifice for the nation. Different orders of blood shedding—the soldier's blood sacrifice and the citizen's blood donation—are analogically transferable (Gell 1992: 316).[31]

If the two different discourses of sacrifice identified by Parry nevertheless in some ways share common ground (Parry n.d.), it follows that it may be possible for reformist social activists to conceptually revisit certain ancient sages and sacrificial practitioners in order to "reform" them into sacrificial exemplars of the new order of social service—this being in line with established trends in religious and nationalist reform in which "the new is turned into something old" (Singer 1972: 399). A key example of this is found in the work of the Delhi-based Dadhichi Deh Dan Samiti (Dadhichi Body Donation Society) which engages the mythic sage Dadhichi—as described in the *Brahmana Purana* and hymns of the *Rig Veda*—as a Sanskritic figurehead for the promotion of body donation in order to ensure a supply of cadavers for dissection by medical trainees. Said to have sacrificed his bones in order that Indra, king of the gods, could use them to slay Vritrasur, the demon king, the samiti declares Dadhichi's action to have been the originative sacrificial body-gift to society (*samaj*). His is the prototype it claims to reanimate through facilitating body donation.[32] The samiti thus exploits the extensible potential of sacrifice, enrolling it in order to demonstrate that Hinduism was always a religion of utility.

Shiva, like Dadhichi, is enlisted as an exemplar of sacrifice for society by the Shiv Shakti blood bank, which employs myths and iconography associated with the god in its attempts to solicit donations.[33] The blood bank's founder, Dr. Banerwal, proselytizes blood donation in visits to Haryana villages in which he tells his audiences: "At the beginning of time, when the ocean was curdled, two substances were produced: poison and *amrith*—which makes you live forever. Someone had to take the poison and it was Lord Shiva who said: 'I will take the poison so others can have *amrith*.' This philosophy is behind blood donation also—you donate blood so others can live. Shiva worked selflessly for others— and he is the god worshiped the most in India. So with this philosophy, it was easy to approach rural people: if you don't know how to do worship (*puja karna*), the best way is to donate blood and the worship is automatically done." The point about worship is emphasized visually by the huge Shiva painting at the blood bank entrance, and also by the current director Dr. Arora's own definition of his blood bank as a temple: "It is better to donate blood than to go to the temple and worship god. Rather than rituals in a temple, god will be happy if you donate blood. We treat the blood bank as a temple. We show the same respect to the blood bank to reflect the feeling that blood donation is equal to worship." Selfless service as worship is a familiar reformist idea and activity. The equation made by Banerwal between drinking poison and giving blood is emblematic of the dilemmas of donor recruitment in India: the "appeal" of sacrifice is seen by some recruiters as key to increasing voluntary donation. However, the view of blood donation as an activity of irreversible depletion (that is, of very real personal sacrifice) also works to hinder an increase in donation activity.

As spaces frequently perceived—as Nehru stated of dams—as working "for the good of mankind," it is perhaps not surprising that blood banks have, for some donors and blood bank personnel, assumed temple status, with blood donation a modernist brand of puja. One Delhi advertisement for blood donation declares, *rakt-dan sach puja hai*—"blood donation is the true worship"—as opposed, it might be inferred, to the "less true" forms of worship enacted in temples. Several donors I met at camps told me that when something eventuates that they had earlier wished for, they go to a blood bank and donate as a way of giving thanks. Such cases recall the "common practice among Hindus of pledging a part of themselves (usually the hair) to gods in periods of danger and redeeming themselves by offering that part when the danger is gone" (Das

1983: 455), though here is it "useful" blood rather than "useless" hair that is offered. Endless similar examples could be given. I shall restrict myself, however, to a comment made by a student I met at a Delhi University camp: "You are sitting in a temple, you are sitting in a gurdwara, you are sitting in a mosque. But by merely praying there do you think that blood is getting into the dying body of a patient?"

Nehru proclaimed his own substitutive ennoblement of the temple in reference to another project of social utility. The blood bank in some ways is the dam's successor as exemplary temple of utility, and the frequent attributions of temple status constitute one way in which blood donation is itself manifested as a religion of utility. The reception area of Delhi's Rotary blood bank houses a visitors' book containing the following inscription: "This is a place of pilgrimage. Those who give and those who receive, both will participate in a yagna-sacred ritual of life-giving." As this example illustrates, utility does not disenchant religion but is itself sacralized.

Conclusion

A donor recruiter in Delhi recalled to me how recently in her blood bank a lady had had tears streaming down her face as she lay donating. The recruiter's enquiry as to the cause of the lady's distress revealed that her son had died exactly one year earlier as a result of a car accident. Three people had given blood to try and save him. She felt a large debt to those people and on the same day, one year later, she was, she said, saving somebody else's child. This analogical repetition and conversion of wasted into productive blood extraction is a formula that we will encounter again in chapters 4 and 5. Significantly, the lady said that she had decided not to go to the temple with the rest of her family where they were shedding "crocodile tears"—she was actually doing something. In the "active" focus of rakt-dan lies its reformist superiority.

The alliance between reformist Hinduism's characteristic focus on action over reflection and campaigns to solicit blood donation is clearly present in the following poem. Its author, a technician at a Delhi blood bank, presents us with another forceful indictment of conventional temple gifts as inferior to the active seva of rakt-dan:

If you go to [the sacred rivers] Ganga, Yamuna, on pilgrimage
Which sin (pap) are you able to get rid of?
Having given an offering in temple or mosque,
What happiness and peace are you able to obtain? . . .
To get rid of your sin and to feel remorse for them
I will tell you a method (upaye).
To be able to give true happiness and peacefulness to another person

I suggest to you a method.
Come to this temple (*is mandir me a jao*).
The strong you will not find, though weak ones you will.
In their prayers they will say this:
If you can give willingly through your heart
We will accept red water (*lal nir*).

Sin can be removed, the poem suggests, through rakt-dan in the modernist temple of the blood bank. Caution is required here, for the removing of sin does not inevitably entail its transfer to another or its physical expelling; removal here could just as well refer to the "erasure" of sin (*pap*) through meritorious acts that would restore the rightful karmic balance. Taken together with the earlier data on mortuary rituals in Haryana, however, the poem does appear to give further credence to the argument that even as reflectively productive giving appears to substitute for and ennoble conventional giving processes, features of classical dan reemerge in striking ways. The point is straightforward: social utility as aim and target of reformist giving does not render classical dan evanescent—rather, the category of dan enlarges, coming to serve several different purposes at once.

The conjunctive structure of the gift's volition, with donors giving to society, to humanity, to the nation, to remove sin or to accumulate blessings—perhaps all at the same time, or perhaps in a divided sense with doctors, for instance, seeing use-value where a donor might see discarded inauspiciousness—is likely to be helpful in persuading people to give blood.[34] Conjunctive volition arises from the exaptation of existing giving structures—their enlistment as a means of effecting new outcomes—helping avoid ruptures in people's experiences of giving, allowing habitual aims to be accomplished even as "in-need" society is made present. Like medieval *bhakti* (devotional) movements that assimilated more than they discarded, thus effectively disarming any radical opposition (see Sen 2003: 18), the conceptual retentions that help structure reformist giving appear to inoculate it against the occurrence of serious misgivings (see also Watt 2005: 71).

The conjunctive volition informing these giving practices differentiates them from most of the examples provided by Haynes in his study of earlier efforts to introduce reform in Surat. There, the Indian elite "did not abandon older forms of gifting such as religious donations. Rather they diversified their charitable patterns, plunging themselves into new philanthropic ventures while continuing to express their devotion to their deities through sizable commitments of capital" (1987: 341). The difference lies in the ability of rakt-dan to mean more than one thing. Diversification is critical here also, but not in the sense of simply adding philanthropic giving to an already existing, mainly religious, charitable repertoire. Rather, in parasiting the existing repertoire, blood donation partakes of the procedures it enters into, and thus comes to encompass in itself the striking volitional diversity that Haynes attributes to separate practices.

Though the existence of several aims within singular giving actions may lessen the potential for rupture in people's giving experiences, and ultimately help to establish blood donation's wider acceptance, the conjunctive volition informing this emergent dan may in addition lead to some very problematic consequences. I have referred several times to Parry's study of mortuary gifts to Brahmin priests in Banaras. These are usually of money as a surrogate for a cow or a bed, and may transmit and thus remove donors' sins (1994: 123–132). The recipient *pandas* are thereby rendered "cess-pits," many living in "a perpetual state of moral crisis" (ibid.: 123). As I noted above, there is limited but nonetheless suggestive evidence that in certain circumstances the expelling of sin, as identified within forms of classical dan, surfaces in certain contexts as an aim of rakt-dan. Bearing in mind Parry's analysis, such an understanding would appear to make blood donation attractive to precisely those it most needs to repel (those who have "sinned" in the conventional senses of engaging in sexual promiscuity or drug use). Non material "karmic" sin potentially coalesces here with actually transmissible infection. If both the nonmaterial accumulated sins of past actions and medically detectable infection were transmissible through rakt-dan, the attempt at removing the former would heighten the risk of the transmission of the latter—with obviously destructive consequences for recipients. This casts in a new light Parry's observation that dan is "saturated with the evil consequences of the donor's conduct" (ibid.: 129). If the transfer of "sin" documented by Parry is understood by his informants literally to result in leprosy for recipient "cess-pits," the practice is still ultimately treated by the anthropologist as a "cultural idiom" (ibid.: 136), and understandably so. The personnel involved in collecting, treating, and testing donated blood, together with transfusion recipients, however, are in an analogous and yet profoundly different sense to Parry's informants, also vitally concerned with the gift's purity or otherwise. The retention of the "sinful" aspect of classical dan within the modernist context of rakt-dan might result in other literal transmissions of infection.

According to numerous blood bank personnel and several of his devotees whom I met in Mumbai, the Maharashtrian guru Narendra Maharaj encourages his followers to give blood at mass donation camps organized by his *seva dars* (service volunteers) precisely in order for them to remove their sins (*pap*). A Delhi-based blood bank doctor provided me with a more detailed example. She told the story of a Sikh man whose wife was suffering from mental illness. He was told by his Sardar Ji (Sikh guru) to give three gifts from his body as a means of restoring her sanity. As a Sikh, he did not consider giving his hair. He subsequently attempted to give blood at a Delhi blood bank on three consecutive days. Three months, however, is the officially sanctioned length of time meant to elapse between donations. The man was recognized by blood bank personnel attempting to give for a second time on the second day and barred from making further donations (though this is no guarantee that he did not subsequently attempt to donate his blood elsewhere). As in the Haryana-based mortuary rituals already discussed, there is the strong suggestion here that he was attempting to give three gifts of medically utilizable blood as a means of removing the inauspiciousness afflicting his family (cf. Raheja 1988: 154). These examples show that the retention of an attribute associated with classical dan within a giving mode extended from it can have potentially lethal consequences for recipients, a relationship explored further in the next chapter.

The conceptual and practical interdependence between voluntary blood donation and religions of utility that I identified in this chapter, though significant, should not deflect attention from the fact of the multiple and diverse extensions and parasitings that are under way that are not directly related to religion. Some of these evince a "hyperbolic utility," some are more restrained and austere: Venkatesh's desire to die a premature death in order to maximize his body's postmortem usefulness is an example of the former tendency. Similarly, the Dera Sacha Sauda demonstrates that it is possible to pursue both a maximizing ethos premised around utility and an excess ethos that destroys utility. But SUGAM's expansive redefinition of Valentine's Day demonstrates that it is by no means only the giving structures associated with classical dan that are being parasited. Virtuous utility has found many "host agencies."

The following two chapters deepen my exploration of the relationship between voluntary blood donation and "religions of utility" through a focus on two north Indian devotional orders in the sant tradition: the Sant Nirankari Mission and the Dera Sacha Sauda.

4

Devotion and Donation

One of the most striking features of blood donation practices in contemporary India is the embrace of voluntary blood donation as a key focus of organized spiritual service by major devotional orders associated with the north Indian sant tradition. These orders have emerged over the last fifteen to twenty years as some of India's highest-profile proselytizers of blood donation as a critical act of service to humanity, world, and nation. The two devotional movements on which I focus—the Sant Nirankari Mission in this chapter and the Dera Sacha Sauda in chapter 5—are both presided over by living saints, commonly known as *satguru* (literally "true master"), who are worshiped as gods. Like the Radhasoami movement studied by Juergensmeyer (1991, 1995) and Babb (1986), these two spiritual organizations have emerged out of the sant heritage, "the creed of the saints, a tradition associated with such figures as Kabir and Nanak" (Babb 1986: 17).[1] This chapter is based principally on data collected from my attendance at twenty or so Sant Nirankari donation camps in various locations across Delhi. I also attended a celebration in honor of the guru's fiftieth birthday, a huge annual gathering of Sant Nirankari devotees (*samagam*) in Delhi in 2004, and several weekly worship gatherings. I draw additionally on the voluminous literature generated by the movement.[2]

My focus in this chapter is the origins and character of the Sant Nirankari Mission's engagement with blood donation. I explore the striking ways in which devotional blood giving activities interact with devotees' understandings and lived experience of sacrifice and the attainment of spiritual reward. The latter parts of the chapter examine devotees' conceptions of the gift's content: since it is devotees' spiritual qualities and what I term "viscous love," reified in their donated blood, that many see as providing recipients with transformative transfusions of spirit, I reconsider the classic South Asianist theme of the spirit of the gift as it surfaces in a novel biomedical context. I also focus on the complex assimilation of allopathic substance provision to a universalizing theology (the latter being an attribute of many devotional orders [Fuller 1992: 173] and of modernist Hinduism in general [Sharma 1998]), and ask the key but hitherto overlooked public policy question: might religiously inspired blood donation produce blood that is medically unsafe for transfusion?

The Nirankari Mission, which began organizing regular blood donation camps in the mid 1980s, was as far as I am aware the first spiritual organization to do so. Analyzing this vanguard movement thus permits a view of the origins of devotional blood giving in general. In Delhi the Nirankari Mission collaborates with the Red Cross blood bank to collect as much as 20 percent of the capital's voluntarily donated blood.[3] Its many places of worship (*satsang bhavans*) form a vital resource for the Red Cross team, which makes regular collection visits to satsang bhavans both within and beyond the city, especially during the lean summer months. At this time, when schools and colleges are closed, the blood of students, Delhi's other main source of blood, is replaced in blood banks by the blood of devotees. Leaflets advertising the Mission enumerate the awards it has received from the Red Cross for "highest donors provided by the NGOs," "outstanding performance in the year 1999," and so on. It has also received awards from the Delhi State AIDS Control Society and from the Association of Voluntary Blood Donors, West Bengal. The Mission remained loyal to the Red Cross during the time of my fieldwork, except for the odd occasion when it arranged camps with other blood banks in order to punish the somewhat lackadaisical Red Cross team for its late arrival at camp venues. Late arrival means less collection time, resulting in the collection of fewer units—an occurrence dismaying to the Sant Nirankari hierarchy, which seeks to maximize collected units in order to demonstrate both the scale of the movement's largesse and also the impressiveness of the guru's ability to mobilize his devotees. Late arrival may also lead to unfulfilled donor expectations. As I demonstrate below, devotees can become extremely anxious about whether their donation will be accepted by blood bank doctors and technicians, feeling that failure to donate will debar them from receiving the guru's blessings; physical disqualification from donation is thus experienced as a declaration of devotional or spiritual unfitness.[4]

The Nirankari Mission forms part of a wide, broadly inclusive sant tradition that crosses formal Hindu–non-Hindu "community" boundaries. It was evident at all the events I attended that devotees hail from a wide variety of caste and class backgrounds. But although I met many devotees who were clearly both of high-caste background and advantaged economically and educationally, the majority of devotees I encountered were poor Hindus and Sikhs: typically small stallholders, bus drivers, construction workers, or domestic servants. Members of the visiting Red Cross team tend to view the guru as the protector of his disadvantaged devotees for whom he (in the shape of the Mission) provides subsidized medicines and foodstuffs. In addition, an insurance arrangement is in place whereby the blood bank provides free blood to needy devotees and their families in return for the units of blood the Mission supplies to the Red Cross. The movement claims to be anti-caste and egalitarian, and it would indeed truly be a scandal if a high-caste devotee refused to consume postdonation refreshments (or *prashad* as devotee-donors call them) along with other devotees. Although hierarchical inequality is a feature of all devotional orders, with the guru always being "recognized as superior by disciples whom he initiates" (Fuller 1992: 164), there is a level of equality among devotees themselves, who demonstrate this by touching each other's feet as a mark of humility, a feature of Nirankari life that does not respect gender or caste conventions and which for this reason often arouses comment among outsiders.[5] As one otherwise very admiring donor recruiter said to me: "In India you should only touch your in-laws' feet, or your husband's, but over there grown men touch the feet of young girls!"

The most controversial aspect of Sant Nirankari religious life, however, relates to devotees' worship of a living human guru. This is a highly problematic issue in religious organizations connected to Sikhism. Guru Gobind Singh in 1708 proclaimed himself the final living Sikh master, designating the text that has become the central devotional focus of orthodox Sikhism, the Guru Granth Sahib, as the next and final guru of Sikh tradition. The book thus replaced living gurus as the focus for devotional veneration (McLeod 1996, 1999; Uberoi 1996). The Nirankari Mission's heterodox worship of a living guru was thus one of the chief reasons for violent clashes that occurred between the Sant Nirankaris and orthodox Sikhs in the late 1970s and early 1980s. These clashes, as I show below, played a crucial role in the establishment of blood donation as a key attribute of Nirankari religious experience.

The Sant Nirankari Mission is distinct from the Nirankari reform movement founded by Baba Dayal (1783–1855) in order to counter the *sanatan* (traditional) Sikh view that God is periodically incarnated in avatars. Dayal instead promulgated a conception of God as singular and formless (*nirankar*), emphasized the need to read Sikh sacred texts, remember God's name, and to remove notions of ritual impurity surrounding childbirth and other ceremonies (Oberoi 1994: 193–194). The original Nirankari movement is no longer visible as a major organization, and when Indians now speak of Nirankaris it is likely to be the Sant Nirankari Mission to which they are referring.

Founded in 1929, the Mission is flourishing in India, with around 1,000 local branches and several million devotees, and worldwide with branches in Australia, Canada, the United Kingdom, and the United States.[6] Like the Punjab (Beas) division of the Radhasoamis (Babb 1986: 17), the Nirankari Mission combines elements of both Hinduism and Sikhism, enjoins devotees to seek "god-realization" through a living spiritual master, and regards itself not as a conventional religion as such but instead as a "wholly new and unique religious dispensation" (ibid.: 205); and, like the original Nirankari reform movement, the Mission espouses a conception of God as formless (nirankar): "All are equally blessed by the True Master with the same divine light. To Nirankaris, religion is a means to complete union with God Almighty, Nirankar" (Sagar 1994: 18). Perhaps most important of all is the concept of gyan (spiritual knowledge). Devotees receive gyan from maha-purush (great humans) within the Mission, or on rare occasions from the satguru himself—Baba Hardev Singh. Devotees then qualify as "saints"—even the common devotee attains sainthood on receipt of gyan. Gyan must not be openly disclosed, but from many conversations at blood donation camps and other Nirankari gatherings, it seems to refer to "soul-connection," the "eye of connection," the unity of all humanity, and the fact that all humanity has the same Father so is bound together as one in kinship.

There are two main strands to the Nirankari universalism hinted at here: first, all those who receive gyan become saints and effectively attain enlightenment. Devotional worship in India ideally allows the devotee, whatever his or her background, to make spiritual progress and even to achieve salvation without renouncing the world. Devotionalism thus universalizes the objective of acetic renouncers (Fuller 1992: 165). Second, the central Nirankari doctrine of universal brotherhood (sarvbhaumik bhratritva) is reflected in basic principles such as (1) "Do not believe in any casteism. Everyone is born as human being," and (2) "Religion essentially means God-realization and love for every human being" (Social Welfare Vibhag n.d.). I argue below that there is an important correlation between the universal directionality of anonymously donated blood (given for anyone, without distinction) and the second form of Nirankari universalism identified above, and that this correlation helps "endow [devotees'] understanding of inherited doctrine with personal experience and conviction" (Laidlaw 2004: 102).

The Origins of Nirankari Blood Donation

Proclaiming the Nirankaris and the guru an affront to true khalsa Sikhism, Sikh extremists assassinated the present Nirankari guru's father—the preceding guru, Baba Gurbachan Singh—in 1980, and according to devotees, it was this event that inspired the inauguration of Nirankari blood donation activities. In comparison with the Radhasoamis, the Nirankari Mission has been incautious in its relations with mainstream Sikhism. Whereas the Radhasoamis have "not been so brazen as to claim a direct association with the Sikh tradition" (Juergensmeyer 1991: 86), the use of identifiably Sikh symbolism and vocabulary by the preceding Nirankari guru, Gurbachan Singh, led orthodox Sikhs to consider that the Nirankaris were making an intolerably blasphemous claim in not accepting Gobind Singh as the last living Sikh guru. This prompted a series of hostile exchanges, brought to a head in 1980 with the assassination of the guru.[7] Prior to this event, orthodox Sikhs had been ordered to refrain from food and marital relations with Nirankaris.

Many devotees I spoke with found it painful to recall these cataclysmic events of the late 1970s and early 1980s. Though theirs is avowedly a religion of love, many devotees at the time, I was told, sought to exact a terrible revenge. As one elderly devotee informed me, "When Baba Ji died the people all said [to the successor guru Baba Hardev Singh], give us an order. Command us to do something [violent] so we may also have the sentiment (*bhavna*) of sacrifice (*tyag*)." Laxshmi, a *sevadar* (service volunteer), told me, "When Baba Ji sacrificed his life for humanity, we were very much hurt. We said, you just tell us and we'll kill those people." What happened next has passed into Nirankari lore. "The people went to Baba Ji to say we should take revenge (*badla*), and he said, we will definitely take revenge, but by love (*prem*). Our revenge is to donate blood for the needy persons."

The Mission thus seeks to convert the martyrdom of its guru from an experience of victimhood into one of self-initiated ennobling virtue, attributing to the successor guru himself the aphorism which is now used as an exhortatory slogan about the transformation of violent bloodshed into spiritually meaningful donation: "Blood should flow into veins (*nari*), not drains (*nali*)." Recalling the examples given in chapter 3 of sacrifice extensible-to-utility, the phrase also serves to rhetorically elevate the Mission above petty everyday violent disturbances, the contrast between veins and drains drawing attention to distinctions between the peace-loving Nirankaris and other religious communities such as extremist Sikhs as well as Hindu and Muslim "fundamentalists" that are wedded to violent outrages.

Devotees' acts of blood donation therefore explicitly refer back to the precursor guru's blood sacrifice. Each controlled Nirankari blood donation commemorates and reenacts—to a greater or lesser extent depending on the age of devotees and their emotional involvement with the originating events—an earlier uncontrolled spillage of blood. As the public address system announced at one donation event I attended: "After He [Gurbachan Singh] had sacrificed his life, *lakhs* [hundreds of thousands] of people wanted to be included in the sacrifice. They all wanted an opportunity to do something. Baba Ji [Hardev Singh] said [of Nirankari blood donation], 'You are talking of one Baba Ji [i.e., the predecessor guru, Gurbachan Singh], but I have produced thousands of Baba Jis for you.'" Devotees' request to exact revenge on Gurbachan Singh's murderers was granted in a radical displacement from an initial desire to generate deficits into an aim of replenishing them. The succeeding guru directed his devotees' anger into a process of "spreading love" (*pyar bantna*) through which sacrifice was "democratized"—made inclusive and participatory.

A further important point concerning the origins of blood donation activity among the Nirankaris relates to the other kind of offering made by

devotees: that of money. At the weekly worship gatherings I attended in Delhi's
Patel Nagar, a *maha-purush* (great man), dressed in white, sat silently on the
dais, with devotees approaching him throughout the service to touch his feet
and leave money offerings. The Mission does not demand a tithe, but there is
undoubtedly pressure to give as much as one can. My friend Sudhir, who had
only recently begun a new job in a software company when the present guru,
Hardev Singh, turned fifty in 2004, gave the guru his first month's salary as a
birthday gift. With the Mission's inauguration of donation camps in 1986,
money was joined by blood as a critical devotional currency. Devotees, as I mentioned above, are generally from unprivileged backgrounds. Recalling Watt's
(2005: 76) argument that the performance of social service as charity in early
twentieth-century India began to "democratize" giving, making philanthropy
accessible to those to whom it was previously a somewhat remote and abstract
concept, it seems reasonable to propose that one of the reasons that devotees
have adopted blood donation so enthusiastically is that it allows them to
actively participate in an area of Nirankari religious life that had until that point
been problematic for them. My experiences at camps suggested to me that the
devotees most eager to donate blood were indeed of very modest means.

Coleman (2004: 436) compares the circulation of words and the circulation
of money among Swedish "Word of Life" Protestants: "Sacralized words have one
considerable advantage over money . . . : they represent an inexhaustible
medium, so that the logic of superabundance of verbal consumption is comple-
mented by an equal abundance of production." In donating blood, devotees are
similarly able to offer a gift that does not cost money and which, as I show below,
is understood to return to them either through the guru's blessings or as an
aspect of the body's physiological processes. Like the utterance of words, there
is the sense in donating blood that one is giving without losing anything; hence
the ability of the poorest devotees now to make offerings.

Although in some ways blood donation clearly does involve a move toward
the democratization of religious gifting, enfranchising those for whom the offering of money poses difficulties, the reality is that the nutrition of economically
disadvantaged devotees will almost invariably be poor, and thus their hemoglobin levels too low for their blood to be considered medically valuable. This way,
a person's relative poverty is registered in the quality of his or her blood.
A healthy hemoglobin level requires a balanced diet that includes foods rich in
iron. Widespread vegetarianism is thought to be a contributory factor to the
generally low levels of hemoglobin in the subcontinent (Mehta 2000: 34). But
the Jains of Maharashtra and Rajasthan are prolific vegetarian blood donors,
suggesting that poverty more than the absence of meat may be the critical
factor. Low weight, anemia, and a history of hepatitis (often resulting from
unfiltered drinking water) are all problems experienced in higher proportions
among the poor, and they are also the main factors leading to ineligibility to

donate blood. Anecdotally, through discussions with doctors and my own experiences at camps, it is clear that Nirankari devotees are far more likely to be disqualified from donating than other sections of the population. I illustrate below the anguish experienced by some devotees on being disqualified. There results the unfortunate paradox that those who in my argument would be the most eager to donate are, by virtue of their poverty, the least eligible to do so. In this way, the tests performed by medics on prospective donors also test their socioeconomic status.

As was noted in chapter 1, the relationship between voluntary blood donation and class is complex. The transition from paid to voluntary donation partly represents an upward transition in the class derivation of donated blood. And yet the Nirankari case appears to suggest a countervailing movement, with blood donation seeming to promise the democratization of religious gifting. At the same time, however, donation activity is revealed to be grounded in exclusions made on the basis of relative wealth, with the tests administered by medics on prospective donors producing vivid demonstrations of India's social inequalities.[8]

Seva and Refraction

What of the relationships between the important triad of actors involved in devotional blood giving: devotees, the guru, and the collecting blood bank? The project of voluntary blood donation relies heavily on religious institutions, and no religious institution is more consistent or prolific in donating blood than the Nirankari Mission. Recruiters recognize the power and intensity of the relationship that exists between gurus and their devotees and attempt to enlist devotees' regard for their guru for their own collection ends. Recruiters realize that if they are able to persuade particular gurus to endorse blood donation and hold camps in their devotional centers, they can cut down on the difficult and laborious task of issuing generalized appeals for blood donors from the population at large: once the guru is motivated, recruiters assume, his devotees will automatically comply. As one Mumbai donor recruiter told me: "I use all the god men. They [donors] have respect for god men. . . . I use these stupid sects to do my job." A less contemptuously expressed, but just as instrumental view was conveyed to me by Dr. Debasish Gupta from the government body, the National AIDS Control Organization (NACO): "Religion is one of the important factors in India that we must tap for voluntary blood donors." This reflects the prevalent view among proponents of social change in India—articulated more than a century ago by Swami Vivekananda—that they must pursue their projects through active engagement with its religion. It also suggests a conception of gurus' devotees as "donor banks." India is the land of "vote bank" politics, where different caste and religious groups are seen to vote in elections en masse as single entities (see Khilnani 1997: 79). Donor recruiters similarly treat gurus' devotees as convenient "donor banks," a shortcut method of acquiring blood; the recruitment of one (the guru) constitutes the mass recruitment of his many followers.

I emphasize, however, that this is not merely a story of recruiters' appropriation of the guru-devotee relationship in order to fulfill the requirements of medical utility. The story, rather, is of the mutually facilitative interdependence that exists between a Mission which, as I show below, appropriates voluntary donation as a means to enrich and transform the experiential basis of its religious life, and an embryonic voluntary donation that appropriates the devotional relationship as a critical source of its materia medica.

Recruiters' enlisting of the devotional relationship depends upon the interplay of several directional intentionalities. Though the guru and the Mission's literature declares that blood donation is service of humanity (*manav seva*), devotees also see blood donation as a way to serve their guru. In fact, it makes sense to view the guru as the transcendental recipient of their donations. Devotees' orientation to the recipients of their donations is thus bifocal: well aware that their donations in fact travel to abstract "humanity," it often appears that the focus of devotees' giving is more the guru than actual transfusion recipients. The apparent prioritizing of the guru is so insistent that it can often seem as though devotees' motivation is singularly focused on the guru.[9] But in fact devotees' orientation toward the recipients of their donations is bifocal, the gift arriving with its recipients through a dual movement: principally offered to the guru, the guru is an agent of multiple refraction (he refracts the gift to "humanity"). There is thus a productive interplay between centripetal and centrifugal directional intentionalities: centripetally directed toward the guru (from many to one), the transcendental focus of the gift multiply refracts devotees' offerings to "humanity" (the gift is centrifuged from one to many). The gift thus travels both to and through the guru toward "humanity," and is for one and for many at the same time—gifts to the guru are simultaneously gifts to "humanity" (see Figure 1.2).

The important role of seva (service) activities, performed by devotees for gurus, has been noted by anthropologists studying guru-led movements in India (see Babb 1986; Juergensmeyer 1991; Warrier 2003a, 2003b). Mayer (1981: 158–159) explains that devotees do the seva of a particular deity or guru. This may be termed centripetal seva—seva with a specific directional intentionality, that is, seva oriented at a guru or deity as target. Classically, guru seva involves ministering to the guru "by performing the work of a menial, by massaging his feet, and by writing down his words" (Mayer 1981: 158–159). For Nirankari devotees, participating in Mission construction works, preparing food for devotees, or offering part of one's salary also counts as guru seva. Warrier (2003a) found that despite the Mata Amritanandamayi Mission's professed humanitarianism, devotees of the Mission's presiding guru, commonly known as the Mata, conduct seva as an aspect of their devotion to her, and not humanity. Seva is thus performed "not as altruism but as panegyric" (Warrier 2003a: 279). Nirankari blood donation seva is comparable insofar as the guru's glorification and the securing of his blessings is an important motivation; this, it is true, can sometimes lead to the conceptual effacement of actual transfusion recipients by the figure of the guru as transcendent recipient. But actual recipients do figure in Nirankari devotees' bifocal calculations as the eventual receptacles of their donations. For example, we shall see how devotees seek through their donations to change as much as save transfusion recipients. The point is that devotees' donations are not aimed in a transparent way toward "humanity," but travel in a more oblique way to it through the guru who assumes the refractive role of both recipient—of devotees' donations—and benefactor—of "humanity."

What appears on one level to be the very specific focus of devotees' seva activities is thus not an impediment to a newly abstracted voluntary donation for anyone but actually enables it. This highlights the important role of the guru in repersonalizing the gift. From one perspective, the policy switch from replacement donation to voluntary donation represents a move from personalized to depersonalized giving. The Nirankari guru, and I would suggest gurus in general, however, steps in as a repersonalizing factor to mediate the transition from "specific" replacement to "abstract" voluntary donation. Devotees' gifts thus turn out to be both specific (centripetal) and abstract (centrifugal) at the same time.

Devotee-donors are aware that they are supposed to be acting as public-spirited doers of service to generalized "society" or "humanity"—that this is the Mission's official policy. At the same time, however, they are achieving a much more familiar goal: being accepted as deliverers of service to a blessings-conferring guru who persists as the personal recipient of their gifting, despite his exhortations that it is idealized, impersonal society which should form the focus of their gifting. All this is to say that one cannot simply work backward, deducing from the impersonal effect of the gift, the giver's impersonal motivation in giving it. Or, as Mosse (2004: 644) puts it, "The effect of things does not explain their properties." These abstract points acquire ethnographic substance through the examples below.

Trials of a Devotee

It might appear that devotees' donation of blood is merely indicative of the "extensibility" (Miyazaki 2005) of guru seva; that devotees who already give portions of their salaries, become sevadars (uniformed servants of the guru), or help in Mission-sponsored construction works (cf. Juergensmeyer 1991: 141) have simply been presented with an additional method of serving their guru and attaining his blessings (*ashirvad*). The violent origins of the new practice, however, along with its enactment, which I outline below, as an austerity and a means to "convert" recipients, suggests that blood donation holds a unique position among the repertoire of Nirankari service activities. As Juergensmeyer (1991: 142) correctly remarks, guru seva is the modern analogue of traditional sacrifices and oblations. This observation is particularly perspicacious in reference to blood donation seva.

At several otherwise rather austere Nirankari satsang bhavans—decorated only with photographs of satgurus past and present—there are large painted pictures of the monkey god Hanuman. Hanuman is the ideal *bhakta* (devotee), performer of pristine service to the god Ram (see Alter 1992b: 198–213). He is pictured in these Nirankari venues with an open chest, torn apart in order to reveal Ram and Sita in his heart. Ram's wife Sita had challenged Hanuman to abandon his body given that it was not inscribed with Ram's name and therefore "useless" to him (ibid.: 209). Ripping open his chest, he revealed the corporeality of his devotion.

This was, of course, a centripetal devotion—directed at the specific target of Ram. Daniel Gold recounts the devotion of Gorakh, a *nath* yogi, to his guru Matsyendra.[10] Gorakh procured food for his hungry guru in exchange for both of his eyes. Similarly, in founding the khalsa, the "pure" Sikh order, Guru Gobind Singh demanded that five volunteers offer him their lives. These stories demonstrate "the disciple's ardent desire to serve" (Gold 1987: 175, 176). In return for their corporeal devotion, devotees attain "vision" or new and profound spiritual insights. Sometimes, such as in the case of Guru Gobind Singh, or Abraham and his son in the Old Testament, it is merely devotees' willingness to sacrifice themselves that is being tested—there is no actual shedding of the sacrificial victim's blood; in fact boons are awarded to them. In the Nirankari case, the satguru does not demand sacrifices for himself but for humanity. As noted above, however, devotees feel they are giving to both entities—to the satguru, and through him to humanity. There is thus, to some extent, a disjuncture between what the guru demands and what devotees feel they are delivering. Devotees experience the need to demonstrate the corporeal "innerness" of their devotion to their guru as part of an "archive of inceptive moral knowledge" (Allen 1989: 48) and absorb blood donation into this moral expressionism.

Hanuman is also a manifestation of *shakti* (the life force, power), a quality that is acquired directly through devotion and self-control (Alter 1992b: 207). As was noted in chapter 1, Indians widely hold blood donation to induce physical weakness. That devotees donate with such commitment and discipline should not, however, be taken as a sign that they, unlike the majority of Indians, have been persuaded by donor recruiters to abandon such "superstitions." Rather, devotees give regardless or even because of the dangers involved as an expression of the innerness of their devotion. And just as devotion resulted in shakti for Hanuman, many devotees I spoke with feel protected from the ill effects of extraction by the blessings of the satguru, believing that true devotion results in a replenishment of substance that would not otherwise occur.

What transpires, in other words, is divinized replenishment. At one Nirankari camp a donor told me: "If we give blood to others, God gives us again this supply. The blood comes back to us, given by God." At the same camp, another devotee, having donated, declared: "I feel fresher and well. Shakti has come from Baba Ji's blessings. We pray for more blood so we can give again." Another devotee expressed the view that "In seven days God (*ishvar*) replaces the blood. If we give something to anyone, that thing gets less. But it is the power of God (*ishvar ka shakti*) that more is produced." It is not that these devotees differ from the majority of Indians in viewing blood donation as a safe activity, but rather that they see themselves as being exempt from the ill effects that would ordinarily ensue. As another donor told me: "We give with the blessings of His Holiness. He gives us the power (*shakti*) to give blood." Another devotee stated: "We must have trust to do this because it affects the health. It is Baba Ji's inspiration. If he says give blood, or jump from the sixth floor, we follow his path and he protects us." And again: "Everyone here has the feeling that no one can touch us with the grace of Guru Ji." One devotee, an ayurvedic doctor, declared that he had engaged in *simeran* (remembering god) as he donated:

> It is not my blood. When we give he supplies (*deta hai*) us with the best quality (*gun*). I feel a continuous flow of energy in me when I donate blood. Energy is coming to me and I am absorbing this. Some cosmic power (*suksham-shakti*) is coming to me. Always energy surrounds me and floats around me, and when I donate it enters me. When we supply energy to others we regain the power from our satguru Baba Ji. It regains energy and it makes healthy blood (*svasth khun*) and for a whole year I don't get sick. When I give blood I feel a prayer in my body and that prayer makes my body healthy.

The view that the satguru or ishvar replenishes the donor's blood is reminiscent of Warrier's findings (2003a, 2003b) among devotees of the south Indian guru Mata Amritanandamayi: devotees attribute phenomena as mundane as having enough petrol to get home to the Mata's miraculous powers. It also resonates with the notion of qualitative karma according to which one's karma "comes to fruition in a way which bears a poetic similarity to the action which initially brought it about" (Laidlaw 1995: 358), not falling ill being seen by some donors as the qualitative effect of their helping others to recover from illness.

The devotional relationship is critical to these attitudes, with many devotees seeing themselves as exceptions to the rule of blood's irreversible depletion by virtue of their devotion to the satguru. That Nirankari devotees donate blood creates an interesting "rationality effect" (Das 2004: 251), for it makes it appear that they subscribe to the claims of donor recruiters and doctors that blood donation is a perfectly healthy activity. But blood donation is not a transparent action. Despite not subscribing to recruiters' claims, devotees nevertheless feel that donation enhances *their* health, but only insofar as this is a reward for submitting themselves before the trial of donation. Like Hanuman, devotees' replenished shakti results from the strength of their devotion and discipline in the face of something that many see as an ordeal.

There were various ways in which devotees' concerns about the physical perils of blood donation became apparent. For instance, one camp I attended was not conducted in the usual setting of a local satsang bhavan but had been transferred for reasons of space to a nearby school. Separate rooms were used for registration, hemoglobin testing, donation, and refreshments. The organizers had displayed only one photograph of the satguru and this was in the donation room—the point in the process at which devotees most felt the need for the protection of their guru's divine image (*darshan*) (see Babb 1986: 16; Fuller 1992: 59–60). At other camps I attended sevadars (service volunteers) would hold the hands of devotees as they donated.

Devotees' assumptions about the ill effects of donation are assuaged not by the "scientific" view of donation's safety but through their involvement in a devotional apparatus through which replenishing shakti will be fed back to devotees—to the extent that health may even be enhanced—as a spiritual reward which doubles as proof of devotional fitness. This aspect of devotees' approach to blood donation can be further illuminated with reference to Cohen's account of surgical operations in India and their relation to the nation-state. He writes that "A person is hailed through the family planning operation as a pre-modern and precapitalist breeder, for whom appeals to modern or bourgeois asceticism will be inadequate" (2004: 171). Sterilization thus "produces a citizen-body that acts *as if* it were modern" (ibid.: 167). The giving of blood, like the operation, produces modernist effects: where sterilization eliminates "frenzied" reproduction, the donating body evinces confidence in the claims of medical science about donation's harmlessness to the donor. Many devotees, however, are hardly committed to this tenet and yet continue to donate *as if* they had "undergone a transformation of reason" (ibid.: 166).

Dangerous Blessings

Further evidence that devotees' blood donations are, in transcendental terms, intended as gifts to the satguru is that for devotees it is Baba Hardev Singh rather than the eventual transfusion recipient who is posited as the principal source of the blessings accruable through donation. It was common during fieldwork to hear non-Nirankari donors presage the blessings that would later be granted by the recipients of their donations. Recipient-derived blessings are in addition stressed by donor recruiters—"Give blood, get Blessings," as one Indian Red Cross slogan puts it rather bluntly. As I noted in chapter 2, such blessings may obtain not only from the transfusion recipient (the primary recipient), but also from the donation's secondary recipients—the dependents and descendents of the primary recipient. Donors imagine the myriad lives their donation may impact upon and prospectively calculate the accruable blessings in accordance with these expanded horizons. For Nirankari devotees, however, it is the guru that is in devotees' sights as principal target and conferrer of blessings.

I suggest that devotees' attempts to attain the satguru's blessings may have significant implications for the quality of donated blood and therefore also for health policy in the region. Recruiters who seek to activate devotee "donor banks" as a shortcut to motivation fail to consider that devotees in turn activate blood donation as a shortcut to improve their own spiritual statuses—this being in such a manner as to imperil the safety of the gift.

The head of Nirankari service activities, Brigadier Sham Sheer Singh, whom I met many times at different camps, told me that "elsewhere people get paid, but it is all voluntary here." When I met Mandeep Singh, a Nirankari sevadar, at a function to celebrate the fiftieth birthday of Baba Hardev Singh, he similarly sought to distinguish what he sees as the nonremunerated blood donation conducted by Nirankari devotees from the remunerated donation practiced elsewhere: "We give blood for our Guru Ji—no money, just blessings." The claims to purity of intention made by Mandeep and the Brigadier on behalf of the Mission imply disapproval of remunerated donation.[11] As was explained in chapter 1, paid donation is now illegal in India. Payment, however, persists as an "incubus" within replacement donation, with relatives too frightened to donate paying "professionals" to donate in their stead. The chief problem with paid donation is the incentive that payment gives donors to conceal information that would, if truthfully revealed, disqualify them from donating. Infection rates are thus higher in remunerated forms of donation.

So Mandeep Singh and the Brigadier both contrast nonremunerated Nirankari blood donation with the remunerated donation they see as taking place elsewhere. The problem is that devotees' wish to obtain the spiritual remuneration of blessings gives them just as much reason to hide potentially disqualifying information as monetary payment does for "professional" donors. A blood bank attached to a Delhi government hospital recently installed CCTV cameras in order to deter professional donors who are reported to have threatened to kill the doctors who refused to bleed them. This is an extreme example, but the pained and protesting reactions of Nirankari devotees to medical disqualification (due to inadequate hemoglobin levels, high blood pressure, recent jaundice or malaria, and so on), which I catalog below, demonstrate a similar desperation to give. I shall argue that the reason for this is that devotees come to construe a biomedical criterion designed to filter out potentially infected donors as a criterion publicly distinguishing unworthy from worthy devotees.

Titmuss (1970: 130) notes the view of one policy analyst that the paid blood donor is the "avid donor"—so keen to give that he conceals personal information. Nirankari devotees, like the wrestlers competing to serve their gurus described by Alter (1992b: 211), and the lay Jains described by Laidlaw (1995: 332) who forcefully press food on renouncers, are also avid donors. Titmuss in addition provides examples of remuneration in kind such as free meals, free medical care, or days off work, all of which call into question the supposedly nonremunerated nature of voluntary donation. Thus money, though paradigmatic, is not the only kind of payment a donor may receive. What Titmuss fails to mention— understandably, given that his study is focused principally on the United States and Britain—is spiritual remuneration. In Indian devotional contexts I think it legitimate to add blessings to Titmuss's list as a further source of danger to the safety of this particularly vulnerable form of gift.

The Brigadier is proud of devotees' avidness, pointing to the distressed reactions of disqualified devotees as evidence of the Mission's successful inculcation of the ethos of donation: "At our camps there are often queues of donors! Old people come and learn that at sixty-five they can no longer donate and they shed tears. Children come and ask, 'Why can't I give?' Menstruating women or women with low hemoglobin, they all want to give and they shed tears: 'Why not?! I want this opportunity!'" The Brigadier's description of Nirankari donation fervor is certainly accurate, with devotees' enthusiasm being especially remarkable given most Indians' strong aversion to the idea of donating their blood.

Devotees' donation fervor was abundantly apparent at each camp I attended. At one in Uttam Nagar, a woman wept on being told of her disqualification on grounds of low hemoglobin, exclaiming: "Why? Take my blood! Take my blood or I can't go home. Baba Ji says give blood, I must give blood!" At the same camp, Naresh declared to me that he feels "too much happiness when it comes out. If someone asks me for blood I say, 'My body is waiting for you.' If more is required I say, 'Please, I am ready—take from my body again.'"[12] At a Nirankari camp in Chandigargh, a seventy-five-year-old man attempted to give blood. When told that donors must be under sixty, he said: "My blood must be taken! Others must live at my expense. What am I? What am I? Take my blood; take my blood, why don't you take my blood?" In an attempt to calm him down, a blood bank technician eventually pricked his finger to produce a drop of blood. He then proceeded to sit down with the other donors in the refreshment area, proclaiming himself very happy. (Pricking the fingers of rejected devotee-donors to produce small quantities of blood is a pacification technique practiced by many doctors. It allows disqualified devotees to say they too have bled for their guru on what they call his day of donation.) At another camp I met thirteen-year-old Samdisha, a Nirankari since birth. She told me defiantly: "I've been fighting the blood bank because I want to give blood but I am not allowed." The qualifying age is eighteen.

At a camp in Kalkaji, New Delhi, a couple in their fifties were both declared ineligible. The man had recently undergone bypass surgery and the woman had recently suffered from jaundice. To the Red Cross doctor who disqualified them, they said: "You are rejecting us but we will donate today at another blood bank. Today is my guru's day of donation (*dan ka din*)." The exasperated doctor turned to me and said, "They think I have come here only to reject them. But we do it because it is bad for them as well as the one who receives the blood. They will suffer too." Later at the camp, a female devotee was disqualified because of her low weight. She protested, "I want to donate! Why do you reject me?" Beginning to weep, she said, "Baba Ji will not bless me. It is the command (*ardesh*) from satguru. We have to donate."[13] Later on, after her finger had been pricked to produce a small quantity of blood, she said to me: "If I donate it will be useful for my career and for my life because I will get blessings (*ashirvad*) from my Baba."

While attempts by some devotees to give blood despite being declared unfit suggest that helping recipients can sometimes carry less importance than the act of donation itself and the ability thereby to amass spiritual credit, the possibility must be recorded that part of the reason some devotees attempt to donate despite being declared medically unfit may have less to do with the prioritizing of the accumulation of blessings over the welfare of recipients than with their lack of familiarity with the biomedical reasons for disqualification. I show below that devotees see their blood as being made up largely of spirit, love, knowledge, and intentions—entities that they would see as being ennobling rather than harmful.

And yet, many devotees are well educated and certainly aware of the risks attached to the donation of infected blood. A point proceeds from this which relates to asceticism: as the above example demonstrates, the screening process is designed to eliminate not only donations that would harm recipients but also donations that would harm donors. Donating blood in the possession of such knowledge carries a suggestion of physical self-denial. In fact, it would appear that some donors actually welcome the thought that their physical frailness may make blood donation physically taxing or dangerous for them. They are thus inclined to treat blood donation as an austerity like those practiced in the form of fasts and other meritorious acts of ascetic discipline. For Jaipur Jains, writes Laidlaw (2002: 321), asceticism is a kind of "enlightened self-interest," with the practice of seemingly self-denying austerities in the present ensuring the self's future spiritual purity and advantage. So too, perhaps, with some Nirankari blood donors. Attempts made by physically frail devotees to donate are, of course, viewed negatively by medics. However, if your priority is to achieve spiritual benefits through meritorious acts of bodily austerity, such a situation may appear as a welcome opportunity. This can be seen as a disjuncture at the heart of the collaboration between blood banks and devotional orders, and is a reminder that interoperability does not equate simply with harmoniousness.

As I noted in chapter 1, recruiters acknowledge that "meanings" associated with blood donation must proliferate to make possible its interweaving with the narratives of diverse donor constituencies. The proliferation of blood donation's signification, however, possesses the built-in danger of producing "bad meanings." From a biomedical viewpoint, the case described in chapter 3 of a Sikh man donating on consecutive days in an attempt to expel his family's ill fortune was an example of problematic proliferation, and so too is the Nirankari treatment of blood donation as physical austerity. From an analytical viewpoint, however, it is clear that devotees are in the process of turning the "modern" biomedical seva exploits of the Mission into a rich complex of devotional activities irreducible to simplistic "alien imposition" narratives.

The striking emphasis on blessings among Nirankaris generates a correlatively pronounced fear in debarred devotees of missing out on their bestowal. Juergensmeyer (1991: 142) notes that the Radhasoami devotee "offers seva as worship and praise, and perhaps hopes for blessings in return." Nirankari devotees appeared to me more certain of the blessings amassable through seva. As Rohit, a bus driver, put it to me: "By giving blood we serve Baba Ji, and we know Baba Ji will return the favor multiple times." Devotees are left in little doubt on this matter by the guru himself. At a memorial camp staged in 2004 on the date on which his father Gurbachan Singh was assassinated, Hardev Singh declared: "Do good to others and forget about it. Don't expect anything in return." Later he said: "Those who benefit others—God benefits them." The reasoning I think is clear: as the Red Cross slogan declares, "Give blood, get blessings." The only difference is that in this instance they are seen to derive principally from the satguru rather than from transfusion recipients.

So some devotees at least would seem to locate the gift's efficaciousness as much in its ability to secure blessings for themselves as in its medical effects. Where donation is a means to an end other than helping the person into whom the donor's blood is transfused—whether that end is the receipt of blessings, money, purer blood or whatever—blood donation is shorn of the sense it carries of being a transaction with another (the transfusion recipient), instead enacting what could be called an "amoral relationality" (Strathern 1997b: 145). Since in such instances recipients in a sense remain unimagined by donors, what results is "recipient-concealment," a logical consequence of which is the suppression by donors of their personal medical histories. A striking example of exactly this was provided to me by Dr. Chaudary from a government blood bank. She recalls that at one Nirankari camp she attended, a young boy was laid on her table:

> He was in his early twenties. He had a big scar on his abdomen. I just happened to see the scar because I couldn't find a vein on the side he was laying. So I went over to the other side, to see if there was a better vein, and I noticed the big scar, and I asked, what is this? He was silent. I asked again

and he said he had had multiple operations for an incisional hernia, the last being just two months earlier. But he said he wanted to donate on this day for his guru. I had to reject him. They [devotees] hide their histories.

When it became clear to me that money and blessings were, in respect of return, equivalent currencies, with devotee donation in some respects resembling a spiritualized variant of paid donation, I asked two blood bank doctors if they had ever checked the Transfusion Transmissible Infection (TTI) status of "devotee blood" against blood from the general population. Neither doctor had done so. Nor did they accept my suggestion that this might be a valuable thing to do. It is easy to see why such data might prove unwelcome—the Nirankaris, after all, are indispensable providers of "voluntary" blood in the capital. Revealing anecdotal evidence on this matter from another context, however, was provided to me by Cecilia Tan of the Singapore Blood Service, whom I met at a Kolkata conference on voluntary donation in 2005.[14] The Buddhist population of Singapore annually celebrates *vesak* day, the Buddha's birthday and a Singaporean public holiday. Local Buddhists consider that double blessings may be secured for good works conducted on this day: "Buddhists organize blood donation camps only in this period. We have observed that when you have such a motive to donate blood, there is peer pressure to donate from Buddhist groups, with some donating only for double blessings. Because of this there is increasing incidence of positives [infected persons] giving blood. We have tested more HIV positive blood from these occasions."

As was mentioned in chapter 2, an idea widely held in India and shared across numerous ethno-religious boundaries is that merit resulting from charity performed at particular times or places can be multiplied. Though the Singapore example shows that this is not a phenomenon restricted to India, it is further evidence that time and space in the subcontinent are "not uniform and neutral, but have properties, varying specific densities, that affect those who dwell in them" (Ramanujan 1989: 51). Such context sensitivity appears to produce in donors an increased ardor to donate blood at particular times or places in order that they secure the multiplied merit available on those occasions. This can result in recipient concealment.

The Singapore example shows that when religious devotees are treated as convenient donor banks, blood banks collect a higher than average quantity of contaminated units. Similarly, I have presented evidence that the blessings Nirankari devotees think are multiplied on their specific donation days may be understood as a spiritual form of remuneration which generates donors just as avid as those that Titmuss and other policy analysts have found to produce the highest infection rates. The expectation of blessings securable through donation shows how returns can surface as "incubus" within a "nonremunerated" system supposedly immune from them.

Blood services across the world require prospective blood donors to undergo a physical examination before being allowed to donate, with acceptance of the gift frequently being considered by donors to provide "confirmation of physical well-being" (Dalsgaard 2007: 107). Although such a confirmation is also provided in the Nirankari case, there is the further question of moral well-being; for if, in Indian contexts, "a whole and perfect body is both a sign of one's moral state, and a prerequisite for making sacrificial offerings to the gods and ancestors" (Parry 1994: 171), then rejection clearly has implications that are far from being merely physical. In his study of blood donation in Denmark, Dalsgaard (ibid.: 102) argues that acceptance of the gift may be considered a form of reciprocation to donors. For the Nirankari donor, a positive adjudication comprises the counter-gift of confirmation not only of physical well-being but also of a moral status fit for making offerings.

Nonacceptance is therefore highly problematic. Laidlaw (1995: 152) states that, for the Jain renouncers he studied in Jaipur, "The body is used as a tool, or a weapon, in the ascetic project of improving the condition of the soul, and the effects of this are indicated in turn by the body's aptitude in performance of these rites." For Nirankaris, medical disqualification reveals the body's inaptitude for the performance of blood donation, an inaptitude that throws into question the condition of the soul. To continue the Jain analogy, the gifts of food given by lay to renouncer Jains are "expressions of devotion," and "the more the renouncer accepts the better the regard she is showing for the family." In accepting food, renouncers make a judgment on householders' general moral probity (ibid.: 320, 322). In a parallel manner, physical disqualification is experienced by many Nirankari devotees as moral ineligibility.[15] Like Jain renouncers picking over and examining the food offered to them for signs of excess or unacceptable qualities of luxury, doctors' pronouncements of eligibility are a kind of judgment upon devotees' moral or devotional probity.

One devotee-donor stated of a disqualified devotee: "This is an examination. He [the ineligible devotee] was instructed [to donate] by the satguru, but the doctor is not permitting him. The satguru is testing him. Maybe he won't come again to donate, maybe he will." Another devotee, Anil, told me, "over here, after donation, a lot of happiness occurs. Baba Ji considered us [those successful donors sitting with him in the refreshments area] worthy of giving blood." The painful logical accompaniment of this, for some devotees, is that physical ineligibility must be understood as moral unworthiness.

Corporeal Capture

By considering now the gift's affective and spiritual content, these observations can be taken further to explore questions about the significance of blood transfer as an operation with moral as well as physical consequences for recipients as well as for donors. Devotees conceptualize their donated blood as a vessel for the conveyance of their moral and affective qualities of love and *gyan* (spiritual knowledge), which they see as forming the basis for patients of transformative transfusions of spirit. As was argued above, Nirankari gifts are structured by the interplay of centripetal and centrifugal directional intentionalities, with devotees having a bifocal orientation toward the recipients of their donations. I have so far concentrated on the ways in which their gifts travel *to* the guru, with actual recipients seemingly reduced to circumambient image. I now explore how devotees' blood travels *through* the guru to "humanity." Blood donation for devotees is a multilayered volitional act. It is in devotees' envisaging of the gift's actual content that the transfusion recipient comes clearly back into view—perhaps less as the focus of their philanthropic endeavors than as the target of their transformative love and spirit, with the emphasis being as much on changing recipients as saving them.

Konrad (2005: 117) has argued persuasively that in the British system of ova donation, donors can take "effective action from out of the uncertain knowledge set up by the conditions of anonymity." It can be argued, likewise, that devotee-donors similarly engage actively with the anonymous structures of voluntary blood donation as a means of disseminating their "spirit" into unknowable locales, thereby generating a sense of continual spiritual expansion. To elucidate these points, I build on recent anthropological works on the theme of the spirit of the gift in India. I also show how the issue of religious conversion emerges in a novel way in this domain of medical utility, not in the familiar manner of patients converting to the religion practiced by the providers of their treatment out of a sense of necessity or indebtedness, but through the unique properties of the treatment procedures themselves.

As I noted above, Baba Hardev Singh's response to the assassination of his father was to proclaim the need for his devotees to "spread" their love.[16] The verb *bantna*, to spread, was used frequently by devotees in discussion with me—most often in reference to love (*pyar*). Devotees espouse several different ideas about the relationship between blood donation and spreading love: blood donation is often described as "love in action" (love for the guru, humanity at large, or both together), or as a process through which devotees' love is reified in transmissible substance for circulation and propagation. Love, in the latter view, is in the blood; affect is tangible. Furthermore, in attaching itself through transfusion to recipients in order that recipients attach themselves to the Mission—a process I delineate below—disseminated love possesses the quality of viscosity. In referring to the adhesive qualities of the gift, I employ the term "viscous love."

Nirankari literature sees expansion of the Mission as congruent with or as a condition for the creation of universal brotherhood among humans. The satguru conducts "salvation tours" around the country and abroad in order to "spread grace," fortify the organization, and attract new devotees. As he said on a tour of eastern India, the enlightened person "spreads love, peace and brotherhood through his life. May God bless us so that the number of such people may increase in the world, so that by following the teachings of saints and attaining God-realization there is love and brotherhood in man's life. May every man spread the fragrance of love and peace—such has been the cherished wish of all saints and sages. Otherwise, human welfare will remain only a far fetched dream!"[17] While I was in Delhi, devotees were circulating among themselves a series of e-mails and text messages called "Gems of Truth," said to emanate from the satguru. One such "gem" is titled "Acceleration, Propagation" and reads: "In the plains, a vehicle runs fast. However, while crossing mountains, it slows down. Lest it should come to a halt, we accelerate the speed. Similarly, knowing that ours is the Dark Age (Kali Yuga), there is a need for accelerating the pace of propagation of Truth to cross the mountains of ignorance." For the Mission, then, its growth is of paramount importance as a condition for the practical realization of its theology of universal brotherhood which would constitute the redemption of this dissolute age.

While the guru's salvation tours are reputedly extremely successful in attracting new devotees, devotees themselves can be important agents of expansion. Several unmarried devotees declared to me their intention of marrying outside the Mission in order to introduce their spouses to it. My friend Sudhir told me: "I want to marry a non-Nirankari girl. I want an unhappy girl so that I can show her *nirankar* [formless god] and make her happy." Though this practice results from personal initiative rather than official policy, it demonstrates that the logic of expansion works on several levels. A further method of achieving the end of expansion derives from the adhesiveness of devotees' gifts. This adhesiveness gives blood donation expansive potential as a subtly transformative means of contributing to the growth of the Mission.

Issues of religious conversion are fraught with controversy in India, as elsewhere (see Copley 1997; Robinson and Clarke 2003; van der Veer 1996). In this case of spiritually transformative transfusions, the term "conversion" is somewhat awkward since, as stated above, the Mission does not regard itself as a religion and it does not request new recruits to renounce their prior religious identities. The word "conversion" is perhaps unable to reflect adequately the subtlety of a transfusion imbued with the potential to insinuate itself into the spiritual life of the recipient. The role of substance in instantiating involuntary conversion "beneath the skin," however, is a pronounced theme in Indianist scholarship (Arnold 1993; C. Bayly 1988; Froerer 2006; Jones 1976), a fact that increases the difficulty in avoiding the term. The use of an allopathic treatment technique to draw recipients into the Nirankari fold I term "corporeal capture." "Capture," like "conversion," perhaps does a disservice to the professed beneficence of devotees' aims, but it would be difficult to think of any kind of missionary who did not regard his or her aims in a beneficent light. Devotees rarely referred to the spiritual transformation of recipients as the principal aim of their donations (these being primarily attaining the guru's blessings or contributing to the welfare of humanity), but Nirankari donations can and do have several aims. Mission literature states that through blood donation, devotees "are able to establish blood relationship with other human beings" (Sant Nirankari Mandal 2003: 20), but makes no mention of what devotees, at least, see as the expansive potential of blood donation in effecting the spiritual transformation of recipients. Corporeal capture takes place in an indistinct zone of ideation, somewhere between official Nirankari doctrine and devotees' own conceptions of donation.

As was noted above, devotees' donated blood spreads their "viscous love," which attaches itself to recipients so that recipients become attached to the Mission. As one devotee put it, "The recipient will get the gene of a Nirankari and join our group. We can join to his body so he can join this mission." Jagdish explained to me that "we feel love always. We feel love inside and the genes in our blood become loving genes. This loving blood will go to others and affect them so they will also follow truth and love. People will come closer to us. We spread our love to mankind." In other words, doctors—unawares—are transfusing affect and spirit into recipients. In a quite literal rendering of Sathya Sai Baba's description of donated blood as "spiritualized liquid love," my friend Sudhir tells me that what he sees as he lies donating is love leave his body through the attached tube and enter the blood bag. Neera, an elderly female devotee, told me: "If there is some sugar in a box, from that box you won't take out chilies, and from a box with chilies in you won't take out sugar. If you have good knowledge (acha gyan) then your blood is also good. If you have daily satsang you are full of god's knowledge, your blood and your heart is pure, and that's why the doctors take it from us."[18] This assertion that doctors select Nirankari blood for the moral qualities contained therein portrays biomedicine as a project of moral perfectionism. Though I heard no other expression as clear as this, it is quite true that devotees—in assuming that their donated blood encodes transfusable affect—treat blood donation precisely as just such a project.

Many Nirankari devotees express the view that their exteriorized body parts "carry the influence of the person, or may even create new persons" (Konrad 2005: 45). As was noted in chapter 1, it is well known that throughout India bodily secretions are thought to possess transformative potential as powerful agents of personal and spiritual transfer. Blood is often considered a particularly potent medium. Daniel (1983: 28) reports that the villagers of Kalappur, south India, understand karma to be transmitted between generations through blood. Cooked food is an additional conduit.[19] In addition, psychobiological qualities (kunams), which "permeate every organ and every aspect of the body," are exchangeable through the sharing of food and sexual intercourse (ibid.: 32).

A calm person will, for example, become hot-tempered as a result of intercourse with a hot-tempered person, and vice versa. It is of course interesting that issues of "conversion" and "capture" have arisen in a novel biomedical context, but in the light of these observations, we should not be overly surprised by devotees' claims about the affective and spiritual qualities of their donated blood.

Given their status as "saints" who have received gyan, it follows that devotees envision their affective qualities as being morally elevating for recipients. One devotee stated that this was the satguru's explicit aim: "He had a vision that the blood of saints will change the thinking of those people to whom the blood is given because the blood of these saints [devotees] is tuned to the super-soul (*paramatma*)."[20] The same devotee then reframed these thoughts in a spiritual-cum-genetic idiom: "This is gene theory. They are the smallest bodies in existence, but they have all the qualities in them, good and bad, and we believe that by knowing paramatma—which is kind, loving, and merciful—these genes will change the behavior of recipients. Their bad qualities will go when the blood is taken." Another sevadar declared: "When our blood flows into the nerves of those who are not god-realized, they also will feel like knowing god. Our beliefs and experiences are in our blood; they will take our good feelings."[21] Prakash expressed a similar view: "The person who has bad intentions—his blood will not heal spiritually. But our blood will inspire and transform them to work for the people and to love their neighbors." For such devotees, what is officially a physically remedial activity is clearly also a vehicle for spiritual healing. Rakesh, an ex-soldier, emphatically elided the moral content of Nirankari-derived transfusions with conversion to the Mission: "Soul power (*atma-shakti*) is in the blood. The patient will definitely become Nirankari." Clearly, "the propagation of objects"—the circulation of Nirankari blood donations—"means attachment to new people" (Strathern n.d.). And likewise, according to devotees, the attachment of objects to people means the propagation of the Mission.

The role of "substance" in Indian religious conversion has been recorded by Jones (1976: 131), who notes that if a Hindu ate with a Muslim in nineteenth-century Punjab, there was a danger that he would be excommunicated and thereafter be treated as Muslim. That the eating of beef was synonymous with becoming Muslim helps account for the logic behind the fact that Muslims reconverting to Hinduism were made to eat pork to "prove" and validate their new status (ibid.: 203). As part of Arya Samaj purification rituals (known as *shuddhi*), those readmitted to what it saw as the Hindu fold would distribute purified food at meetings of reconciliation (ibid.: 133). Further, the final spark that precipitated the 1857 Indian Mutiny is widely believed to have been soldiers' belief that the cartridges provided by the British had been greased with fat from cows and pigs (C. Bayly 1988: 180). The soldiers, writes Malleson, "had been told that the object of their foreign masters was to make them all Christians. The first step in the course to Christianity was to deprive them of their caste.

This end would be accomplished insidiously by the defilement to be produced by biting the greased cartridge. . . . Having become out-caste by their own act, they must, in despair, accept the religion of their masters" (1987: 67).[22] This highly charged politics of substance is by no means a relic of the nineteenth century: Froerer (2006: 52) notes that on International Women's Day in 1999, a gathering of Hindu and Christian women was organized in remote Chhattisgarh at which a group of Hindu women refused to eat, apprehensive that the food "would turn us into Christians."

Of course, the provision of treatment in order to "convert" beneficiaries is a familiar concept to many Indians—this is how Christian missionaries are said to (and almost certainly do) bring about conversions from Hinduism. Activist Hindutva groups protest against and seek to counter such "bribery," engaging combatively with what they see as the Christian dilution of the Hindu fold in competitive practices of conversion and reconversion. The method of the Nirankaris, however—if it can be called a method—is very different, for it is through the transfusion of charged substance, say devotees, that effects of spiritual transformation are produced. It is not through indebtedness created by the provision of treatment, but through the innate properties of the treatment itself that a disposition toward the Mission results.

Lambert (2000: 78) provides evidence from a predominantly Hindu village in Rajasthan that "caste boundaries are selectively maintained through restrictions . . . according to the limits of commensality."[23] It follows from this that the disruption of restrictions might produce disruptions in essences, which, as S. Bayly (1999: 312) following Madan (1991) notes, can be "simultaneously both innate and alterable." The Nirankaris put a related intimate logic of substance and transformation to work in order to create an opposite, universalizing effect—they want to be related to everybody, to draw anybody toward themselves through the enactment of blood donation as a mode of corporeal capture. The very means of preserving particularity and distinctiveness—restrictions on flows of substance—is subverted by the Nirankaris and made to open up onto the universal in another striking example of exaptation, the operating of existing social structures in order to effect new outcomes.

The vital point about the relationship between the Mission and voluntary blood donation is this: the former seeks to "centrifuge" its viscous love to anyone without restriction. The latter seeks to "centrifuge" the narrow directional focus of replacement donations (given for someone) through promoting the wider directionality embodied by voluntary donation (given for anyone). The relationship is one of mutual facilitation with the fashioning of what could be termed a centrifugal alliance: the large quantities of blood provided by devotees helps realize the project of voluntary donation for anyone; this centrifuged mechanism of provision in turns makes the Nirankaris' viscous love motile and expansive. Blood donation enables their love to travel.

The anonymity of voluntary donation is critical to the alliance. Donors in a voluntary system do not know to whom their donations will travel. Whatever the imbalances and asymmetries of actual provision by blood banks to recipients (the Red Cross does not charge for patients in government hospitals, and certainly does not discriminate along caste or gender lines, so can thus make a good claim to universal provision), from the point of view of the donor, the anonymous conditions of voluntary donation produce a universal directionality. It is this directionality, formed out of the anonymity of voluntary donation, which maps onto and becomes coextensive with the professed universalism of the Nirankaris, and which is used by the Mission to mechanically transgress community restrictions and distinctions and thereby to transcend itself and so realize its theology. As the satguru told devotees in 2002, "God-realized persons have a different point of view. They treat every fellow being as the image of the Almighty and make no discrimination between one person or the other. . . . The donation of blood gives you the best kind of blood relationship. Since the noble act is done in the name of humanity, it goes a long way to strengthen the feeling of universal brotherhood."

The anonymity of voluntary blood donation thus provides a universal directionality which, in being enlisted by the Mission, endows its doctrine of universal brotherhood and connectivity with tangible force and experiential dynamism. Through blood donation, devotees "spread" their viscous love in a universal fashion, without restriction, an allopathic treatment technique utilized as a method of "capture" viewed as moral perfectionism. Devotees' blood, as it were, is sent into the distance while bringing distances up close.[24]

Beyond Sinfulness

The above observations prompt a reflection on the Indianist debate about the "spirit of the gift." The paradigmatic content of the gift in Indian anthropology is "sin" or inauspiciousness (Parry 1986; Raheja 1988). The gift is often characterized as a vessel of expiation; in the village of Pahansu in Uttar Pradesh inauspicious gifts are endlessly given with the effect of reinforcing the dominance of a particular caste grouping (the Gujars) (Raheja 1988); in Banaras, funerary gifts "corrupt the recipient body and soul, and result in untold misfortune unless proper expiatory steps are taken" (Parry 2000). Parry (1986: 460) noted that variations upon this concept of the gift are widespread in India, and in recent years several studies have borne this out, while at the same time seeking to refine Parry's and Raheja's explanations regarding the gift's dangerous properties (Laidlaw 2000; Mines 2005; Osella and Osella 1996; Säävälä 2001; Snodgrass 2001).

In an important challenge to Parry's definition of the spirit of the gift, Laidlaw (2000: 630) declares that the gift's spirit or "poison" is "not some unique or mysterious substance found only in gifts." What Parry took to be a specific feature of Indian dan was really a manifestation of "the dangers attendant on social interaction in general." Laidlaw (ibid.: 629) gives the examples of cooked food, cloth, and detached parts of the body as "powerful media for the flow of bio-moral qualities between persons." As I mentioned above, in devotees' employment of voluntary donation as a mechanism for providing access to others' bodies, devotees pursue a closely related logic to that which lies behind caste restrictions in some villages, but in order to produce the opposite effect of unrestricted spiritual relatedness. This is in line with Laidlaw's argument, "the gift" being a context for transmission of "spirit" rather than a unique manifestation of transmission.

One devotee told me: "We have seen so often that if someone takes water from a sangat [attendee of satsang, fellowship of the true], this person becomes attracted to the Nirankaris. We donate blood through our Guru Ji. Our blood will go to you and the same spiritualism will be inspired in you also." The capacity of shared water to effect similar changes to blood donation suggests it is less a property of the gift that transforms recipients than of propinquity in general. A further example was provided to me by a devotee who practices homeopathic medicine: "My patients are all happy because my cosmic energy is all around me when I give them the medicine. They do not get cured from others; from me they cure very easily. The medicine in my hands takes my atmic-waves [soul-waves]. I say, Nirankar, bless them with your divine power (shakti), and later, they all want to become Nirankaris." Once again, the ability to "capture" new devotees is not conditional on dan but results from a more generalized social adhesiveness.

The case of Nirankari blood donation, in addition, demonstrates that gifts do not necessarily poison or pollute. However, of the anthropologists I cited above who have engaged with the earlier work by Parry and Raheja, only Laidlaw (2000) and Osella and Osella (1996) acknowledge that Indian gifts' bio-moral content could be anything other than negatively valued.[25] Devotee-donors obviously understand their spiritual qualities to be reified in their blood donations, but where Parry's gifts morally imperil recipients, Nirankari donors suppose that their gifts will do the reverse, enhancing the moral and spiritual status of patients. This is not a contradiction: Parry's model at least implies the possibility of the reverse effect, for if gifts from mourners to Brahmins are imperiling because "saturated with the evil consequences of the donor's conduct," gifts from those who are of elevated, even enlightened status, such as "saintly" devotees in possession of gyan, might well be "saturated" with the morally edifying consequences of the donor's conduct. In this light, Parry's priests, in emphasizing the sin they accumulate from donors' gifts, reveal less that the gift is an exemplary means of sin removal than their own pessimistic view of their fellow Indians.

Mines (2005: 72) notes that in order to dispose of negative moral qualities in the village in which she worked in Tamil Nadu and in Pahansu, the Uttar Pradesh village studied by Raheja (1988), these qualities are often "transferred from persons to objects and then on to other persons." In Pahansu, for example, "transfers are effected through simple ritual procedures . . . such as circling an object around a person's body to remove an illness or other negative quality and then transferring it to another person or place" (Mines 2005: 68; Raheja 1988: 85–86). Negative moral qualities are thus made finite and disposable through their objectification. In the Nirankari case, however, there is no hint that they lose or are emptied of what they pass on. This once again connects Nirankari gifts of blood to more general themes of contagious social contact. For example, when the saliva of a sacred teacher is transferred to worshipers "as a source of grace and power" (S. Bayly 1989: 52), there is no suggestion that the sacred teacher is himself emptied of grace and power.

Laidlaw (1995: 294) has questioned analyses that strive to identify a single Indian ideology of dan. In line with this, rakt-dan's multiplicity can help us see the multiplicity of dan in general. In the Nirankari case, devotees see their gifts as morally elevating for recipients. But this, it should be emphasized, is a finding specific to the Nirankari experience of blood donation. For I have also noted a strong resonance between a blood donation thought to expel corrupting cells and forms of classical dan, which also remove the donor's impurities or sins: in both cases the ideology of the gift's *purity* is compromised by virtue of the fact that it is also *purificatory*; and in chapter 3 the example was given of a man donating blood to remove the inauspiciousness afflicting his family. Moreover, the "official" ideology of dan as a pure gift—"a voluntary and disinterested donation made without ostentation or expectation of *any* kind of *this*-worldly return, whether material or immaterial" (Parry 1989: 66)—is reflected in the legal definition of rakt-dan as a nonremunerated mode of giving, and is actively mobilized by doctors for whom the promotion of unreciprocated giving is a means to ensure the safety of donated blood. Diverse conceptions of dan compete with each other in rakt-dan, which is a dan in formation. Different parties imbue it with qualities associated with different sorts of dan, and the differences between what rakt-dan is imbued with are the differences that characterize dan more generally. As Corbin (1986: 30) said of definitions of violence: as much as possible the meaning of Indian gifts should be a variable to be investigated ethnographically and not a constant to be built into the definition.

Conclusion

This chapter has added the pursuit of blessings to Titmuss's list of returns that can compromise the safety of donated blood. Devotees donate blood as guru seva and receive blessings from the guru, the transcendental recipient of their gifts. This is not to say, however, that devotees do not give to "humanity." They do so in a very particular way whereby their blood is donated both to and through the guru to others. Their gifts, structured by this perspectival duality, travel simultaneously to one and to many. The highly particularized institution of guru seva is thus consolidated, even as it facilitates the reform of blood giving according to an abstracted philanthropic template.

While recognizing that purified concepts of altruism and self-interest are inadequate in accounting for the multiplicity of motivations harbored by Nirankari devotees, there remains the problem that a safe blood donation system is premised on complete separation between compassion and self-interest. If obtaining blessings, health benefits, or any other kind of "return" reduces recipients and their welfare to "circumambient image" (Greenblatt 1996: 282), or epiphenomenon of the act of donation, there can result grave consequences. Incentives, whether material or spiritual, can endanger the quality of the blood supply. Here I write from an inescapably biomedical perspective in the hope of seeing a safer system of blood provision. In "A Note on [Derrida's] 'Faith and Knowledge,'" Anidjar (2002: 40) writes: "religion counts, again; it accumulates returns and thus returns." Though somewhat homogenizing, the statement is suggestive in the case under consideration. Should devotees' propensity to "count" returns lead blood banks to call a halt to their arrangement with devotional orders like the Sant Nirankaris? I think not, but steps do need to be taken to reformulate in the minds of devotees the triadic relationship between merit, act, and effect. This can be shown through presenting an example from another context which suggests that it is not counting per se that is the problem, but the particular manner in which some Nirankaris count.

The following citation, from an article on attempts to encourage blood donation among Buddhist monks and novices studying at a temple school in Chiang Mai, Thailand, suggests that if returns are correlated with the effect rather than with the act of donation, they might actually help to ensure the safety of donated blood:

> Before a statue of the Buddha, they vow to respect their blood as "community blood" and look after it on behalf of the community or anyone who may need it in the future. As monks and novices, they already practice celibacy so there is little or no risk of infection. . . . In this way, they are not only assuring a supply of untainted blood, but are also applying traditional values and culture, and indirectly encouraging youth and community members to abstain from any behavior that could put the "community blood" at risk of infection. And, in accordance with their tradition, they are accumulating merit that could help them in this or future lives.[26]

In this example, what I term "donation asceticism"—the requirement of constant moral and physical commitment from donors in order to protect their as yet undonated blood, which is held in trust for future recipients (see Copeman 2006: 117–119 and chapter 8)—is brought into line with the ascetic restraint demanded of Buddhist practitioners. The taking of a solemn vow not to endanger their blood, made before a statue of the Buddha, is directly comparable to the tenet contained in a French voluntary blood donor's code which exhorts signatories "to remain worthy of being a Voluntary Blood Donor, respecting the rules of morality, good behavior and solidarity with human beings" (Ray 1990: 69).

The article suggests that merit ensues less from the specific act of donating blood than from ensuring the safety of transfusion recipients. This implies that merit would result from refraining from attempting to donate if, for example, the donor had recently suffered from malaria or hepatitis. In the Nirankari case, it could be that a concerted effort on the part of the Mission hierarchy and blood banks to conceptually redirect the attainment of merit away from the act of bleeding itself to ensuring recipients' safety could foster the provision of healthier blood.

5

Blood Donation in the Zone of Religious Spectacles

Established procedures–doing things carefully, methodically, predictably–
would become the heart of a safe system of blood use and exchange in
the postwar world.

Thomas Laqueur, "Pint for Pint"

The day will come soon when every child in this world will have the name
of Sacha Sauda on his tongue.

http://www.sachasauda.com

The "Medical Marvels" section of the *Guinness Book of World Records, 2005*
includes such entries as most fetuses in a human body, most surviving children
from a single birth, most operations endured, and most hand amputations on the
same arm. Also included is the achievement of a north Indian devotional order in
collecting most units of blood in a single day: the 12,002 450 ml units collected by
the Dera Sacha Sauda, says the book, "is the equivalent of 67 bathtubs of blood!"[1]

Through the Indian media and forms of government communication,
blood donation has over a number of years been formulated as a critical idiom
for the articulation of ethical and patriotic citizenship (cf. Addlakha 2001: 154).
Guru movement and political party adherents vie to donate the most blood in a
kind of national league of virtuous beneficence. The successive setting and surpassing of world records has turned the collection of blood by religious movements in India into something akin to a system of "alternating disequilibrium"
as described by Andrew Strathern (1971: 222), one group achieving the record
and being dominant until another group breaks it, and so on.

This chapter explores the phenomenon of the staging of record-breaking
'mass' or 'mega' blood donation camps. The Dera Sacha Sauda devotional order
has twice broken the world record for most units of blood collected in a single
day, first in December 2003 on the death anniversary of a former guru (attracting
15,432 donors), and then again—breaking its own existing record—in October

2004 as part of the mortuary ceremonies of the present guru's father (17,921 donors).[2] Founded in 1948 and based on the outskirts of the city of Sirsa in Haryana state, the Dera Sacha Sauda, like the Sant Nirankari Mission discussed in chapter 4, emerged out of the north Indian sant tradition and is headed by a revered spiritual master. My concern in this chapter is to show how record-breaking blood donation activity allows what claims to be a restrained and austere devotional order, opposed to *tamasha* (spectacle) and "show off," to enact spectacles of donor excess, with the utility of blood donation helping sanction and sanctify the taboo. I also explore efforts on the part of the Dera Sacha Sauda to redefine what counts as a "miracle," and discuss the vanguard role of the devotional order in instituting blood donation as a high-profile mode of political protest in contemporary India. As a means of redressing grievances, we shall see that blood donation possesses an interesting and highly ambiguous relationship with Gandhian protest styles.

A Catalogue of Claims

The breaking of blood donation world records is characterized by a remarkable inflationary spiral. In 2001 the world record for most units collected in a day, held by a U.S. university, was 3,000. Then in 2002 the Mumbai-based Limbdi Ajramar Jains collected 10,000 units in a day and the next year 12,000.[3] Before regularizing and reducing the scale of their camps in response to requests from donor recruiters (see chapter 6), the Sant Nirankaris collected 5,000 to 6,000 units annually on April 24 (Human Unity Day—the day on which in 1980 the present guru's father was assassinated). The devotees of the Maharashtrian guru Narendra Maharaj claim to have collected 6,500 units in 2003, more than double the U.S. record. The Youth Congress tried and failed to break the Guinness record in 2003 on the death anniversary of Rajiv Gandhi (Copeman 2004: 140–141), though it did manage a place in the less prestigious *Limca Book of Records*. The *Limca Book of Records* is India's own soft-drink sponsored version of the Guinness enterprise, which, according to its Web site, "since its first edition in 1990, is aimed at showcasing 'India at her best' before the world community, and reviving the spirit of excellence and pride among Indians."[4] The *Limca Book*, notes Lal (2002), "largely whets the appetites of those Indians who are not manly, bold, or lucky enough to make it into Guinness' compilation of world records. . . . [Limca record holders] can nonetheless satisfy themselves with the thought that they hold some record in India."

A news report of a Congress camp staged in Delhi in 2005 captures well the aggrandizing function of camps, demonstrating in particular the way one person may take on credit for the donation efforts of many:

> If it was meant to be a show of strength, then the Delhi Pradesh Congress
> Committee president, Ram Babu Sharma, certainly had his way on

Saturday. Not only did the blood donation camp organized by the DPCC in memory of the former Prime Minister, Rajiv Gandhi, at Talkatora Indoor Stadium register a record number of donors but the Member of Parliament from Amethi, Rahul Gandhi [Rajiv Gandhi's son], stole the show with his sudden appearance on the scene leading to a commotion as Congressmen jostled for catching the eye of the young leader. . . . The very fact that senior AICC [All India Congress Committee] leaders . . . took part in the program and donated blood indicated Mr. Sharma's hold.[5]

The novelist Gore Vidal's (1997) term "altruistic megalomania" is apt in referring to such performances of "conspicuous extraction." The report's use of the term "record," however, seems less apt: 2,146 units are reported to have been donated—nothing like a world record. The "record" here refers to the DPCC having never before collected such a quantity of blood at a single event. It is thus evident that the clamor for "records" results in organizations making record-breaking claims for the somewhat obscure differentiating features of the events they stage; and, since each occasion is inevitably unique in some way or other, every public performance comes to be "record-breaking." Many examples of this trend can be given: at a camp I attended in a Lord Ayyappa temple in Delhi, the organizers claimed to attendant press reporters that they had broken the world record for most women donors—indeed it was the claim in advance of the camp that a record was to be shattered which persuaded large numbers of press reporters to attend what was in reality a rather routine collection event. A former director of the Sathya Sai Baba blood bank in Puttarparthi informed me that it had attained the world record for receiving blood donations from the highest number of nationalities. And a couple from Mohali made it into the *Limca Book of Records* in 2004 after each donating forty-one times over thirteen years: "Looking proudly at his certificate Jaswant said, 'It's God who has given us the power to achieve this record.' "[6] I could go on.

Though this catalogue of claims demonstrates that it is by no means only religious movements that compete for records, it is they who have actually entered the record books, and who are playing an increasingly important role in the provision of blood in India. Currently dominant in this system of alternating disequilibrium is the Dera Sacha Sauda with its camps of 12,000 and 17,000 donors, respectively, each of which attained world record status. Hopkins (1901: 158) described competitive fasting in India, whereby creditors starve themselves to force the hand of debtors who are in turn obliged to starve, as "a sort of stomach-duel." Guru-led devotional movements do something comparable with blood donation, competing with each other to attain world records and primacy in the national league of virtuous beneficence in what may be termed vein-duels.

English (2005: 10) argues that prizes act as "effective institutional agents of *capital intraconversion*" through which transactions and conversions can be negotiated between different forms of capital: economic, cultural, political, and so on. Through the achievement of Guinness world records the Dera Sacha Sauda guru "cashes in" the symbolic fortune of having many devotees who worship him as a god and who unquestioningly follow his directives, the external recognition of a world record serving to establish synonymity between his name and incomparable munificence, and to circulate this resonant name throughout the world. The world record is thus the transfigured capital of the guru's control over his devotees' bodies. I return in the next chapter to the issue of the "deployability" of gurus' devotees.

Supercharity: The Mass Camps Controversy

The claims listed above reflect both what Lal (2002) calls India's "national obsession" with world records and also religious movements' concern with the quantities of seva they perform.[7] The Guinness world records achieved by devotional orders for most blood collected in a single day combine the two concerns, with countable feats of seva being propelled "into the pages of what the West calls 'history'" (ibid.). Examples provided by McKean demonstrate the ways in which the Divine Life Society in Rishikesh makes seva enumerable. At the Society's 1986 Centenary Celebration, the guru Chidananda took pains to list the numbers of patients treated at the society's clinics (McKean 1996: 250). The society's adherents are also encouraged to keep a "spiritual diary" in which they should note not only how many lies they have told per day and how many hours they have spent in "useless" company, but also how long they have spent in "disinterested, selfless service" and how much they have given in charity. This exercise, the society claims, produces "quick progress" and "marvelous results." Devotees are thus encouraged "to mould for themselves identities that conform to criteria which can be enumerated and evaluated" (ibid.: 218). The Divine Life Society is not unique: there is a longstanding propensity for devotees and the spiritual organizations to which they belong to enumerate and quantify the seva they perform.

In an extension and externalization of this logic so that it comes to structure relations between orders rather than simply being internal to them, the hyperbolic numbers necessary for the surpassing of world records allow devotional movements to achieve dominance in the system of alternating disequilibrium and so have their seva activities writ large, thus guaranteeing a high degree of media attention, with this, in the case of the Dera Sacha Sauda, contributing to the glorification of the guru. An official Dera Sacha Sauda publication assures the reader of its blood donation activities: "That a Guinness World Record was also created in the process was sheer chance" (Dera Sacha Sauda n.d.a.). English (2005) terms the varying ways in which award recipients affect to disdain the awards they receive, "strategies of condescension." During my stay at a Dera

Sacha Sauda ashram in Sirsa, I was given access by a camp organizer to a file of photographs and mementos documenting the movement's two record-breaking camps. The file revealed the extent to which the organization had engaged in the determined, painstaking task of collecting artifacts of verification, such as signed letters from medical officers confirming their participation, necessary to establish for the Guinness authorities that the camps qualified for the world record. Also dispelling the notion that the world record attempts had not been planned, I saw a printed e-mail sent in advance of the 2003 camp to the compilers of the *Guinness Book of World Records* requesting clarification of the rules and of the collection figure the organizers needed to surpass. The movement's emphasis on "sheer chance"—its strategy of condescension toward world records—is necessary because of its own "official" stance against "show off" and spectacle. Indeed, the puzzle is that all these record attempts exist in tandem with a taboo on exhibitionistic seva. I return to this matter below.

Devotees I met in Sirsa were less diffident than the official literature. Virtually all were unabashedly delighted at the movement's achievement: "It means Pita Ji's [the guru's] name is in there; he has entered the *Guinness Book* and can become world famous. We are ready to do anything for his sake." At a satsang (worship gathering) in Sirsa, a devotee declared to me: "Our aim was to get into the *Guinness Book* and we did it! Everyone will know Pita Ji now."

Lal (2002) has noted that a tenth of all correspondence the *Guinness Book* receives is Indian, and he links the phenomenon to Indians' "propensity towards numbers": "the Indian imagination is particularly drawn to taxonomies, numerology, and the sheer play to which numbers lend themselves. The Hindu *Puranas* contain the most complex concatenations of numbers, and numbers have been critical to such enterprises as divination, ritual sacrifice, literary compositions, construction of genealogies, cosmogony, and astrology." Lal claims that the outlandish nature of Indian world records represents "a counter-hegemonic force to modern orthodoxies about development, production, competition, and modernity." He juxtaposes the ideology of the *Guinness Book*, informed by a competitive spirit and a drive to raise productivity, with Shridhar Chillal of Pune's record for the world's longest fingernails, five of which together measured 205 inches. Hence, argues Lal, one of the ways Indians engage with an ideology valorizing productive utility is through setting world records of discernible disutility: "Chillal would appear to have made himself quite useless: one cannot be certain how he prevents his manicured hands from being grazed by objects, how he dresses himself, or how he attends to his other daily needs."

Lal (2002) sees in records such as Chillal's a relation to productive modernity consisting of both "homage and parody," noting that the "freakishness" of Indian records such as furthest "backwards running" and most time spent on one leg embarrasses and disturbs those Indian elites which cherish narratives of Indian progress. As I show in a moment, Lal's argument is certainly not without insight as regards blood donation records, but its somewhat celebratory tone (in terms of these records' supposed "subversion" of productive norms) needs to be qualified by a recognition of the extremely problematic basis of much Indian world record seeking, especially when the records are of a medical nature (as they very often are). The subject populations for medical world record seeking are frequently made up of the bodies of the poor, for "beggars can't be choosers" when it comes to the quality of treatment—when it is something to be treated at all. As I noted in chapter 3, Sacha Sauda doctors engage in a "cost-benefit screening analysis" of pilgrim-patients with eye tests conducted in a matter of seconds. One may well conjecture whether the startling speed of screenings, with the inevitable deficiencies of care this entails, might be for the aggrandizing purpose of surpassing yet another world record. Furthermore, it was recently reported that a surgeon in Tamil Nadu attempted to make it into the *Guinness Book* "by performing 50 hernia operations in 24 hours at a private hospital in the state capital, Chennai. He was trying to beat the world record of 41 hernia surgeries in 13 hours 41 minutes and 19 seconds."[8] It seems unlikely that patients knew their operations were being performed in haste for the purpose of achieving the record. It was also reported that a fifteen-year-old schoolboy recently performed a caesarean section because his parents, who run a hospital in Tamil Nadu, "wanted their son's name in the *Guinness Book of World Records.*" The boy had apparently been performing such operations from the age of twelve.[9] Referring to the schoolboy's reported feat, a spokeswoman for the *Guinness Book* declared: "This is not a record that the Guinness World Records would endorse, as we wouldn't want to encourage bad medicine practice." No doubt this is true, but it nonetheless endorses mass blood camp world records.

Lal's argument is nevertheless instructive in regard to doctors' ambivalent response to record-breaking blood donation camps. While the donations made in them are indeed on one level "productive," the immoderation of such enactments frequently results in wastage and disutility. Mass camps are in consequence highly controversial. As one of the elites to which Lal refers, Indian doctors are perturbed by and extremely critical of the excessive donation of blood at mass camps. At the same time, however, doctors are dependent on these movements for their blood supply and so felicitate them at awards ceremonies, lavishing their gurus with thanks and praise—thus revealing the conflicted nature of their professional selves.

The mass camp is an interesting interface between intersecting and yet divergent imperatives. Doctors profess a commitment to pure medical utility and are averse to wastage. An ethnographic account from the United States highlights how physicians allocate kidneys according to a criterion of likely wastage by "noncompliant" recipients. Doctors experience "fear of waste," and patients who "waste" a kidney via noncompliance commit a moral transgression for not taking the doctors' scarcity dilemma seriously enough (Gordon 2000: 365, 367).

Wastage as taboo possesses a similar stature of transgression within the Indian biomedical community. As was seen in chapter 3, devotional orders like the Dera Sacha Sauda and Nirankari Mission make a reformist correlation between utility and virtue, with the Dera Sacha Sauda in particular exalting blood donation as the substitutive ennoblement of wasteful feasting and pind-dan. The reform of giving practices among devotional orders would appear therefore to consist of a move toward the principles of medical utility. And yet we know that these movements' officials and devotees seek to maximize donations in order to demonstrate both the intensity of their own devotion and the scale of their guru's largesse. And further, the system of alternating disequilibrium requires feats of supercharity through which, like North American potlatch ceremonies in which rival chiefs seek to vanquish each other's names through crushing expenditure, preeminence in the national league of virtuous beneficence is attainable. So while the gift is certainly now "useful," and to that extent "reformed," the conditions are also in place for the production of a surplus of blood, some of which inevitably remains unused—thus transgressing the taboo on wastage.

The North American potlatch ceremonies described by Boas (1966: 93) involved the destruction by chiefs of blankets, canoes, and coppers in order to make their names "grow."[10] Mass camps share with potlatches these agonistic and name-growing aspects. Disturbed by the material ruin wrought by potlatches, the Canadian government legislated against them. Doctors likewise condemn one-time mass camps for being pointless and wasteful, seeking to convert them into events of predictable regularity. But as I have noted, the blood donation camp is an interface between several different imperatives. While the Dera Sacha Sauda may ostensibly have moved away from "wasteful" devotional activity toward practices of virtuous utility, from the point of view of doctors, utility-valorizing organizations such as the Sacha Sauda smother utility in their quantitative embrace. Conflicted doctors hardly know whether to encourage or to attempt to suppress such unrestrained donation episodes.

The institutional move away from replacement toward voluntary donation necessitates the centrifugation of directional intentionalities: donation to someone must become donation for anyone. Doctors and recruiters further require that the temporally delimited donation activity signaled by one-time mass camps undergo what might be termed temporal centrifugation. Hanson (1997) claims that socialist time regimes existed in a tension between "rational" and "charismatic" temporalities, the former routine and predictable, the latter spectacular and unpredictable. In India, replacement donation is the prototypical one-time donation, but "voluntary" mass camps, staged on the deaths of gurus, or the death anniversaries or birthdays of significant personages, are similarly irregular and delimited. Recruiters therefore aim to temporally centrifuge one-time "charismatic" donation activity in order to imbue it with a more "rational," routinized temporality (cf. Whitehouse 2000).

For example, in much of India blood stock levels trace the population's episodic surges in patriotic sentiment, with countless camps being organized on India's Independence and Republic Days (August 15 and January 26, respectively). One Mumbai recruiter, Vinay Shetty, told me: "When people call me to arrange a camp for these days I say, please do not. People don't only fall sick on 15 August when we want to give blood. There is a major surge of patriotism on these days. We also say you should be patriotic, but throughout the year."[11] In an effort to temporally "uncontain" delimited donation activity, Shetty has devised a poster intended to trigger the emotions of prospective donors. It depicts an Indian soldier in battle, with the slogan in Marathi: "Not everyone can join the armed forces and defend the country. Do the next best thing—donate blood four times a year."

Mass camps, which involve the bleeding of thousands of devotees in a single venue by multiple medical teams, are a particularly vivid and controversial example of charismatic donation activity. As I noted above, they are controversial because doctors demand a "rational," more repetitive temporality of giving that avoids wastage. Doctors I spoke with disparaged mass camps as being "like circuses." One recalled a mega camp he had attended: "It was a frenzied donation . . . it was a mass frenzy. We need small, regular camps. It is not reasoned." At the annual conference of the Indian Society of Blood Transfusion and Immunohaematology (ISBTI) in Chennai in 2004, a doctor gave a lecture titled, "Mega-camps: A Critical Review." At such camps, according to the speaker, there is an increase in adverse donor reactions due to inadequate donor care, many extractions produce "quality not sufficient" units (that is, bags are not properly filled so as to save time and extract more units), and excessive collection results in 13.6 percent wastage through expiry. These negative consequences result, said the speaker, from camp organizers' fixation with "some stupid magic number." The Indian propensity toward numbers similarly vexed nineteenth-century intellectuals such as James Mill, who saw "Hindu numbers"—such as the 17,064,000 years during which the Creator transformed itself from "neuter to masculine, for the purpose of creating worlds"—as signs of the "rude and imperfect state" of the Hindu mind. Hegel, too, felt that numbers in India "have not the value and rational meaning which we attach to them" (cited in Lal 2002). The doctor's criticism of mass camps shows that representatives of "progress" remain exasperated by irrational number usage in the subcontinent.

I have been arguing that interoperability characterizes the relationship between north Indian devotional orders and projects to foster voluntary blood donation. While each entity contributes vitally toward the fulfillment of aspects of the other's phenomenal and practical existence, I have emphasized that their interdependence is equally marked by "jolts and disjunctions" (Pinney 2005: 270), such as Nirankari devotees' desire for blessings and view of donation as an austerity, which might produce blood that is medically unsafe for transfusion.

A further disjunction between the imperatives of doctors and those of devotional orders relates to the size, structure, and regularity of camps. As was argued in chapter 1, blood donation may be considered a boundary object which, though the immediate cause of the coordination activities of blood banks and devotional movements, in no way guarantees the bridging of the perspectives and understandings of the different collaborating parties (Wenger 1998: 107). For example, recruiters and doctors' dual requirement of securing an adequate number and the safety of donations causes them to simultaneously embrace and attempt to order the unfolding plurality of priorities and meanings associated with blood donation. The case of the mass blood donation camp is exemplary in demonstrating that coordination between different communities of practice does not necessarily mean convergence or agreement.

Utility as Sanctioning Device

The Dera Sacha Sauda has since 2003 proudly held the Guinness record for most blood donated in a single day. The data on which this and the following sections are based was chiefly gathered during my stay in a Dera Sacha Sauda ashram in Sirsa in November 2004.

As with the Nirankaris and Radhasoamis, the guru is of pivotal importance as devotional cynosure of the movement, and the institution of guru seva is strikingly prominent. Recalling Sathya Sai Baba's Sarvadharma symbol, made up of symbols from the principal world religions, the spiritual master's name, Guru Maharaj Gurmeet Ram Rahim Singh Ji, combines linguistic inflections from several religious traditions.[12] When addressing satsang (worship) gatherings, the guru sits beneath conjoined Hindu, Sikh, Muslim, and Christian symbols which, through a contrivance of directing lines, appear to emanate from the figure of the guru, thus depicted as these religions' incarnate union.[13]

"Dera"—the extended residential site of an influential figure—has similar connotations to "ashram," while "Sacha Sauda" means literally true deal or dealings, and is an allusion to the fact that monetary gifts from devotees are not accepted by the organization, which claims to be fully autarkic, owning extensive lands in Haryana and in other states on which its resident "sadhus" work "eighteen-hour days." From the produce of the land, the movement runs a supermarket; it also manages a petrol pump, a biscuit factory, and one of its ashrams houses a revolving restaurant and boating lake, said to be for the benefit of the hundreds of thousands of pilgrims who annually converge on the site.[14] Strong disapproval of monetary donations is expressed in all the literature it produces and in satsang gatherings by the guru himself: "Man . . . wants to bribe God. Man does not understand that God, who made this world, and made this entire universe, can he not make your few small rupees? Just think about it! But nobody thinks!"[15] Satsang orations consist of many such exposés of supposedly exploitative religious practices—the offering of money in temples, but also the donation of funds to high-profile, media-savvy gurus such as Sathya Sai Baba.[16] Demanding that devotees be reflexive and critical ("Use your mind!"), the guru constructs himself as their honest protector.

Dera Sacha Sauda devotees are predominantly working- and middle-class Hindus hailing from towns and villages in Haryana and Rajasthan, though there are also many Sikh adherents, and the gurus have all, thus far, been of Sikh origin.[17] The organization claims to possess more than a million devotees and thirty-eight ashrams throughout India, though most of these are in the north of the country. Like those of the Radhasoami tradition (Juergensmeyer 1991), Dera Sacha Sauda teachings emphasize the importance of reciting sacred words (*ram nam*) for the achievement of transcendence. The guru exhorts devotees to abstain from alcohol and meat, to be faithful in marriage, never to lie and, as was noted above, never to make religious offerings of money. The group also expounds a strong anti-ritual message: "Dera Sacha Sauda does not believe in any kind of false practices, false pretensions, misguidance or any kind of show off which has nothing to do with spiritualism and those ritual practices which take you away from your real goal."[18] In my discussions with them, devotees repeatedly drew attention to the absence of distracting "rituals" (*rasmen*), something they saw as one of the movement's key defining features. Instead, they argued, it is through the more direct method of *guru-bhakti* that spiritual progress results. The movement's professed aversion to ritual and "show off" (*tamasha*) situates it in a reformist tradition that has been determined to undermine "superstitious ritual."[19]

From one angle, the Dera Sacha Sauda is a prime example of a religion of utility, as discussed above in chapter 3. As was also noted in that chapter, the guru extols offerings of medicine and blood because they encode usefulness and non-convertibility. This encoding of donated blood results from the assumption that only those who need them receive transfusions.[20] Money, however, is proscribed because it can be put to any kind of nefarious use and therefore encodes not usefulness but dangerous ambiguity: "O! You give a donation of money and say it is given to God. Does God sign on that?" The guru valorizes the cow not because it is a physical abode and amalgamation of the gods as espoused in classic Hindu texts, but because of its utility: "Animals are ahead of humans in many ways: the body of the cow is used after death [i.e., for leather], and while they are living their dung is also used [for fuel and manure]. Their bones are also used (*khad*). But out of these, nothing is used (*kam ana*) of a human being."[21] Blood donation, however, makes a human being useful and is thus "really a great donation and God must bless you for this."[22] The point I wish to underline here is that the guru's exaltation of blood donation on account of its usefulness is a means by which devotees can do what the movement supposedly bans in the name of its austere brand of purified, "reformed" religiosity: that is, give gifts and conduct spectacular ritual. "Virtuous utility" both sanctions and sanctifies the taboo.

But there is a further difficulty for the Dera Sacha Sauda. Gifts that encode utility, unlike gifts of money, certainly possess virtue, and doing lots of this "good thing" is therefore surely acceptable, nay admirable behavior. And yet, as Sathya Sai Baba puts it: "Service should not be exhibitionistic. You must seek no reward, not even gratitude or thanks from the recipients."[23] Ann Gold (1988), Laidlaw (1995), Cohen (1998: 170), Mayer (1981), and others have documented the widespread suspicion and policing of intention that surrounds acts of seva and charity in India. In the eyes of Hindu villagers in Rajasthan, "anonymous donations to strangers made in distant pilgrimage centers are considerably more meritorious than ostentatious charities undertaken at home" (A. Gold 1988: 9). As was noted above, the Dera Sacha Sauda's ostentatious charities are indeed frowned upon by doctors. This is perhaps as much for their "exhibitionism" as for their destruction of use-value. The movement's spectacular, much-reported camps appear to enact a version of blood donation precisely contrary to the revered category of *gupta-dan*, a gift given in secret, and therefore immune from the "immediate reward of an increase in the donor's public status, and people say that because of this the unseen reward which comes as merit or good karma will be greater" (Laidlaw 1995: 297). The movement's "conspicuous extraction" seems in fact to resemble what for Jains in nearby Rajasthan is the most degenerate form of dan—*kirti-dan*: "a gift given to earn fame" (Laidlaw 1995: 296).[24]

As was noted above, the Dera Sacha Sauda engages in "strategies of condescension" toward the records it attains—this is one way in which it seeks to demonstrate that its gifts are not given to earn fame. The anonymity of blood donation provides the guru with a further means of making the same claim. At a satsang I attended in Sirsa, he stated: "Sometimes when doing seva for others you get pride (*ghamand*), but when you donate blood you do seva without knowing where it is going—there is no pride. Blood donation is the best seva because you don't get pride and you [unknowingly] help many people." In locating virtuous secrecy in the absence of contact between blood donor and transfusion recipient rather than in the setting of donation, the Dera Sacha Sauda can publicize its great feats of dan and seva while claiming to conform to the highest standards of nonattachment and humility. Donors at Dera Sacha Sauda camps are bled under the media spotlight, and yet, argues the guru, their donations are given to persons unknown to them and therefore resemble the "donations made to strangers in distant pilgrimage centers" which for Gold's villagers in Rajasthan is the mark of charity's virtue.

A New Order of the Miraculous

The Dera Sacha Sauda also uses its attainment of world records in order to generate an aura of the miraculous. As a strategy it is dependent upon efforts to redefine or reform what counts as a miracle. The guru, as I have noted, seeks to portray himself as a debunker of fake and exploitative religious practices, and his demystifying ire extends to miracles. In one satsang oration he stated:

> Some people sit in heat, a lot of heat. With fire all around, they sit in the middle. People are surprised! Wow! This is a big show and a big drama. Our body can bear heat, a lot of heat. . . . Keep the fire at a distance and go to it inch by inch, and someone or other one day will become quite fit to go near the fire. What's the big deal? . . . Saints hold satsangs in which they don't put on any spectacle (*tamasha*) where they touch a thing and it becomes a ring (*anguthi*), where rice will come, or ashes (*rakh*) materialize. This is the work of a magician, not of a saint. "I'll make you live. I'll kill you." The saints can do it, but they don't do it. They are one with God and it is not impossible for them to persuade God to do something. But they don't go against the will of God. They remain under His orders.[25]

The reference to ash is probably a thinly veiled criticism of Sathya Sai Baba, who famously produces sacred ash (*vibhuti*) from his wrists (see Babb 1986: 164). Juergensmeyer (1991: 82–83) notes the differing views on miracles (*chamatkar*) within Radhasoami communities: some masters disclaim miracles completely, while others claim to be proficient in them. Some devotees argue that their masters are quite capable of performing miracles but that they "prefer not to meddle in the laws of nature." This claim to be capable but unwilling is somewhat similar to the Sacha Sauda guru's position, though it is God's laws rather than those of nature that he wishes to refrain from violating. Laidlaw (1995: 69–77) documents similar attitudes among Jains in Jaipur, for whom the laws with which miracles interfere are those of karma.

A conventional view of miracles, which would expect them to consist of transformation, cure, or paranormal materialization—that is, infringements of the laws governing the universe, whether their provenance is nature, God, or karma—would be unlikely to consider the performances of the Dera Sacha Sauda as in any way miraculous.[26] Its "miracles" neither violate nor threaten to compete with a rule-governed cosmos but instead are fully consistent with it. My concern here is with "reformed" and "participatory" miracles—miracles of magnitude and quantity, mobilization and organization.[27] The events and objects I describe achieve miraculous status by way of the superlatives used to describe them. Further, these miraculous feats of provision, far from materializing rice or rings, are "useful for society"—their "demonstrable utility" (Ssorin-Chaikov and Sosnina 2004) is virtue's guarantor.

Devotees I met in Sirsa expressed wonder at the Dera Sacha Sauda's miraculous achievements, and would point out to me with pride the many guru-inspired constructions in the area and the "world records" they signify. For such devotees, Sirsa and its environs is a sacred landscape sanctified by externally provided prizes. Several Delhi-based doctors who had been invited to Haryana to take part in the camps also described the events as being miraculous. One doctor told me: "Baba Ji created a miracle. He made 16,000 people donate blood in one day—it's definitely a miracle. Nowhere in the world could anyone make 16,000 people give blood in one day. Jesus and other spiritual masters did miracles in their own times based on the needs of society at the time. Jesus had hungry devotees—all of them needed to be fed, and the food multiplied. Similarly, Hazoor Maharaj created a miracle based on the needs of society."[28] The doctor's argument reflects the guru's emphasis on social utility: unlike the "useless" materializations of ash or rings he criticizes so acerbically, Hazoor Maharaj's miracles are miracles of virtuous utility that are performed "for society." What might be termed the reform of the miraculous is thus connected to the reform of giving and ascetic practices in the direction of social utility outlined in chapter 3. In that chapter I discussed cases where the pledging of "useful" blood seems to have supplanted the pledging of "useless" hair as a means of averting misfortune. In the province of miracles, too, "useful" blood defeats tawdry ash as the more virtuous spiritual material.

The movement thus attempts to create an aura of the miraculous through the performance of feats of improbable scale that attain external recognition as "record-breaking." A Sacha Sauda publication titled *Believe-Me-Not: Simply Incredible!!* (n.d.a.) introduces the order's Ray of Hope mobile hospital, an operating theater on wheels, described as moving "with medicine and benediction." An "astounding creation," constructed by order of the guru, it is reported to hold the Limca record for "world's smallest hospital." In addition, the Shah Satnam Ji Cricket Stadium, named after the preceding guru, is announced in the publication as being "A miracle in 42 days." I was informed by several devotees that a claim has been lodged with the *Guinness Book* for speediest ever construction of a cricket stadium. The same publication draws the reader's attention to the Shah Satnam Ji General Hospital of 175 beds, which it says "was constructed in merely 17 days under Guru Ji's divine guidance. . . . Guru Ji's energy is infectious as on average, every room came up in merely 45 minutes. . . . By creating these vast and beautiful abodes each in a few hours and days, Hazoor Maharaj Ji has made the world wonder-struck."

Speed and quantity are the primary attributes of this new order of the miraculous. The point is underlined by the example of "A miraculously huge 'Ajooba' [miraculous or wonderful] washing machine," described under the heading "What a wonder it is!": "The washermen [in a Sacha Sacha students hostel] urged Hazoor Maharaj Ji, and He gave instructions about this wonderful washing machine [which] has the capacity of simultaneously washing 1,000 clothes within half an hour only." The repeated use of variants of the English word "wonder" is apt in that it is wonderment inside the bounds of natural law that is the hoped-for foundation of these "miracles," wonder, in Greenblatt's

(1996: 276) definition, being "the power of an object to stop the viewer in his tracks, to convey an arresting sense of uniqueness, to evoke an exalted attention." It is not only the movement's own literature that refers to its achievements as wondrous feats; local news reports documenting the record-breaking 2004 blood donation camp classified the event in similar terms: "The blood donation camp organized in the pious memory of Shri Magghar Singh, the venerable father of the bethroned saint of Dera Sacha Sauda . . . established a new world record. This camp, organized in the small village of a population of 2,000 was nothing less than a miracle."[29] The cycle of the washing machine and the sevadars' construction of the hospital, just like devotees' superabundant collection of blood, evoke an exalted attention through their performance of impressive quantitative feats within improbably short spaces of time.

I referred above to the official position of the Sacha Sauda that the achievement of the Guinness world record for largest ever blood donation camp was "sheer chance." I suggest that the movement's strategy of condescension toward world records is necessary not only because of its official stance against spectacle but also because meticulous planning is hardly congruent with the spontaneity and artlessness meant to characterize miracles. The Believe-Me-Not publication thus seeks to create an a posteriori sense of "as if spontaneity" (Ssorin-Chaikov 2006: 363) in order to draw a veil over the painstaking preparation required to stage camps on such a scale.

What is clear is that the Dera Sacha Sauda, a devotional order that exists in a constant state of emergency, epitomizes a "culture of rush" (Lewin 1985), as conceptualized by Ssorin-Chaikov (2006) in his analysis of the birthday gifts given in 1949 to Joseph Stalin. Just as some of the birthday gifts were destroyed in the rush of erecting exhibition halls to demonstrate the nation's largesse and the love inspired by its leader, the Sacha Sauda's compulsion to break the world record within the stipulated time limit of twelve hours resulted in pressure being put on doctors to under-bleed devotees, and consequently, in the abundant production of "quality not sufficient" units. The Sacha Sauda culture of rush is a feature of the charismatic temporality referred to above, being starkly at odds with the routine and repetition that doctors would like to see structure the giving of blood. The rush of devotees to give blood and other forms of guru seva fashions the as if spontaneity and compressions of time that lie at the heart of the Sacha Sauda's new order of the miraculous.

So with respect to miracles, as well as tamasha and the giving of gifts, it is utility—particularly the apparently transparent utility of blood giving—which lends its virtue to and thereby sanctions that which the guru otherwise lambastes. Its occurrence firmly within the bounds of natural law grants this variant of miracle a somewhat insecure status, which makes all the more important the construction of an elaborate discourse of spontaneity. Having focused hitherto on the enabling function of blood donation vis-à-vis the movement's proclivities toward the spectacular, I turn now to the camps themselves, exploring what they can tell us about the internal devotional logics of the movement.

The Remembered Village Camp

In October 2004 a world record-surpassing Dera Sacha Sauda blood donation camp was staged in Sri Gurusarmodia village in Rajasthan as a feature of the mortuary ceremonies of the present guru's father. I was not present, so draw on the recollections of devotees I met in Sirsa, and also on photographs provided to me by my guide in Sirsa, a co-organizer of the camp and member of the organizational hierarchy. This was a unique camp, with thousands of devotees and a multitude of medical teams converging on the usually quiet village in which the guru's father had resided. Photographs depict the camp's inauguration, the guru joining two ribbons together—a conscious inversion of the familiar ribbon cutting ceremony which is meant to represent the need for unity, not separation.

The fervor evinced by devotee-donors seems comparable to that which I witnessed at Nirankari camps. As a Punjabi devotee told me: "When the doctors saw the amount of donors, they touched the feet of Baba Ji and started weeping. But when the doctors started to run out of blood bags at about 1 P.M., some donors became angry—'Why are you not taking our blood?' Some donors were very devoted and gave blood twice.[30] On that day I donated one unit, but my heart wanted to donate three. I said [to the doctors], 'If you have the capacity, please take one more, one more unit.'" A female devotee declared that at the camp she had felt "just as happy as at the birth of my son, just as happy as at his marriage." An important feature separating the Dera Sacha Sauda experience from that of the Nirankaris, however, is the presence of its guru as the camp's cynosure, and, for reasons that will become clear, it is here I think that the main interest lies.[31]

Dera Sacha Sauda publications contain photographs of the "Holy royal family members" at the camp in postures of performative humility such as distributing refreshments as prashad to donors. The guru's presence is electrifying. Photographs depict rapt donors, mid-donation, gazing at the guru in the posture of *namaskara*. "Rays of blessings" (*ashirvad ki kirne*) come from the upturned hands and eyes of the guru, say devotees. Other photographs depict the guru blessing the extractive needles prior to insertion into devotees and touching with his hands devotees' outstretched arms; one photograph shows the guru's medically unqualified son performing an actual insertion. At a camp conducted in Delhi by the Sawan Kirpal Ruhani Mission, an offshoot of the Radhasoamis, one devotee told me he had not at first intended to donate for fear of the harmful physical consequences, but when the guru arrived—granting, as it were, the gift of appearance—they exchanged a glance, and the donation "just happened." This underlines the importance that donors attach to the guru's presence.

His visibility to them and theirs to him, I suggest, is a critical issue in devotees' willingness to donate.

Three main factors help explain the importance of the guru's presence. The first is darshan, the exchange of vision between worshiper and worshiped, which is linked to the second: blessings. Darshan is an important feature not only in the worship of temple gods but also in *guru puja*. As I mentioned above, blessings stream from the guru's eyes and hands, and as was noted in chapter 4, apprehensive Nirankari donors view pictures of the guru as they donate for protective purposes. Pictures of the guru can and do provide his darshan, but have a lesser effect than direct visual exchange in the guru's presence (Babb 1986: 76). In the Radhasoami tradition, the eyes are "energy centers and energy transmitters; hence the meeting of eyes between master and devotee is a moment of dramatic spiritual interaction" (Juergensmeyer 1991: 84).[32] As was seen in chapter 1, energy is precisely what many Indians think blood donation drains them of. It is thus not surprising that devotees, many of whom remain unconvinced by recruiters' claims about the safety of donation, seek a direct connection to the guru's replenishing vision as they donate. Shakti, as it were, simultaneously exits and enters through veins and eyes, respectively. Devotees "drink" energy through their eyes (Vidal 2006: 5), even as it drains from the prick in their arms.

The third factor relates to the guru's omniscience, and its implicit questioning by devotees. Dera Sacha Sauda devotees say their guru travels through past, present, and future, seeing everything. Babb (1986: 178–179) too notes that Sathya Sai Baba performs miracles of omniscience: aware of everything, he knows the thoughts of his devotees even before they tell them to him. I suggest, however, that though this is indeed what devotees profess to believe, the requirement of the guru's presence at camps—in order, as it were, that he may record and reward devotees' donations—may be gauged by their unwillingness to donate elsewhere. This signals, of course, devotees' intuition that their donations will not be recorded and consequently not rewarded when enacted at a distance from the guru's physical presence.

Sirsa's Shiv Shakti blood bank, located close to the Dera Sacha Sauda ashram, encounters this difficulty. In a discussion with its director, who had collected blood at both of the Dera Sacha Sauda's record-breaking camps, I was told that when his blood bank required blood on a day-to-day basis, devotees were reluctant to come and donate: "And next time when I appeal to the *sadh-sangat* [followers] to please come and donate in my blood bank, they will not come. They never come when we actually need the blood. It hurts me. Instead they collect blood only in these mass camps where most of the blood gets wasted." Several doctors in Delhi also complained to me that the same devotees who would rush from their homes in Delhi to Sirsa to give in mass camps rarely respond to doctors' requests to come to Delhi blood banks to donate when stocks are low.[33]

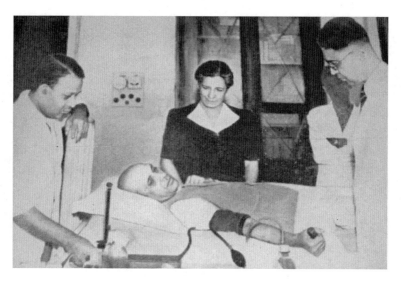

Nehru donating blood, 1942.
Photograph displayed in Shiv Shakti blood bank, Sirsa (see chapter 3).

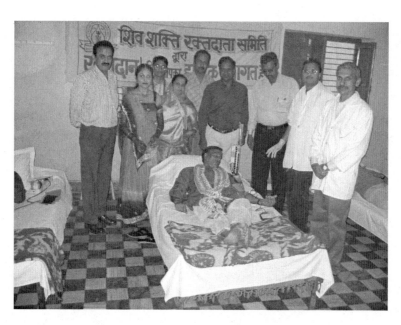

Father of the bride donates blood, Sirsa (see chapter 3).

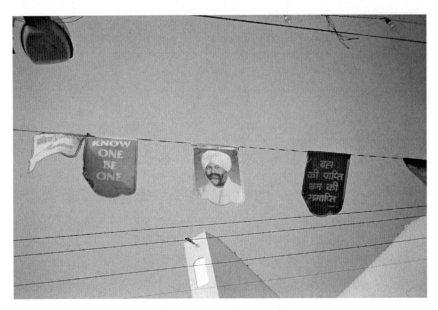

Image on flag of Sant Nirankari guru Baba Hardev Singh (see chapter 4).

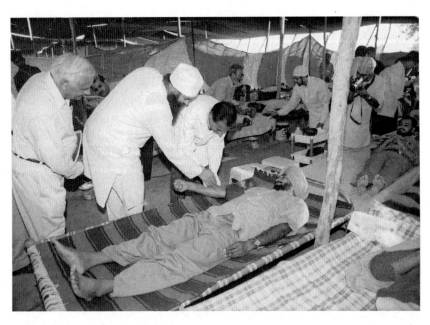

Dera Sacha Sauda spiritual master Hazoor Maharaj Ji blesses the needle as the doctor inserts it into a donating devotee, October 2004 (see chapter 5). The three Dera Sacha Sauda photos are courtesy of Guru Ji Sant Gurmeet Ram Rahim Singh Ji Insan, Chief of Dera Sacha Sauda Sirsa (Har).

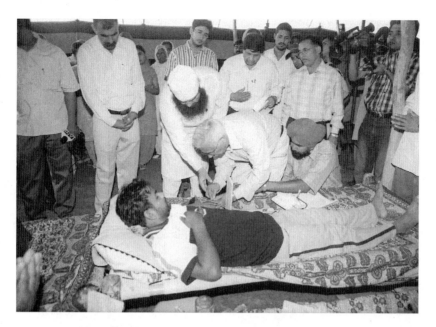

The Sacha Sauda guru blesses another donating devotee.

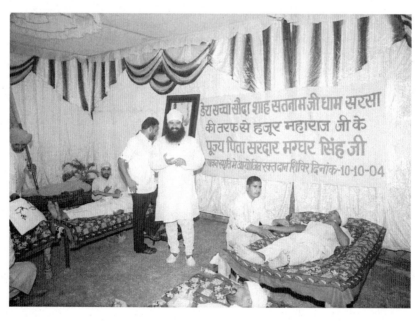

Hazoor Maharaj Ji before an image of his late father, Sadar Magghar Singh, in whose honor the Dera Sacha Sauda's second world-record–breaking camp was organized in October 2004.

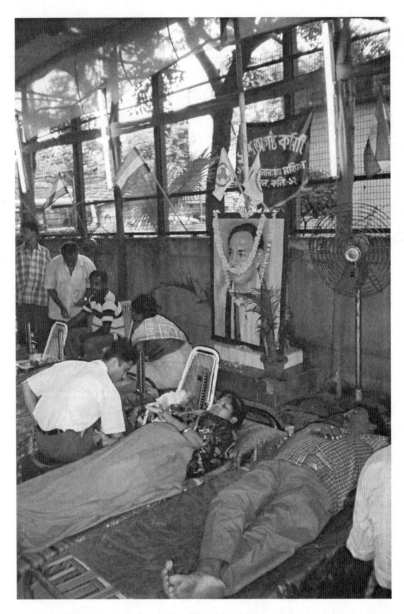

Congress activists donate blood in Kolkata on August 20,
the birth anniversary of former prime minister Rajiv Gandhi.

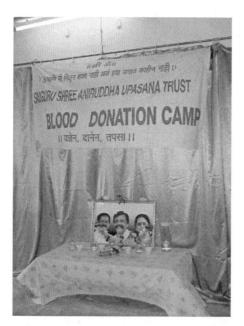

Garlanded image of Mumbai guru Aniruddha Bapu, his wife, and his brother-in-law at a blood donation camp organized by his devotees (see chapter 6). The trinity is probably meant to recall that of Ram, Sita, and Lakshman.

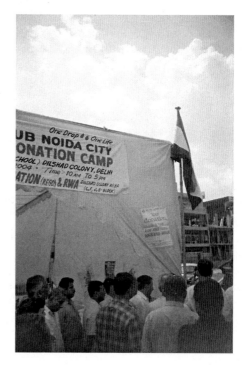

The Indian tricolor is raised at a blood donation camp on India's Independence Day (August 15), Delhi (see chapter 5).

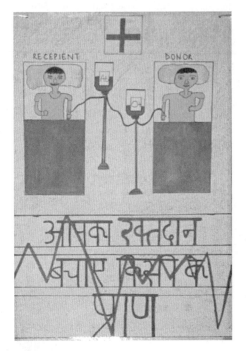

A school student's poster at a blood donation camp at a Delhi school. It reads: "Your blood donation saves someone's life."

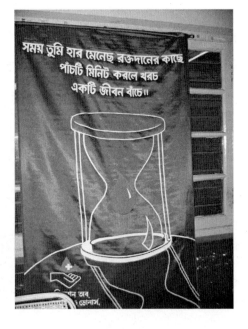

An Association of Voluntary Blood Donors, West Bengal banner advertising the temporal effects of blood donation. It reads: "Time is defeated by blood donation. If you spend only five minutes you can save a whole lifetime."

In the often grimy and uninspiring environment of a blood bank, the donating devotee's guru is likely to seem far off and remote and is certainly inaccessible for the purposes of darshan. Guru and devotee, as it were, remain invisible to each other. In contrast to the guru's presence at Dera Sacha Sauda camps, the private setting of a blood bank is far removed from the guru's immediate presence and there are likely to be no other witnesses than the blood bank staff—one therefore cannot be sure of obtaining his blessings. Though devotees of different persuasions frequently profess that their gurus constantly watch over and protect them, as well as keep a record of both their meritorious and unmeritorious actions, anxieties nonetheless exist over whether anonymous or "hidden" meritorious acts are really documented and recognized by their masters.

Coleman (2004: 432) has noted in reference to Swedish Protestant revivalism that spiritual transactions in the context of generalized exchange can act to test adherents' faith. The observation also has validity in Indian contexts. Warrier (2003a: 274), for instance, notes that for devotees of the Mata, individual recognition from the guru is extremely important, giving them "much-needed assurance that the Mata is aware of their every little act of service." Dr. Bhatia of Delhi's Rotary blood bank, a Sathya Sai Baba devotee, recalled to me the querulous thoughts he harbored after donating blood in a hospital blood bank in the 1970s on his guru's birthday: "I am lying on the bed recuperating. Now my monkey mind on the one hand is saying thank you Swami for fulfilling my desires and letting me donate on your birthday. On the other hand this same mind questions Swami: do you know that I have donated blood? On the one hand I considered him the divine incarnation, and on the other hand I was questioning him—does he know that I have done this?"

To draw on terminology employed by Boyer (1999) and Whitehouse (2004), devotees' belief in their guru's omniscience is the theologically correct position. When, however, the theologically correct position is seriously challenged there is recourse to what Whitehouse (2004: 189) calls the intuitive default position. I suggest that in the present case, the theologically correct position comes under strain when devotees are asked to donate blood in settings removed from the guru's person. Since their master is not physically present in the private setting of the blood bank, devotees have recourse to the intuitive default position, which is that their guru may not be aware of the meritorious actions performed therein. My suggestion that devotees' reluctance to donate in blood banks results from their feeling that this is a setting in which meritorious actions are likely to go unrecorded recalls the argument that the spatio-temporal context sensitivity that marks devotional giving can provide the basis for "recipient concealment," the varying properties of time and space acting as a bar to continuous or need-based helpfulness. Or to put it differently: that heightened merit is available at certain times and places appears to lead to the continuous rhythm of need becoming subordinated to a more irregular rhythm of meritorious maximization.

Just how central "looking" is within the movement may be clarified by a parallel example. Greenblatt (1996: 282), writing of the visitor's experience in art galleries, defines "enchanted looking" thus: "Looking may be called enchanted when the act of attention draws a circle around itself from which everything but the object is excluded, when intensity of regard blocks out all circumambient images, stills all murmuring voices. To be sure, the viewer may have purchased a catalogue, read an inscription on the wall, switched on a cassette, but in the moment of wonder all this apparatus seems more static." As I showed above, the enchanted looking of Sacha Sauda blood donors similarly "draws a circle around itself," the intensity of their regard for their guru leading to the exclusion of the "circumambient image" of transfusion recipients. This enchanted looking was vividly demonstrated at one of the satsangs I attended in Sirsa. At its commencement, the then-current Hindi film song "Bale Bale" (Wow! Wow!) was played at high volume, and it was to this soundtrack that the guru made his entrance. He was accompanied by a small deer.[34] Many male devotees, of varying ages (though no women), stood up and danced frenetically, all the while agitatedly pointing their fingers and arms forward toward the guru. As the guru took to his throne, his palanquin jerked forward and began to move steadily, on a rail track I think, bisecting the crowd in a kind of local royal progress, enabling even far-off devotees to gain close-up darshan. As the palanquin moved past them, so devotees would adjust their gaze and deportment by degrees so that the guru was always before them. Having reached the far side of the satsang hall, the palanquin swiveled round and began to slowly return to the front, at which point I saw the guru flick a switch on his altar, causing a further rotation so that he was once again facing his devotees. It was a more benign manifestation of the enchanted looking which "draws a circle around itself" at Sacha Sauda blood donation camps and which contributes to the concealment of recipients. Gathering the gazes of his devotees as he progressed through the crowd on his palanquin, perhaps the guru was considering the next prestigious project of provision to which might be applied their exalted attention.

Donating Blood to Redress a Grievance

A set of critical events in May 2007 highlight the extent to which blood donation has developed into a multilayered expressive act both within devotional orders and beyond. A global presence has been the aim of the movement for a number of years, but its ambition was achieved in a manner it would neither have sought nor ever envisaged. "Cult Leader Sparks Sikh Riots with 'Guru' Stunt" was the headline in the British *Independent* newspaper on 21 May 2007. The allegation was that the Dera Sacha Sauda guru had, in an advertisement in a local newspaper, impersonated the tenth and—according to orthodox Sikhs—final living Sikh guru, Guru Gobind Singh. Gurmeet Singh was reported to have been shown administering nectar (*amrit*) to devotees in the manner (and dress) of Gobind Singh. As was noted in chapter 4, relations between sant movements headed by living gurus and orthodox Sikhs are tense, given the status for khalsa Sikhs of Gobind Singh as the final of the living Sikh gurus. The alleged ritual and sartorial imitation of Gobind Singh by the Dera Sacha Sauda guru precipitated violent clashes in Punjab in May 2007, which left at least one dead, and many more injured. News reports proclaimed the situation to be "perhaps the most serious law and order crisis since the militancy days," a period of threat and instability that began in the late 1970s with the Sikh-Nirankari clashes and which continued into the 1980s with agitations for a separate Sikh homeland.[35] Indeed, the parallels with the Nirankari controversy of several decades before are striking, with the Sacha Sauda now taking the place of the Nirankaris as the orthodox Sikh object of opprobrium.

News reports commented on the hard line taken against the devotional order by the Akal Takht, the primary seat of Sikh religious authority, based at the Golden Temple in Amritsar, and by various factions of the Sikh nationalist political party, the Akali Dal. Some Sikh organizations called for suicide squads to "carry on the task of uprooting all Sacha Sauda deras in Punjab," while the Akal Takht somewhat more measuredly demanded a *bandh* and protest marches in addition to the closure of all deras in the state.[36]

The Dera Sacha Sauda guru, under intense pressure, eventually made a not very fulsome apology for the offence caused, which was rejected by the Akal Takht *jethedar* (spiritual leader), who "quoted the 'Gurbani' (religious scriptures), saying that even the Guru, who was bountiful in pardoning, would not accept anything from a person whose spirit did not reflect a mindset suitable for a religious way of life."[37] The marches and boycotts continued for a time, but after several weeks an uneasy calm descended, which has largely persisted until the present time of writing.

What was not reported in the international news coverage was that the Dera Sacha Sauda staged a blood donation camp in order to protest against the Akal Takht's decree (*hukamnama*) that its ashrams in the Punjab be closed. One Indian news article quoted the Sacha Sauda's senior vice chairman: " 'The question of vacating deras does not arise at all.' . . . Prithviraj told a gathering of followers immediately after Sikh priests gave a fresh ultimatum to the Punjab government to shut down all deras in the state. He said the group will protest against the *hukamnama* in a peaceful manner with its followers donating blood and organs after death."[38] A television news report documenting a camp in Sirsa on May 21 at the height of the tensions quoted a devotee: "We believe in non-violence, following that we have organized this blood donation camp. We hope the central government and the judiciary will definitely do justice."[39]

This usage of blood donation as a mode of protest alerted me to what is in fact a wider emergent trend in India, that of giving blood as a form of contestatory behavior. Blood donation has, in fact, been incorporated into the repertoire of protest techniques throughout the country.

It is clear is that the Dera Sacha Sauda's episodic enactments of conspicuous extraction enable the movement to achieve a number of different things, from the spectacles of excess and miraculous materialization it officially repudiates, to renown and preeminence among the devotional orders in the national league of virtuous beneficence. As was noted in chapter 3, on the death of the present guru's father the movement conducted rakt-dan as the substitutive ennoblement of pind-dan, in what might be termed the contrastive achievement of virtue ("useful" vs. "useless" giving, this-worldly vs. other-worldly giving, and so on). This provides a helpful starting point for beginning to understand how blood donation has come to possess purchase for the Sacha Sauda and others as a mode of contestatory behavior. The Dera Sacha Sauda's giving of blood was unlike the styles of protest called for by Sikh organizations in two important respects: First, in contrast to the Akal Takht and Akali Dal-inspired protests which took the form of bandhs, marches, and even calls for the deployment of suicide squads, the Sacha Sauda's protest behavior was demonstrably "socially productive"; and second, in contrast with orthodox Sikh threats of violent bloodshed, Sacha Sauda devotees also shed their blood, but *nonviolently.*

The Indian repertoire of protest techniques has been and continues to be the subject of much criticism among social reformers in modern India. Nehru, for instance, criticized hunger strikes and bandhs in the 1950s as "obsolete" political methods: "I feel that the time is gone when we could solve our problems in this way in India or anywhere else" (quoted in Chakrabarty 2007: 37). The bandh attracts criticism as being a particularly unproductive style of contestatory behavior. Indeed, bandhs have been officially proscribed since 1998 (though they still occur with great frequency).[40] A recent newspaper editorial disparaged bandhs as "fully paid holidays" which cause misery and destruction.[41] Another declared that they "demean the very cause they are supposed to promote" and spoke of the unfortunate vortex effect of calling a bandh: "another bandh to protest the first bandh, followed by a strike by the people against whom the first bandh had been called." The writer proposes alternative, "more effective" modes of protests such as the wearing of black armbands and, if the protest is in response to an atrocity, a fund to help the victims. Significantly, blood donation is also suggested as a more constructive way than a bandh to express discontent.[42]

The "positive action" of the Sacha Sauda's blood donation protest thus contrasted with the bandhs called by Sikh bodies, the latter being a mode of protest frequently scorned as being benighted and self-indulgent. Protest blood donation may in consequence be considered a style of protest congruent with the reformist agenda of virtuous utility and, to reengage the vocabulary of chapter 3, as being the substitutive ennoblement of key existing styles in the protest repertoire such as bandhs, marches, and fasting. Other examples support this view. For instance, members of the United Forum against Consumption of Liquor in Hyderabad are reported to have "constructively" donated their blood in protest against the preponderance of "anti-social" liquor shops and bars.[43] Of particular interest is the Oasis NGO, based in Vadodara, Gujarat, which organizes workshops for "character building" and "healthy living," and which in 1999 conducted what it termed a "constructive *dharna*" in protest at a "smear campaign" against it: "Managing trustee Sheeba Nair said a blood donation camp was organized . . . as Oasis wanted to keep away from rallies, slogan shouting and bandhs, the usual modes of protest."[44] The example corresponds with those presented in chapter 3: whereas in that chapter it was forms of gift that were subject to reform via blood donation, here it is the dharna that is renovated via exactly the same means. Just as the gift must add to "in-need" society, so must protest enactments.[45]

What the Oasis example underlines so well is that blood donation, in contrast with bandhs, disruptive rallies, and so on, is as a protest form the antithesis of civil disobedience. After all, blood donation is something the government persistently (if somewhat ineffectively) enjoins Indians to do. Whereas bandhs potentially disturb state functioning (witness Nehru's comments above), blood donation is a state-loving mode of protest. What has been termed "avoidance protest" consists of "dissatisfied groups seek[ing] to attenuate their hardships and express their discontent through flight, sectarian withdrawal, or other activities that minimize challenges to or clashes with those whom they view as their oppressors" (Adas 1981: 217). On one level, the Sacha Sauda's protest blood donation did indeed reproduce the logic of avoidance protest insofar as it probably did help minimize clashes; and yet unlike strikes (*hartals*), nonpayment of taxes, and election boycotts, protest blood donation constitutes an extreme positive engagement. I do not suggest these other protest styles are not politically engaged—the manner of their engagement takes the form of disruptive avoidance; blood donation, however, engages not through avoidance but through intensified involvement; that is, through the active pursuit of civic virtues. Unlike "abstemious acts" (Haynes 1991: 276) such as fasting and strikes, then, where the structural logic is one of closure and subtraction, blood donation subtracts (from veins) only in order to make an addition (to "society"), and hence is structurally open and engaged. Blood donation extends the body into the world, while fasting withdraws the body from it.

The Sacha Sauda blood donation protest was not overtly directed toward the state, though it was probably designed to impress several different audiences, including state governments. What is the logic of a blood donation protest when it *is* directed at the state, given that blood offerings, far from disrupting state functioning, actually contribute to it? An example would be the blood donation protests, discussed below, of medical trainees agitating against state reservations in medical training institutions. Blood donation as contestatory behavior in disputes with the state, it might be suggested, draws the state into a close embrace by doing exactly what the state wants, with control being exerted through overbearing compliance and suffocating propinquity rather than disobedience. This model of protest bears a resemblance to what Appadurai (1990: 97) has termed "coercive subordination," the attempt here being to neutralize or control the intentions of the state through exalting it with gifts of blood. Gifts of blood in protest may thus be seen as a kind of stockpiling of a physical form of moral asset—the attempt is to store virtue and/or to force on others a moral debt redeemable through redress to the grievance in question. Nandy (1970: 72) rightly points to a distinction between "formal means of demand articulation and protest" such as recourse to the law and "extrasystematic pressures" such as fasting and bandhs. The interesting thing about blood donation protests is that they appear to hang midway between the two means of demand articulation. Of course, blood donation protest is not a "formal" means of redressing a grievance, but neither is it at all "disobedient" or antithetical to state systems; quite the reverse. It bridges, in this respect, systematic and extra-systematic forms of demand articulation.

The second contrast I identified above concerns modes of bloodshed. At the height of the tensions in May 2007 a pro-Sacha Sauda blogger ("samiinsaan") wrote: "The followers of DSS are expressing their dissatisfaction by donating blood but bad tempered people are flowing the blood of innocent people."[46] Recalling the Nirankari donation of blood in response to the assassination of the present guru's father ("Blood should flow into veins, not drains"), the Sacha Sauda's positively reconstituted blood shedding enabled the movement to achieve virtue contrastively. To quote again "samiinsaan": "They [Sikh protesters] are forgetting ... that Respected Sri Guru Gobind Singh Ji has given the swords for saving [the] helpless, not to make the blood shed out of helpless people. These terrorists have taken the lives of many innocent people in the last decade when there was demand of Khalistan. . . . Again same scene is in Punjab, whereas on the other hand Dera Sacha Sauda devotees are proving themselves to be *real Sikhs* by donating blood, by giving their kidneys, bone marrow and eyes after death. Even some devotees are donating their whole body for the sake of humanity" (my emphasis). "Samiinsaan" thus provocatively suggests that the Dera Sacha Sauda's protest in the form of *manav seva* makes it really Sikh, whereas the violent nature of the orthodox Sikh response represents a perversion of the true Sikh faith. The claim is also implicitly made that Dera Sacha Sauda devotees' donation of body parts (blood, kidneys, bone marrow, eyes, and even the totality of their bodies) reanimates a consecrated template laid down by Gobind Singh in a way that orthodox Sikhs fail to do. As is well known, Gobind Singh is said in 1699 at the foundation of the khalsa to have demanded that five devotees offer him their heads (Mahmood 1997: 43). But now, says "samiinsaan," it is only the Dera Sacha Sauda that fulfils Gobind Singh's teachings in this respect, with its bounteous corporeal offerings "for the sake of humanity." The contrast thus becomes one between "Sikhs" and *Real Sikhs*—as defined (or revealed) by those who are willing to excavate their bodies most deeply.

The donation of blood as contestatory behavior thus acquires reformist virtue by means of contrast with other forms of protest and bloodshed. What I wish to argue now, however, is that what really gives blood donation force as a mode of protest derives from the ways in which it both reconnects with and surpasses Gandhian styles of protest. (I do not wish in the following to suggest that what I am calling Gandhian protest styles are necessarily exclusive to the Gandhian nationalist tradition. But while Gandhi undoubtedly learned and drew deeply from numerous existing colonial and precolonial archetypes [see Spodek 1971], he also adapted them in all sorts of significant ways—not least in wielding them on a far broader canvas than had hitherto been the case.)

The Gandhian leaders of the merchant protests against British rule in early twentieth-century Surat "emphasized the virtue of acts of abstinence and self-control. Involvement in protest was an act of renunciation (*tyag*), of self-suffering, and of penance (*tapascharya*). . . . Rhetoric stressing the selflessness of resistance essentially confirmed the merchants' sense of the moral rightness of their actions, and contributed to a growing feeling of ethical ascendancy vis-à-vis the British." Central to Gandhian resistance was "the control of personal emotions" (Haynes 1991: 276). As Gandhi (1961: 6) explained, *satyagraha* does not admit "of violence being inflicted on one's opponent, [rather] he must be weaned from error by sympathy and patience." This designation finds a reflection in the account of the pro–Sacha Sauda writer cited earlier, his suggestion being that the blood donation protest was characterized by similar principles of calmness and restraint: "They [Sikh protesters] started breaking *namcharcha ghars* [prayer meeting houses], setting fire to the homes of *sadh sangat*, and misbehaving with the effigies of guru ji and this way hurting the emotions of crores of people who are the believers of Dera Sacha Sauda. . . . On the other hand, the followers of Dera Sacha Sauda are so calm and silent that to protest they organize blood donation camps, filling forms of body parts donation after death, eye donation after death, and donating kidney, liver and bone marrow alive."[47] It was not only "samiinsaan" who connected the blood donation protest with Gandhian styles.[48] So the first association between protest blood donation and "Gandhianism" pertains to the exhibition of restraint and nonviolence.

The second relates to asceticism. Like fasting, blood donation is enacted by and on the protesting self. Moreover, satyagraha—"truth-force"—was conceived by Gandhi (1961: 6) as "vindication of truth not by infliction of suffering on the opponent but on one's self." As was seen in chapter 4, blood donation is indeed considered an act of ascetic self-denial by many Nirankari and Sacha Sauda donors. Therefore, in instances where blood donation protests are performed by populations who understand the action as inflicting suffering more on themselves than on their opponents, the connection to a Gandhian idiom is established all the more forcefully.

The third connection to Gandhian styles concerns the directional orientation of protest. For Gandhi, it was essential that fasting and other modes of protest transcend self-interest—he was unequivocal in stating that fasting should be "for the good of others" (Alter 2000: 41). As was noted above, the protest actions of Surat merchants were similarly pervaded by a rhetoric of selflessness which lent their acts of civil disobedience a sense of "moral rightness" and "ethical ascendancy." The important point here is that blood donation is continuous with this rhetoric while, at the same time, surpassing it, since its "being for the good of others" is built into or made explicit in its enactment in a less ambiguous way than, say, fasting. As Alter describes so well, Gandhi continually downplayed the political utility of the fast; the means (self-purification) were the primary end of its performance: "Our concern is the act itself, not the result of the action" (Alter 2000: 52, 49). And yet, the fast in present-day agitational strategies *is* used as a means to an end: the principles of "self-abnegation" and "impulse-control" are critical tools for the achievement of political potency (Nandy 1970: 72).[49] For all the talk of protest "for the good of others," techniques that foreground self-abnegation remain open to the charge that they simply force the will of the protester upon those with whom he or she disagrees.

Blood donation possesses efficacy here as a protest technique that "self-evidently" produces effects which are "for the good of others," being possessed of a transparency of utility that the protester seeks to harness in order to avoid charges of "coldly calculated blackmail" (Alter 2000: 29). Both the fast and blood donation can plainly be used as techniques of moral suasion for the furtherance of *any* kind of cause—causes that will be perceived variously by different parties as reprehensible, laudatory, or whatever; indeterminacy pervades the potential applications of both techniques. But blood donation differs from the fast in one vital way: counteracting its indeterminacy vis-à-vis protest usages is its predetermined status with respect to its medical usage. Ambiguity on one level is met with clarity of encoding on another. As was noted above, blood donation is proclaimed by the Dera Sacha Sauda guru to be a far greater offering than that of dangerously ambiguous money because of its predetermined usage, and it is this usage which also counts in its favor as a protest technique. Thus, in fulfilling more transparently than fasting the injunction that protest be "for the good of others," blood donation not only connects with Gandhian styles but surpasses them. Bleeding under the spotlight at media-friendly donation camps, the protesting blood donor exhibits his or her beneficent helpfulness with a clarity that the protesting faster would find it difficult to achieve. Even if an observer were to question the validity of the grievance in question, they would likely concur that the means of redressing it were "socially useful and out-reaching rather than inward-turning" (Vanita 2002: 155). This perhaps begins to explain why there are signs that blood donation is the emergent successor to the Gandhian fast as moral suasion technique of preference.

Several examples seem to bear out this argument. When, for instance, in November 2007 trainee medics in Tamil Nadu protested against a year-long extension of their Bachelor of Medicine/Surgery (MBBS) courses because of a new compulsory rural service scheme, blood donation was central to their agitation, for it put on view their legitimating commitment to utility. The protest as a whole consisted of a virulent conjunction of signifiers, with medics not only striking and undertaking a "fast unto death" but also sporting "saffron dress and carr[ying] books on their heads to drive home the point that they have to forego everything if the Centre went ahead with its decision and extended the MBBS course by a year." The critical supplement to these protest styles, however, was the students' donation of blood, given in order "to make it public they were not against rural service but only opposed compulsory service."[50] Thus did they attempt—by means of giving their blood—to preserve their selfless virtue even as they fought for their self-interest. In a similar case in 2006, trainee medics in Bangalore fasted, conducted numerous boycotts, formed a silent human chain, and donated blood in protest against proposals to reserve 27 percent of places in elite medical institutions for OBCs (Other Backward Classes). This campaign, wrote one medic, "provided blood to the needy, irrespective of him being SC/ST/OBC and negated the propaganda of the Government saying that the strike, protests are against public and against patients."[51] Again, blood donation was enacted by medical trainees as a means of demonstrating that they cared about the good of all as a counter to the widespread perception that a dominant group was protesting in order to further its domination.

There are, then, several connective threads that suggest congruence between protest blood donation and protest fasting. Like the archetypal fast, blood donation is suggestive of nonviolence and ascetic discipline. Where it surpasses Gandhian protest is in its making explicit (for purposes of exhibition) the external directional orientation meant to attach to acts of Gandhian protest. Contestatory blood donation thus combines Gandhianism with demonstrable utility in a new and powerful protest mode. Its constructiveness contrasts with the forms of protest that it replaces: hartals, bandhs, nonpayment of taxes, election boycotts, and so on. Its inner logic is not one of avoidance but of intensified involvement in a new combination of systematic and extra-systematic forms of demand articulation. Unlike the threat of dying to redress a grievance (Hopkins 1901), protest blood donation operates through imposing a moral debt to be repaid through redress to the grievance in question. As a still embryonic protest form, it is not possible to say whether contestatory blood donation will fulfill its present promise and succeed the Gandhian fast as *the* virtuous technique of moral suasion. What can be said about protest blood donation, however, is that it vividly attests to the wide range of cultural forms open to reformist renovation by means of the incorporation of blood donation. The Dera Sacha Sauda has been at the forefront of such renovations, as evidenced by its performance of protest blood donation. The movement has also been at the vanguard more generally in exploring blood donation's multiple and diverse expressive possibilities. The following chapter makes this even clearer.

Conclusion

Hansen has recently pointed to "a proliferation of political performances at all levels of [Indian] public life." Some of these performances take the form of "competitive populist schemes," which result partly from successive governments' inability to deliver on their promises (Hansen 2001: 230, 232). Hansen's argument is clearly pertinent to the themes of this chapter. In view of the fact that the central government has failed to put together a well-organized and funded campaign to bolster voluntary blood donation, religious and political groups have been given free reign to fill the gap. This chapter has demonstrated that their exercises in this regard have taken on a spectacular life of their own, being marked by both spiritual dynamism and frenetic competitiveness. The extravagant devotional expressionism that lies behind the phenomenon of record-breaking blood donation camps demonstrates a forceful religious presence within what Hansen (ibid.: 232) calls the "zone of public spectacles." Mass donation camps are undoubtedly an "obsessional theatre" (Barthes 1959: 163) of the highest order.

Alter (2000: 151) has compared Gandhi's intricate bodily experiments to "more straightforward" and less "labor-intensive" large-scale blood donation events: "ten thousand liters of blood as against a drop of semen" he says. The point is well taken. I would not wish to deny that blood donation—in its enactment as a grandiose form of political and devotional expressionism—is in many ways a far cry from Gandhi's complex somatic enactments. And yet, the integration of blood donation into the repertoire of nonviolent protest styles suggests that it might in certain cases be more "Gandhian" than Alter allows. (I further explore associations between blood donation and nonviolence in the next chapter.) Moreover, this chapter has shown that even when conducted on a large scale, blood donation is not particularly straightforward. It is employed as a sanctioning device in enabling the Dera Sacha Sauda to do what its "austere" theology supposedly proscribes: give gifts, conduct spectacular ritual, and even enact miracles. Further, the anonymous relationship between blood donor and transfusion recipient allows the guru to depict his movement's spectacularly publicized blood donations as conforming to the highest principles of secretly given dan.

Anonymity remains an important theme in the next chapter, which shows how the spatio-temporal distance anonymity generates between donors and recipients allows donors to mediate between apparently opposed values of violence and nonviolence. It also considers in greater detail the "gateway" function of gurus in the subcontinent as arch-facilitators of blood collection.

6

Utility Saints and Donor-Soldiers

The aims of this chapter are to complement my account in the previous chapter of blood donation as a nonviolent form of protest through a deepening of the exploration of the relationship between blood donation and violence/nonviolence, and to reflect more fully on the special role played by gurus in the field of blood donation and in Indian society more generally as "gateways" to universal philanthropy and other forms of "modernist" practice. Focusing on further aspects of the biomedical/religious interoperability through which a growing proportion of India's voluntarily donated blood originates, this chapter underlines the pivotal role of guru figures in producing what could be called India's efflorescent biospiritual medical creativity.

I have been concerned throughout this study with the complex moral significance of anonymity, and with detailing the ways in which it is engaged with in innovative ways by voluntary blood donors and made to serve an array of biospiritual and kin-oriented purposes. This chapter seeks to show that as well as possessing striking spiritual and familial implications, the anonymity of blood donation plays a further powerful role in regard to questions of violence and nonviolence.

My argument takes its cue from the valuable historical and thematic overview of violence in India provided by Vidal et al. (2003b), which emphasizes that our understanding of the concepts of violence and nonviolence in Hindu society is hindered when they are dissociated from each other or treated as opposites. Such a view resonates with the material presented here, which shows how, in the contemporary north Indian devotional context, versions of violence and nonviolence may be transformed into each other, mediated between and made to enter into relations of concurrent intimacy and distance by way of blood donation procedures.

Violence forms a major theme in anthropological studies of corporeal donations. Scheper-Hughes's article "Theft of Life" (1996) is typical here. Cohen

(2004: 169) too sees "bioavailability" as being organized at least in part around "authoritarian or piratical forced extraction or seizure." Yet another influential article is titled "The Quest for Human Organs and the Violence of Zeal" (Lock 2000). The present chapter differs in focusing less on the subjection of donors to violence than on donors' own ability to engage in violent activity through giving. I am not seeking to challenge the premise that biological exchange is frequently characterized by iniquities, though the data presented here would seem to caution against a priori assumptions that donors are operated on by donation ideologies rather than themselves being quite capable of both generating and operating donation concepts and practices for particular ends. Rather, the perspective of this chapter is I think complementary to those of Lock et al. in broadening out the range of forms of violence that may be associated with biological exchange. None of this is to say that issues of subordination are not pertinent to guru-devotee relationships and to the way in which devotees are recruited to "voluntary" blood donation. A further aim of this chapter is to delineate the "deployability" of what I term gurus' captive voluntary devotees, recognizing that devotees' creative engagement with corporeal donation practices does on one level form part of a political economy of innovation designed to make Indians bioavailable for extractive purposes.

Donor-Soldiers

As was noted in the last chapter, anonymity is made by the Dera Sacha Sauda guru to serve a very particular purpose: in keeping separate donors and recipients, anonymity enables the guru to claim that the otherwise very public donation of his devotees' blood conforms to the highest principles of secretly given charity. Giddens (1990: 22–26) says of money that it is a "means of time-space distanciation," and the same is true of blood donation: anonymity and the mediating role of the blood bank ensure that this is so. The guru, of course, uses the distanciation effect of blood donation to proclaim that such a mode of giving can generate no pride. Another consequence of money's time-space distanciation, claims Giddens, is that it enables individuals and organizations to act "at a distance." Just as we have seen how Nirankari devotees act at a distance to "corporeally capture" transfusion recipients, I suggest that Dera Sacha Sauda and Nirankari devotees employ blood donation to establish for themselves a role in India's military campaigns. An overt role—for example, enlisting devotees to fight—would be problematic, given that both movements subscribe to tenets associated with the doctrine of *ahimsa* (nonviolence). The donation of blood for the Indian armed forces, however, allows covert military participation, at a distance from actual operations, and may thus be viewed as an action which mediates between violence and nonviolence.

Many I spoke with in everyday conversation and who were of the right age gave blood for the first time when China invaded northern India in 1962 and had given since then only during times of military strife (such as during the Kargil war with Pakistan in 1999).[1] The Indian middle classes in 1962 are reported to have been extremely enthusiastic in contributing to the war effort (Varma 1998: 69)—and one of the ways in which they contributed, judging from the many testimonies I heard, was to give blood in large numbers. Transfusion medicine was developed over two world wars, becoming an important defensive technology (Cohen 2004: 168); early United States blood donors (circa 1950) donated in response to a Red Cross campaign poster depicting an injured American soldier, with the slogan: "Your blood can save him" (Holtorf 2001: 26). The origins of blood donation activity are thus intimately bound up with patriotic action and sentiment, in India as elsewhere (Laqueur 1999: 3). The connection is visible in a variety of striking ways in contemporary Indian blood donation settings. At camps I attended in educational and corporate locations, donors would often say their donation was "for the nation" or showed their *desh-bhakti* (devotion to the nation). As I noted earlier, "freedom fighter" songs from the period of the Independence struggle are also frequently played over a loudspeaker system at such camps; they invariably proclaim the need to sacrifice, to shed one's blood for the country (cf. Parry n.d.).

An interesting analogy is often set up between soldiers and blood donors, leading to the creation of what might be termed a third category: the donor-soldier. On 1 October 2004 there appeared the following letter in *The Hindu* newspaper: "Sir,—Today is voluntary Blood Donation Day. The joy and satisfaction one gets after donating blood is very heartening. Let us, on this day, resolve to donate blood and be 'peace time soldiers.' Colonel R. D. Singh." A Sikh businessman, a benefactor of Delhi's Rotary blood bank, compares donors to soldiers: "In one case the blood doesn't come back—that's on the battlefield. In the other case the blood does come back. But in both cases you shed blood for the country. I love my country so I give blood." Recall the Marathi poster mentioned in chapter 5: "Not everyone can join the armed forces and defend the country. Do the next best thing—donate blood four times a year." Similarly, on All India Voluntary Blood Donation Day, 2004, the National AIDS Control Organization (NACO) placed an advertisement in Delhi newspapers with a picture of an Indian soldier above a montage of faces of individuals of different genders and ethnicities; the text reads: "He gives his blood for his countrymen. . . . So do they! Blood donation is service to the nation. Make a pledge. Donate blood."

On reading the existing literature on contemporary Indian religious nationalism, one could be forgiven for concluding that the only religious nationalism of significance in present-day India is that espoused by Hindu nationalist, and less prominently, Sikh separatist groups. The Nirankari and Dera Sacha Sauda movements, however, are both staunchly nationalist in outlook, without subscribing to a narrow, exclusivist nationalism. Their gurus advocate Nehruvian-style "national integration," continually preach religious tolerance, and Muslims and Christians are counted among their adherents.[2] Devotees in both movements read strong patriotic significance into blood donation. Nirankari devotees proffered some of the most strident depictions of the donor-soldier. Phrases such as: "When I donate blood I feel as proud as a soldier when he is fighting for his countrymen" or "Here we do seva like in the army where you serve your nation; we also are serving the public" were not uncommon. In a leaflet advertising the Nirankari Mission, it is stated that "A special camp was organized for the Army on the occasion of Bhakti Parav i.e. 13 January, 2002 where 604 devotees donated their blood. Pujya Mata Sawinder Kaur Ji [the guru's wife] was among the first donors."[3] During the Kargil war in 1999, the Nirankaris in Chandigargh offered to meet all the Indian army's requirements of blood.[4] It is just such a scheme, with a single devotional order providing all the army's donation requirements, which members of the Sacha Sauda hierarchy told me the movement is currently seeking to establish. Negotiations are under way with the Indian army for the Dera Sacha Sauda to become its sole supplier of blood—so claimed those I spoke with in Sirsa.

A Dera Sacha Sauda publication (n.d.a.) lovingly enumerates the organization's manifold feats of service—its world-record-breaking blood donation camps but also its role in disaster relief operations undertaken in the aftermath of earthquakes and cyclones. In the large section on its blood donation accomplishments, pictures of soldiers giving blood under the benevolent gaze of the guru are given prominence. Another Sacha Sauda publication, *A Saga of Welfare Work for the Sea of Humanity* (n.d.b.), declares of one donation event: "Guru Ji showed his concern for the guardians of the country's frontiers by inaugurating the camp with the Armed Forces Transfusion Centre contingent." I heard numerous devotees air the wish that their blood would be transfused into soldiers in the Indian armed forces. "Guru Ji prefers the army," one devotee told me.

It has been shown that the Nirankari Mission and the Dera Sacha Sauda have both on different occasions sought to become the Indian armed forces' principal or even sole supplier of donated blood. The provision of blood to the military thus seems to have developed as an arena of competition between north Indian devotional orders. Following Mazzarella's (2002: 388) discussion of "cultural enclosure" in which publicly circulating narratives are imagined as a form of "symbolic commons" over which corporate promotional rituals (advertisements and so on) attempt "to proclaim exclusive ownership," these movements' endeavor to found singular relationships between themselves and the Indian army may be understood as attempts to culturally enclose or proclaim exclusive ownership over the available "national capital."

To help shed more light on the militaristic aspects of these movements' engagement with blood donation, I turn to a study by the historian William Pinch of militant asceticism in north India. Pinch discusses images of ascetic patriotism and violence deriving from both sacred texts and actual practice that conceptualize hermit mystics as military strategists and keepers of "magical weaponry" (Pinch 1997: 19). He notes that by the seventeenth century the practice of arms had begun to extend to the Vaishnava and *Nanakpanthi* communities—the latter being followers of Guru Nanak—where previously it had been confined to Shaiva asceticism. Military training and activity also spread into the practices of sant and bhakti movements (ibid.: 17). The orthodox Sikh community, or khalsa, in the Punjab was one of the most significant examples of this extension of militancy (see Fox 1985; Uberoi 1996). As north Indian devotional orders in the sant tradition, each presided over by masters from Sikh backgrounds, the Dera Sacha Sauda and Nirankari Mission are both genealogically related to the general "martial religious culture" that devolved from the "ascetic military culture" that Pinch describes (1997: 11). It is quite evident that devotees of both orders are from the kinds of caste and religious populations that harbor many longstanding army families. Interestingly, the first two spiritual masters of the Beas branch of the Radhasoami movement, closely related to the Nirankari Mission and the Dera Sacha Sauda, had both been soldiers prior to assuming their spiritual duties (Juergensmeyer 1991: 136).

The Dera Sacha Sauda, however, and the Nirankaris to a slightly lesser degree, have incorporated and now espouse certain key tenets associated with a reformist brand of Hinduism. Campaigns to eliminate animal sacrifice—seen as "a barbarity inconsistent with Hinduism's central tenet of nonviolence" (Fuller 1992: 101)—were pursued in the late nineteenth and early twentieth centuries by an alliance of progressive reformists and conservative, mainly Brahmanical neo-traditionalists. Both sets of activists sought to raise ahimsa to the stature of a universal Hindu value. Dera Sacha Sauda devotees too list ahimsa, along with vegetarianism and abstinence from alcohol, as core values.[5] Ahimsa is also a value the movement attempts to instill in others. For example, in working for tribal "emancipation" in Rajasthan, the organization's sevadars are reported to have befriended "the intrinsically violent and hostile populace," who, as a result of these service volunteers' efforts, "pledged to give up liquor, non-vegetarianism and immoral conduct" (Dera Sacha Sauda n.d.b.). The guru is said by devotees to have noted the "tribals'" abject plight while in Rajasthan on a drought relief mission. Shocked by the sight of a young tribal boy killing an eagle with a bow and arrow, the guru is reported to have declared: "If any creature is cut, blood comes out. Don't kill whatever has life. Don't even use words that hurt. Don't hurt any person." Nonviolence is also valorized by the Nirankaris. As I noted earlier, Nirankari devotees initially sought to take violent revenge upon the Sikh extremists who killed their guru in 1980, but were persuaded by the succeeding guru to engage in the nonviolent "revenge" of donating their blood in order to assist suffering humanity: blood should be put nonviolently into veins (*nari*) rather than violently into drains (*nali*).

Comparable Radhasoami attitudes to violence have been documented (Juergensmeyer 1991: 136). Despite its gurus' military backgrounds, Radhasoami teachings unequivocally oppose violence. As the grandson of one spiritual master stated: "We do not kill birds or animals for food, nor are we to kill anything for sport. We practice nonviolence." Though soldiers may take up arms, "if you are sincere and you really do not want to kill . . . there is a guiding force behind you which saves you from such situations."

My suggestion is that for these devotional orders which arose out of a martial religious culture but which subsequently embraced the modern Hindu reformist, or Brahmanic tenet of ahimsa, blood donation mediates between violence and nonviolence. Patriotic blood donation, aimed at soldiers by devotee-donors, allows devotees to play an active role in military affairs while ostensibly maintaining their commitment to nonviolence. The argument remains partly speculation, but it seems legitimate to suggest that these orders, through blood donation, manage to be at the same time detached from and yet profoundly connected to militaristic praxis.

I emphasize that caution is required here. Laidlaw (1995: 155) has noted that the preeminent Jain value of ahimsa does not preclude soldierly action among Jains. Though the Jain version of ahimsa is far more nuanced than that of the devotional orders under discussion, the analogy is illuminating. Alter (2000: 146–147) reports having met a Jain in a train carriage, proud of his role in helping the militant Hindu organization, the RSS (Rashtriya Swayamsevak Sangh— Association of National Volunteers), collect 10,000 liters of blood to aid the Indian troops during the 1999 Kargil war. "More blood than they bloody knew what to do with," laughed the Jain.[6] Intrigued by the Jain's connection with the war effort, Alter notes that the man, being a Jain, could not advocate violence, and yet neither did he advocate nonviolence. Organizing the provision of blood for the Indian army appears here to have mediated between the different imperatives of ahimsa and RSS militarism.

Given the absolute centrality of nonviolence to Jain religiosity, it does indeed seem outlandish on one level that a practicing Jain could ever *not* advocate nonviolence. Not advocating violence, and yet not advocating nonviolence either, and, not fighting, but collecting blood for the armed forces, may represent just one individual's attempt to work through seemingly difficult to reconcile imperatives. And yet, on another level, it could be argued that Jains were the original practitioners of distanciation in regard to nonviolence, even providing a kind of model of what I have been describing for the Nirankaris and the Dera Sacha Sauda. According to Laidlaw (1995: 153–159), Jain attitudes to nonviolence are characterized by an "ethic of quarantine," such that what matters is not necessarily preventing violence from happening (for violence is inevitable and natural), but separating oneself from violence so that it does not attach burdensome karma to oneself. What is important, in other words, is avoiding being violence's proximate cause. Similarly with blood donation: an activity of literal connectivity, by virtue of its anonymity it is also one of disconnection, which allows devotee-donors to avoid the role of proximate cause, and to assume instead a role more inexact, more remote, more supple.

My argument that blood donation seems to allow people who profess nonviolence to nonetheless engage in the arenas of violence from which they are supposedly barred, but from a distance, might therefore help explain why the Sacha Sauda and the Nirankari Mission are both so eager to provide blood for the Indian armed forces, and why so many of their devotees conceptualize their blood donations in soldier-like terms: with theologies emphasizing nonviolence, but with genealogical provenances intimately tied up with militaristic praxis, blood donation mediates between and helps make experientially practicable these apparently divergent values.

Though I have so far emphasized the mediating function of blood donation for several north Indian devotional orders and a Jain RSS volunteer, there is also some evidence to suggest that blood donation has in other contexts become an—perhaps *the*—exemplary "modernist" expression of nonviolence in India. A recent editorial in a newsletter published by the animal rights organization, People for Animals, Calcutta, provides a striking depiction of blood donation as a consummately nonviolent activity. The editorial highlights the plight of the country's sacrificial animals: "Thousands of animals are sacrificed to appease the Gods, all over the country. Certain religious customs and rituals sanction such sacrifices. Incidents in rural areas and major religious centers, even in Metro cities, continue even amongst the educated. But, doesn't all religion speak of love, nonviolence and compassion? . . . Public awareness regarding the non-essentiality of animal sacrifice is necessary." In order to help create this awareness, an animal shelter and hospital managed by People for Animals organized a blood donation camp: "No; it was not just another blood donation camp. The day chosen was significant. It was 11th October, 2004, KALI PUJA. . . . The reason for selecting this day was to create awareness against primitive and cruel practices in the name of appeasing Deities or God Almighty. The slogan was 'If you want to offer blood to the Goddess Kali, give your own, and help to save a human life.' " Like the Nirankaris, People for Animals activists believe in "blood donation for needy victims, not in blood shedding."[7] The occasion was also another striking example of the "making social" of the gift (see chapter 3).

It is well known that Hindu reformist opponents of animal sacrifice have sought over recent decades to substitute vegetarian offerings such as lemons and cucumbers for sacrificial animals (Parry n.d.; Srinivas 1965: 182; Fuller 1992: 102). In the People for Animals example it is the donated blood of humans which is offered to Kali as the substitutive ennoblement of the offering of animal blood. Since animal sacrifice is itself widely thought of as a substitute for human sacrifice (Samanta 1994: 798), there is a sense in which sacrifice has come full circle, with human substance substituting for that of the animals substituting for humans. Through analogy with violent blood sacrifice, blood donation is portrayed as an exemplary nonviolent mode of behavior. The Nirankari response to the taking of the previous guru's life—the violent shedding of his blood—by donating their own blood to help save lives, appears to be a further example of the reflective mobilization of blood donation as the nonviolent response to an act of extreme violence.

But herein also lies the double-edged nature of the relationship between blood donation and violence. As was seen above in chapter 4, the memorial donation of Nirankari devotees' blood not only substitutes for a violent response, it is also the sublimation of the violent response that devotees wanted to make. As Vidal et al. (2003b: 15) note: "That sacrificial violence is euphemized shows that it does not lose all its menacing characteristics, despite its sacralization." Thus, on one level it is certainly true to say that blood donation has become an exemplary practice of nonviolence in the subcontinent, but that is not all. The aspiration shared by the Dera Sacha Sauda and Nirankari Mission to provide blood for the Indian army, along with the memorial origins of Nirankari donation activity and the predicament of the Jain RSS volunteer, show clearly the different ways in which blood donation has come to intercede and arbitrate between conceptions and enactments of violence and nonviolence in the subcontinent.

Gurus as Gateways

Having focused here and in chapters 4 and 5 on the blood donation activities of several guru-led devotional orders, what then of the figure of the guru? I attempt now to locate more precisely the role played by gurus in Indian blood donation activity and also more widely in Indian society. The focus hitherto has principally been on gurus in the sant tradition, but they are part of a much wider landscape of gurus in the subcontinent whose devotees conduct high-profile seva activities, and I have referred frequently to two of them: the contemporary avatar gurus Mata Amritanandamayi and Sathya Sai Baba. To give concreteness to my argument about what I call the "gateway function" of gurus, I consider here the activities of two gurus not yet discussed: Aniruddha Bapu and Saumyendra Nath Brahmachary.

There are of course immense variations between types of guru and spiritual teacher in India[8]—but nevertheless the arguments presented here have broad applicability, with my examples deriving from several different varieties of present-day guru-led movement ranging from those of the sant tradition, to "superstar" avatar gurus like Aniruddha Bapu, to the spiritual leader of a little-known West Bengal community which worships the goddess Haimavati. Each movement recognizes the virtues of utility, and their gurus, as it were, induct their devotees into its ambit. But as I have argued throughout, I do not mean "utility" in any narrowly instrumental sense, but utility as itself a source of rich, new spiritual experience. Shah (2006: 245) has recently asked, "Are sects playing a creative role in Indian society and culture in modern times?" The present inquiry is strongly affirmative in its answer.

There have been a number of attempts to define the various roles of different sorts of Indian guru. Kakar's (1984: 47) contention that devotees are infantilized by their dependence on spiritual masters has been influential and is often quoted approvingly (e.g., McKean 1996: 3; van der Veer 1988: 160–161). The claim that gurus serve to resolve ambiguities and replace "true listening" with "submission" (Badrinath 1993: 46) is reflected, for instance, in van der Veer's (1988: 160) description of devotees' "uncritical, reverential attitude" to Ramanandi gurus. McKean (1996) connects this to what she sees as modern gurus' camouflaging of their own and others' financial exploitation of devotees. In contrast to Kakar and McKean, Warrier (2003b) sees modern avatar gurus like Mata Amritanandamayi and Sathya Sai Baba as forming part of a landscape of religious figures in which choice and flexibility reign supreme, with devotees acting reflectively to revise their religious identities as they see fit. It is not lack or alienation (Kakar 1984; Varma 1998) which leads mainly middle-class Indians to seek "anchorage" in joining such movements, but "the hope of increasing possibilities and multiplying opportunities" (Warrier 2003b: 231). Though I reject none of these approaches, all of which shed light on different aspects of the guru and his or her relationship with devotees, I propose an understanding of gurus that has hitherto received inadequate attention. This is that gurus initiate devotees not only into devotional orders but also into key aspects of modernist practice. They are gateway figures through which devotees pass into an osmotically produced modernity.[9]

The argument was prefigured in chapter 4. The policy shift from the personalized, family-oriented replacement form of blood donation to the depersonalized and abstract voluntary form is mediated by the repersonalizing role of the guru. Devotees give to and through the Nirankari guru to "humanity." This dual directional intentionality causes the gift to travel simultaneously to one and to m/any. The guru"s multiply refractive role is that of conduit, or gateway to universal philanthropy. As Bornstein (2003: 90–91) points out, anonymous gifting to unrelated others is often seen as a feature of Christianity and Western modernity and as something which requires inculcation into those non-Western countries which "lack" it. As was seen in chapter 1, Ramanujan (1989) views modernization in India as a movement toward the context-free. I am arguing that context-free voluntary donation is recontextualized by the guru in a new combination of the personal and the impersonal (cf. Hart 2005: 104) which facilitates devotees' induction into gifting for unrelated others.

Before providing further examples of gurus' gateway function, it is necessary to consider the combination of freedom and compulsion that generates devotees' acts of seva, thereby enabling gurus to become gateways. As was noted above in chapter 4, the donor recruiters I know tend to see gurus' devotees as convenient "donor banks" whom they hail as a "mass body" (Cohen 2004: 166)—rather like Kakar and McKean, they view devotees as lacking in individual reason. Recruiters thus attempt to motivate gurus as a shortcut method of accessing blood. I have also noted that the Dera Sacha Sauda's attainment of the world record represents the transfigured capital of the guru's control over his devotees' bodies. Gurus' ability to extract record-breaking quantities of blood from their devotees is partly explained by Parry's (1994: 80) observation that "The power to bless or curse puts the Mahabrahman [or guru] in a position of strength when it comes to negotiating the size of the offering." The very process that demonstrates the guru's corporeal control over his devotees is experienced by them as the occasion for the attainment of spiritual goals.

The guru's devotees thus constitute his "standing reserve"; a dependent and deployable resource in the projects of provision he initiates.[10] Titmuss (1970: 136) identifies what he calls captive voluntary donors, donors who are "in positions of restraint and subordinate authority who are called upon, required or expected to donate [blood]." In such cases, there is unlikely to be direct force or stringent coercion applied, and yet such donors may be led to believe that a negative response would adversely affect their future in some form or other. For prison inmates, who are perhaps the archetypal captive voluntary donor population, remission of sentence has in both India and the United States been held up as a potential reward.[11] The retention of the word "voluntary" in Titmuss's schema is important because even persons under pressure to donate may, in his words, "be strongly moved by a sense of giving." Similarly for devotees: peer pressure and the prospect of spiritual rewards call into question any idea that donation is "a free, spontaneous act" (ibid.)—and striking examples have been provided of devotees' desperate acts of avid donation—but neither, ultimately, are devotees forced to enter this devotional deal. While devotee-donors are not enough the adequate cause of their actions to be viewed as being active or autonomous, neither are they purely passive—theirs is an active subordination. Hence devotee-donors are a good example of Titmuss's category of the captive voluntary donor, but only inasmuch as they were already captive voluntary devotees.

The osmotic or gateway function of the guru thus depends on the deployability of his captive voluntary devotees. The Nirankari Mission was the first devotional order to regularly collect the blood of its devotees in substantial quantities. Its first camps in the mid 1980s were staged on an annual basis on the anniversaries of the assassination of its former guru, and each of them attracted thousands of donations. This was "charismatic," one-time donation activity, and such radical overcoming of the widespread and deep-seated unwillingness to donate blood in the subcontinent provokes awe in doctors used to dealing with reluctance as opposed to fervor. These same doctors, however, also complain of the wastage that results from such events, proclaiming that camps should be structured according to a more repetitive, "rational" temporality. As one doctor put it to me in reference to the Dera Sacha Sauda: "They don't understand that it's a continuous requirement, not a one-time thing."

The Red Cross in Delhi approached the present Nirankari guru and asked him to stagger and reduce the scale of the Mission's camps. A member of the Red Cross team I spoke with recollected making the request: "From May to August is the lean period because education institutions are closed. Can we have two camps every month between these months? He readily agreed because he wanted to see the blood utilized in a better way. This means they have to put in labor not once but ten times! They worked very hard in various zones." The Nirankaris are now universally praised by doctors for arranging their camps in what one doctor called an "organized pattern": "They utilize properly. They divide by region and they do it every month." The guru, under no illusions as to the extent of his authority and therefore assuming automatic compliance, thus transformed the giving experience of his devotees from a charismatic to a rational temporality. Through the guru's intercession, devotees now give with a reliability which has parallels with charitable standing orders or monthly remittances. Multiple spatio-temporally distributed Nirankari camps have thus replaced the single annual camp conducted in a centralized setting.

This shows that the giving of a useful substance on its own is not enough—the manner of its giving also has to be reformed for the full realization of "virtuous utility." Devotees profess a certain wistfulness about the change, regretting the lessening of the Mission's ability to produce hyperbolic donation numbers—an important capital in the national league of virtuous beneficence. As one devotee told me: "We wish that we could give more but there is not enough storage so we spread our camps out now." Another declared: "We can give much more than this, but Guru Ji says the doctors don't need so much all at once, so now we have fewer donors and more camps." The guru's decision to routinize the Mission's donation activity thus entailed a certain sacrifice: the price paid for its full embrace of virtuous utility is a diminution of its ability to vanquish the names of other devotional orders through tournaments of blood value.[12] The guru is attempting to reveal to his devotees another kind of value (that of virtuous utility).

On one level, this clearly amounts to the ambivalent rationalization of religious practice, but it is more interesting than that. Gurus are not neutral gateway figures: they alter and operate upon the modernist practice which they help facilitate. The fact that it is gurus who valorize and induct devotees into "utility" helps sacralize that utility. This should ward against viewing gurus simply as facilitators of "Westernization." I argued in chapter 3 that reformist giving practices reinforce the existing giving structures they "parasite" through being dependent on them, and the case under discussion presents a comparable picture: philanthropic practice which is universalistic, anonymous, structured by a rational temporality, and encoded with utility comes to fruition through the personal relationship between guru and devotee, as expressed in the "traditional" institution of guru seva. The guru as facilitator thereby presents devotees with a utility dripping with spiritual possibilities and amenable to incorporation within multifarious donation theologies.

This is seen particularly clearly in the case of the Mumbai-based guru Aniruddha Bapu. An avatar guru in the mold of Mata Amritanandamayi and Sathya Sai Baba, his devotees hold him to be, in their words, the "highest percentage" incarnation of Vishnu since Krishna. I attended two blood donation camps in Mumbai organized by the Sadguru Shree Aniruddha Upasana Trust, founded by Bapu, and visited Happy Home, the guru's residence and the Trust's headquarters. So far this book has largely focused on interactions between gurus and doctors as distinct entities. Bapu, however, combines the two roles, as both guru and doctor, having practiced rheumatology in a government hospital prior to committing himself fully to spiritual activities in 1996.

On the face of it, this Mumbai doctor-guru appears to promote and is a gateway to recognizably modernist ideas and activity: he extols forward planning, encourages environmental projects that range from promoting "eco-friendly" Ganpati idols to vermiculture, and his Trust actively engages with "medical utility" in organizing regular blood donation camps.[13] Various populations of the subcontinent have from the colonial era onward frequently been characterized as being immured within the present, with a consequent "inability to think for the morrow" (Parry n.d.; Reisz 2004). Bapu's teachings, which center on usefulness and forward planning, appear to take heed of this assessment, and to offer redress to it, but in a very striking and particular way which calls attention to the role of gurus as non-neutral gateway figures who operate upon the modernist forms of practice they facilitate.

Bapu prophesizes that between 2007 and 2025 there will be untold natural and manmade disasters (*appatti*), brought on by man's wretched moral decline. The world will be seriously threatened but will not end—in 2025 the calamities will cease and *ramrajya*, Bapu's heavenly kingdom on earth, will appear. In his weekly spiritual discourses (*pravachan*) he warns his predominantly middle-class devotees that the frequency of disasters is increasing, ready for the deluge of 2007–2025, and that only devotion to him will protect them from their ravages. Devotees report his warning: "Whoever follows me will survive—those who do not, I don't know."

The "millennial mode of attention," state Stewart and Harding (1999: 286), is "vigilant, anxious, excited, always watching for signs of the times," and similarly for Bapu and his devotees, every disaster is studied and seen as evidence that the events he foretells are gathering apace. Mumbai is particularly prone to bomb attacks, communal riots, and flooding, and it can be no accident that it is here that this theology of disasters has been developed.[14] But disasters worldwide are also examined and scrutinized, with the September 11 attacks on the United States having attained particular importance both as a sign of what is to come and as a demonstrative example of the need to offer bhakti to Bapu and obtain his protection. One United States–based devotee is said to have had a job interview planned in the World Trade Center for the morning of September 11, 2001. In a telephone call to Bapu prior to the interview to ask for his advice and blessings, he is reported to have instructed her to cancel the interview, claiming she would die if she did not. She cancelled it and was "saved."[15]

Devotees evince an acute apocalyptic sensibility: several saw as portentous what was then the recent massacre of Russian schoolchildren in Beslan.[16] When soon after my visit to Mumbai the 2004 Asian tsunami struck the coastal regions of south and southeast Asia, killing many thousands, I received a text message from a devotee stating: "Told you so . . . disasters are going to mount like hell as I told you . . . and the relief and savior is that one and only Lord Aniruddha . . . so start loving him and understanding him very soon." In some instances, it is not clear whether appalling events are being held up as the immoral episodes precipitating the disasters or the retributive disasters themselves. For example, it is unclear whether the notion (described to me by devotees) that children in India and beyond will soon begin asking their parents for genetic proof of parentage would count as a precipitating cause of disaster or a disaster in itself. I e-mailed several Mumbai friends after the bomb attacks on 11 July 2006 to check if they were okay. A Bapu devotee replied: "With Lord Aniruddha's grace I am fine," before reminding me of Bapu's threat: "In this universe, those who come to me, love me and feel that I am their best friend shall survive in the dreaded times ahead." "Keep watching," my friend concluded.

Millenarian theologies are uncommon in the subcontinent, though examples do exist such as that espoused by the Brahma Kumaris.[17] Contrary to claims that millenarian expectations are alien to Hinduism (see, for instance, Hobsbawn 1959: 58), Babb shows that they fit within a standard Hindu cosmology according to which history is organized into epochal cycles (*yugas*), each lasting millions of years. In the case of Aniruddha Bapu and Brahma Kumari prophesying, however, these cycles are speeded up, or "run at high RPM" as Babb puts it (1986: 113). Both movements dedicate themselves to preparing for calamitous times, though Bapu is more precise than the Brahma Kumaris about when exactly the destruction will begin. Whereas Brahma Kumaris prepare through "purifying" themselves through a regimen which includes celibacy (ibid.: 93), Bapu's devotees conduct preparatory seva activities that can be connected with Bapu's status as an incarnation of Vishnu, preserver and sustainer of the world. In particular Bapu encouraged his devotees to set up an Academy of Disaster Management (Appatti Nivarak Dal), which, with contributions from various scientists, engineers, police, fire, and army personnel, has produced a professional-looking publication called *Textbook of Disaster Management* (2002). The academy claims to have trained more than 20,000 of its devotees in disaster management techniques.[18] Among other activities, its disaster management volunteers (DMVs) warn Mumbai citizens of the "plastic menace," promote vermiculture, plant trees, and control crowds during religious festivals. Since there are apparently more Sadguru Shree Aniruddha Upasana Trust branches than police and fire stations in Mumbai, DMVs are reported to work in coordination with the police and fire services, with the former looking after emergency situations until the latter arrive and take charge.

Though Bapu's devotees line up to donate blood in response to bomb blasts, they also donate in preparation for forthcoming disasters.[19] As one devotee told me: "We need gallons and gallons of blood for the disasters which are going to come." At a donation camp another donor informed me that "soon there will be rivers of blood flowing so we are donating to get ready for that." A member of the academy told me: "This [blood donation] is for 2007. 2007 is the crack point maximum. The blood is for our soldiers and our Indian brothers and sisters. So many people are going to die, and we can't help that. But those who survive can take our blood." Another devotee's statement recalled the qualitative view of karma discussed in chapter 4: "Bapu says, if you donate blood for me once, you will never need to take blood, and neither will your next seven generations." With the prospect of an imminent period of bloodshed and disaster, it is easy to see the appeal of this.

Bapu expounds a theology that radically counters perceptions of Indians' "inability to think for the morrow," and its central focus on forward planning and utility seems on one level to be in perfect accord with "scientific modernity." And yet, to say the least, Bapu fosters utility and planning very much on his own terms. As was noted earlier in chapter 3, classical utility may be understood as a doctrine that sees value only in those social activities that promote production and conservation. Conservation is at the heart of Bapu's concerns; just as with any incarnation of Vishnu it has to be. Devotees' environmental schemes and donation of blood are both conservational activities and can be seen as modes through which they partake of their guru's sustaining role and therefore his divinity. Utility and preparation are thus operated upon in a particular way by the guru who advances them. In enacting them, devotees become, as it were, micro-Vishnus. Moreover, the parables of protection I heard such as that cited above concerning the 11 September attacks suggest that, contrary to Warrier's (2003b) argument, well-to-do Indians' adherence to modern avatar gurus can partly be explained by gurus' anchoring and protective function, though I acknowledge that Mumbai's particular proneness to disaster makes it is easy to see why its citizens might more urgently seek protection than those elsewhere. There is more than one orientation to protection presented

here: in embracing Bapu, devotees insure themselves against the coming ravages; in donating blood and qualifying as disaster management volunteers, they
insure others against them too. In addition, these acts for the protection of
others qualitatively "feed back" to devotees, further fortifying them against
impending catastrophe.

To conclude, I turn from a theology of ultimacy to one of immortality.[20] The
Association of Voluntary Blood Donors, West Bengal has enlisted the charismatic religious leader Saumyendra Nath Brahmachary as a blood donation proselytizer. Saumyendra, whom I met on numerous occasions and several of whose
lectures to donor recruiters I attended, heads Dev Sangha, a small West Bengal
community consisting of a few hundred devotees who worship the goddess
Haimavati, mentioned in the Kena Upanishad, and an amalgamation of Brahma,
Vishnu, Shiva, and Durga. After a period in business, and having been desig-
nated the future leader of the Dev Sangh, Saumyendra undertook spiritual training: "I was a blood donor. I was also doing spiritual practices. I asked, how is
blood donation related to my spirit? What is the spiritual basis for doing this? I
realized it is a *sadhana*, a spiritual penance. I can do this through meditation
and reflection and also through blood donation." He explains to both his own
devotees and to donor recruiters that "TTI is not only Transfusion Transmissible
Infection. There is another kind of TTI which is Touch Transmitted Ignition. We,
as individuals, have an existence limited by time and space, puny thoughts.
Even from within this limitation, when we offer this gift of love we join the
stream of eternal life. The blood I gave in the past continues to flow in someone
else. People say blood donation saves the recipient's life, but it does not—it only
postpones their death! It is the donor's life which gets saved. Restricted in time
and space, I donate blood and I elevate myself to immortal existence. It is not
just social service; it's a new form of yoga. We unite with others in eternal life;
through your donations you will reach eternal experience."

This notion of the transcendence of finitude through blood donation was
broached in the discussion in chapter 2 of donors in a sense taking credit for the
future reproductive generativity of saved persons. Saumyendra's idea of a kind
of relational immortality is echoed in the testimonies of British ova donors who
see themselves as acting through recipients to extend themselves in another
form (Konrad 2005: 114). Saumyendra's reference to yoga is particularly interesting. The final goal of yogic practice is samadhi, "a reversal of the flow of time
[and] immortality and transcendence over the entire created universe" (White
1996: 45). Alter (2004) also emphasizes immortality as the ultimate end of yoga.
The guru Saumyendra thus assumes a gateway function in extolling an exemplary practice of medical utility while operating on that utility to saturate it with
associations irreducible to narratives of simplistically rationalized religious and
social practice—in this case blood donation being formulated as an escape
from finitude and an addition to the yogic pantheon. Gurus are the porous

membranes through which, in a kind of spiritual osmosis, devotees pass into inimitable versions of modernist practice both like and unlike those with which we are familiar.

Conclusion

Through identifying in this chapter the "gateway" function of gurus in regard to blood donation and also more widely in Indian society, I have sought to elucidate the central role of gurus in the production of India's efflorescent biospiritual medical creativity. In so doing it has become clear that arguments to the effect that "the values of Western scientific medicine were exported to the rest of the world along with the theory, practice, institutions and social relations of that medicine" (Cunningham and Andrews 1997: 10) are not equipped to shed much light on the recent history of blood donation in India. The gradations and nuances of gurus' donation theologies demonstrate that voluntary blood donation is subject to multifaceted forms of resignification and rearticulation which undermine widespread assumptions that biomedicine in non-Western contexts comprises only a terrain of loss and disaffection. It is helpful to think of biomedical knowledge moving through the guru to devotees, just as devotees move through the guru to engage with biomedical knowledge. I draw here on Ingold's (2006) depiction of an animist ontology of movement according to which living beings move *through* rather than *across* the surfaces and textures of the world.[21] The premise may be extended to forms of knowledge, which also travel through rather than simply across terrain both geographical and conceptual. Indeed, this chapter has shown that the enlistment of gurus as proselytizers of voluntary blood donation and other forms of modernist practice results in a complexly inductive *moving through* rather than a more neutral and simply conceived *moving across* vis-à-vis "the theory, practice, institutions and social relations of [Western scientific] medicine." When entities move densely through, rather than impartially across, then "the properties of the medium through which they move are all-important" (Ingold 2006: 17). And so it is with the guru conduits who transform the "Western scientific medicine" which passes through them to their devotees; the biomedical rendered into the biospiritual.

Practices of medical utility thus come to light as a source of harnessable conceptual material, with all sorts of latent capacities amenable for making abstract spiritual formulae "compelling and experientially present" (Laidlaw 2007). A final striking example attests to this. I quote from a doctor (though "blood donation guru" would perhaps be more apt) whom I witnessed addressing a crowd of potential donors: "Donor and recipient are part of a *mahayagna*.[22] You are praying, you are forgiving—yes! The phlebotomist who gives the prick is causing you pain, but you are not saying: 'Why have you done this?' In a yagna, you pour ghee, you pour *ahutis* [oblations of incense and foodstuffs], and it burns up. So similarly in this *maha-yagna* of voluntary donation, every drop of blood given by the voluntary donor has the highest value of life and starts rejuvenating the dying patient." Donated blood, like ghee thrown into the fire, revitalizes that into which it is placed—the recipient's body—making its life flare up once more. As with Bapu's followers who "preserve and sustain" through the giving of their blood, it is evident here that utility's constituent properties of production and conservation are hardly mere abstractions but rather are key bases for the reinvigoration not only of bodies but also of religious conceptualization and enactment.

If blood donation provides material for the realization of particular devotional and spiritual possibilities, the other side of this biomedical/religious interoperability is the large amount of blood this results in for blood banks. This chapter has identified a further key aspect of this interoperability: blood donation, I have argued, through its properties of distanciation, mediates between and helps make experientially practicable for sant movement devotees the apparently divergent values of himsa and ahimsa. I have not been arguing that logical consistency is achieved or even that it is a goal; rather, my suggestion is that blood donation can enable people to charge their acts with significance without having to reconcile them as being of a piece. The operation of donation as a mechanism of time-space distanciation underlines the point that there is no single meaning of blood donation for devotees. Instead, I have tried to show how a field of ambivalent signifiers is negotiated through this medical practice. Time-space distanciation—the ability to enact agentive capacities from a distance and intimacy at one remove—appears to render experientially practicable the taking on of possibly divergent positions. I return in chapter 8 to the subject of donation and distanciation, demonstrating that it possesses implications beyond moral dilemmas about violence.

In addition to examining how the distanciation function of anonymity enables blood donation to mediate between the seemingly opposed values of himsa and ahimsa, this study has explored the Nirankari enlistment of anonymity as a means of generating a sense of continual spiritual expansion and Hazoor Maharaj Ji's utilization of the anonymous conditions of voluntary blood donation as a means to depict Dera Sacha Sauda donations as conforming to the highest principles of disinterested dan. Having touched upon issues of anonymity and nationalism in this chapter, the following chapter—on blood donation as a means of reinhabiting Nehruvian logics in contemporary India—further explores ways in which the anonymity of voluntary blood donation may be engaged for explicitly nationalist as well as religious projects.

7

The Nehruvian Gift

Given its cultural diversity and religious plurality many were skeptical about the ability of the nascent state, which achieved freedom from British colonial rule in 1947, to live beyond a couple of decades as a democratic nation. On more than one occasion, India has reached the brink of both disintegration and authoritarianism.

K. N. Panikkar, *The Concerned Indian's Guide to Communalism*

The physical incorporation by recipients of corporeal gifts of organs and blood is in a literal sense integrative inasmuch as it enacts a physical connectivity between persons. In India as elsewhere, this connectivity is often subjected to political readings. What I seek to show in this chapter is that in addition to integrative physical connection (i.e., acts of transfusion), the practical processes involved in the gathering and distribution of units of donated blood in India have come to be viewed by various donors, doctors, and other actors as providing anticipatory visions of an integrated nation. Like the rituals of transformation described by Handelman (1990: 23), the choreography of blood donation "pre-views a hypothetical condition and it provides procedures that [it is hoped] will actualize this act of the cultural imagination." This kind of performance, says Handelman, "contains particular futures within itself." Such representations of the nation thus possess a hoped-for generative aspect: rather than fading away once they are done, their purpose is "to impress a mark upon the course of time" (Osborne 2005: 282). What I seek to show here is that medics and donors view the physical processes which constitute what doctors sometimes call "the vein-to-vein chain" as particularly suited to both signify and produce the Indian political aesthetic of national integration. I thus argue that the central Nehruvian ideal of "national integration"—hitherto overshadowed in scholarly treatments by the related concept of "secularism"—has, through complex imaginative processes connected to physical and ideational points of "gathering," retained a strong and enduring presence in the field of voluntary blood donation.

As we shall see, enumeration of the differential components of particular gatherings is a key feature of the integrative narratives that I explore here. Such enumerations devolve from (but are not the same as) a set of enumerative practices enacted in both pre- and post-Independence India through which, in the words of Kapila (2008: 120) "social diversity was imagined and governmentalized along religious, ethnic and linguistic axes." Cohn (1987), Kaviraj (1989), Chatterjee (1996) and others have drawn attention to the importance of enumeration as an instrument of the colonial rule of India. Control took the form of "enumerating the diverse communities which, in the colonial imagination, comprised the society over which they had been destined by history to rule" (Chatterjee 1996: 285). Cohn (1987) notes that caste and religion became the "sociological keys" to the "numerical description" of Indian society. The enumeration of diverse communities continues to be performed for the purposes these scholars describe, the formalization of community distinctions having led to competition between these groupings in seeking access to state resources (Chatterjee 1996: 285). These scholars rightly connect "state" and "statistics" (see Lal 2002), but their monologic focus on the role of enumeration in formalizing what had previously been "fuzzy" communities (Kaviraj 1989), and on the competition between these newly identifiable interest groups, has resulted in a direct and singular equation between enumeration on the one hand and reification and fissiparity on the other.[1] What has in consequence hitherto been overlooked is another important aspect of enumeration: its role in the formation of visions of a differentially composed and yet harmoniously functioning national life.

From the originating blood donation camp, which acts as a means of bringing together people from diverse origins, through to the transfusion, a centering of several diversely sourced units of blood, the chain consists of various points of gathering. Both doctors and donors see "indicative continuities" (Strathern 2005b: 67) between these moments of assembly and the Nehruvian nationalist tenet (to paraphrase Strathern 2006) that heterogeneous societal interests must ultimately be made to fold into a single social field, that of the Indian nation. The focus, then, is on the role of what might be termed "congregative thought" within a variety of Indian actors' imaginings of the Indian nation as a coherently functioning "bounded aggregation" (Segal and Handler 1992: 3). What blood donation allows is the generation of microcosmic integrative images at a variety of scales. The several scales of gathering at which Nehruvian logics are reproduced demonstrates that Nehruvian conceptualizations of national integration do not merely persist within blood donation processes but are being recreated and reasserted through them. As I explain below, the choreography of microcosmic gatherings is a familiar one, but its replication at different levels and locales suggest a new creative thrust at the heart of Nehruvian logics. Given the supposed death of all that is Nehruvian in contemporary India, this point requires particular emphasis.

My depiction in this chapter of the positive productivities of anonymity draws on the work of two scholars in particular, public policy analyst Richard Titmuss and anthropologist Monica Konrad. Titmuss was perhaps the first to consider in detail possible connections between blood donation and integration. Chapter 1 discussed Titmuss's empirically based argument in *The Gift Relationship* (1970) that voluntary donors provide safer blood than paid donors. However, Titmuss makes the far wider social claim on behalf of voluntary blood donation that it provides "opportunities for people to articulate giving in morally practical terms outside their own network of family and personal relationships." His focus on "anonymous helpfulness" directed toward the "universal stranger" was strongly functionalist in its emphasis on "integrative systems: on processes, transactions and institutions which promote an individual's sense of identity, participation and community" (ibid.: 290, 208, 306, 290).

Konrad has provided a powerful critique of anthropological characterizations of anonymity which discount the imaginative possibilities of "not-knowing." Though Konrad (2005: 39–40) finds in Titmuss's work a rare instance of a serious scholarly treatment of anonymity, she questions his functionalist approach, contrasting his integrative project with her own notion of "anonymous sociality," deployed in reference to British ova donation, which is "predicated on relations of non-relations and instantiated as secrets within the gift"—an approach which, she says, "could not be said to be 'integrative' in its social effect." Despite the differences in approach, there is I think profit to be had from combining the two positions: as will become apparent below, Konrad's insistence on the imaginative possibilities of anonymity is strongly backed up by the Indian experience of voluntary blood donation. Unlike Titmuss, my concern is not with evaluating the actual integrative properties or otherwise of the gatherings I document—indeed an interesting and important question, but one that is beyond the province of this chapter—but rather with the prevalence and structure of the idioms of integration employed to refer to them. Donors and doctors would frequently express the hope that the eventual, cumulative outcome of blood donation processes would be "national integration." The purpose of gathering practices, in this view, is to produce national integration. My argument, conversely, is that the ideology of national integration is more discernibly the grounds of such politically composed blood donation gatherings—their very condition of possibility. In any case, an Indian nationalist variant on Titmuss's argument is the very substance of the way some Indians express what Konrad calls "the creativity of non-linkage"—it is in their expectation of donation-induced national integration that the "inventiveness of [their] anonymized engagement" with these procedures lies (Konrad 2005: 6, 243). This chapter thus takes Konrad's arguments about the power of anonymity to a quite different context from that in which they were originally devised, demonstrating their elucidatory potential for issues of nationalism.

Marxist theorist Alexander Bogdanov, a colleague of Lenin, also provided an integrative reading of corporeal donations in seeking to apply blood donation to the principles of communism. Practicing what he called "physiological collectivism," he underwent twelve "revitalizing" transfusions, before the foreign red cells which "litter[ed] his bloodstream with their broken fragments," induced a massive reaction leading to his death (Starr 1998: 76–77). Something of the same collectivist vision can be seen in the slogan that accompanied an international colloquium for the promotion of voluntary blood donation staged in Beijing in 2004: "Many countries, many cultures, one river of life . . . Blood!" Though the world's many countries and cultures may seem to threaten a mire of multiplicity and confusing disparity, there is yet a biological continuum, an integrative filament that cuts across these multiplicities. Blood acts as what Eco (1997: 50) calls "the hint of an anacoluthon, or the block of an aphasia"—a "line of resistance" which grounds the world's seemingly out-of-control diversity and multiplicity (cf. Leder 1990).

Instances of the donation of organs across "distances" and "divides" are often interpreted according to an idiom of integration. Simpson (2004: 851), for instance, discusses highly symbolic corporeal "boundary crossing acts" in Sri Lanka, such as the donation of a kidney by a Buddhist priest to a Christian woman. Turning to India, a recent news report highlighted the capacity of corporeal donations to provoke integrative interpretations on a geopolitical scale. In 2004 a Pakistani child was brought to Chennai for an eye operation during which he received a corneal graft from an Indian donor. The headline read: "Today an Indian eye will blink in Pakistan," the suggestion being that Partition was annulled on the level of the child's body—that the operation represented the covert moral reconquest of a lost territory. After the bomb attacks in Mumbai on 11 July 2006, widely considered to have been carried out by militant Kashmiri separatists, Muslims in the city were reported to have rushed to donate blood for survivors of whatever hue: "Abdul Khan, waiting in line at the blood bank near one blast site at Jogeshwari station, said: 'We don't care whether it's a Hindu or a Muslim who gets our blood as long as we can save them.' "[2] Blood donation was thus employed by donors and news reporters in order to provide a powerfully integrative conception of the nation at precisely the moment the attackers were attempting to call into question such conceptions. Symbolically loaded blood donation across alleged divides is in fact a standard response to these kinds of events, queues to donate providing the basis for a kind of choreography of solidarity and integration. For example, when in September 2002 Islamic militants shot dead twenty-eight worshipers at the Swaminaryan temple in the Akshardham temple complex in Gandhinagar in Gujarat, the director of a local blood bank drew attention to the many Muslims queuing to donate blood to help the Hindu victims, stating: "Blood is such a thing that there is no religion involved. A blood bank creates communal harmony."[3]

Similarly with caste, blood typing and donation have been engaged in attempts to "undivide" caste communities from one another. Caste is widely thought of as a quality inherent in the blood (Fuller 1992: 21). However, since Landsteiner's ABO system of blood groups crosscuts these "primordial" distinctions, it has been imbued by some with the capacity to disrupt them.[4] Parry (1999: 148) notes that when a worker at the Bhilai Steel Plant requires a transfusion, his workmates, of whatever caste, are quick to come forward to donate for him: "every worker knows that when it comes to life and death it is blood group not caste that counts." In a further example, a news report describes the efforts of a health NGO to equip rural Indians with knowledge of their blood type: "How easy it is to look for differences and miss similarities! This was proved when blood tests of more than a hundred women were carried out. Much to their amazement, the women realized that blood groups could differ not only within their own religion or caste but also within their own families, while those they thought had 'bad blood' could in fact have the same blood group as their own."[5] In an analysis of the depiction of blood typing and transfusion in Indian films of the 1950s and 1970s, Cohen argues that traditional caste and religious allegiances are subjected to Nehruvian nationalist "recoding." In the film *Sujata*, for instance, a high-caste couple foster an "untouchable" girl. When the couple's family air misgivings, the foster father demands "they show him under a microscope what caste is and where in the blood it is to be found" (Cohen 2001: 14, 15). Later, when Sujata's foster mother is in need of a transfusion, it is only her foster daughter's "low caste" blood that matches.

In the examples just given, the varieties of person subject to "integration" are known: Pakistani/Indian, Buddhist/Christian, and so on. And yet a key aim of this chapter is to demonstrate how the anonymous conditions of voluntary blood donation, which *disallow* known identities, play an important role in conceptions of integration. Such conditions create a kind of blank page that permits donors to engage in imaginative acts of enumeration in regard to possible future beneficiaries. Thus, rather than disabling integrative narratives, what anonymity enables is the normalizing entrenchment of the boundary-crossing gift. So in contrast to the above examples, the reporting of which emphasizes the exceptionalism of the boundary crossing act by virtue of the differences between donor and recipient being known, anonymity ensures that *every* such corporeal gift is potentially "boundary-crossing." It is the nonavailability of knowledge in respect of to whom one gives and from whom one receives that produces the imaginative spaces of enumeration and traversal to which I have referred. The normative nonavailability of knowledge entrenches and makes nonexceptional the difference-traversing gift.

National Integration

Thus integrative political messages are frequently read into the physical connectivity that characterizes corporeal donations, in different sorts of cultural context. In the Indian variant of these narratives, religion and caste issues come to the fore. Cohen clearly shows that corporeal donations are interpreted by some Indians as a means to undivide the nation, thereby becoming expressions of a Nehruvian vision of national unity. However, Cohen also asserts that the Nehruvian integrative vision, "in cinema as elsewhere, now seems passé" (Cohen 2001: 15). Similarly, the political success of groups espousing Hindutva-based ideologies has led Rajagopal (2001: 272) to view "Nehruvianism" as amounting to a set of principles "observed largely in the breach rather than an active working policy." There is much evidence that lends credence to these arguments, and Sheth (1996: 321) is persuasive in suggesting that "national integration" has in large part been divested of its egalitarian content and infused with a vertical brand of majoritarian nationalism.

The Nehruvian ideology of national integration enjoys a presence of important dimensions in the field of voluntary blood donation, however, suggesting that, though its meaning is contested, it is a more tenacious mode of conceptualization than some scholars allow for. Further, it is not merely from the physical connectivity of blood donation that the ideology of national integration is made physically manifest and potent, but through a powerful combination of anonymity as an imaginative canvas and a series of moments of gathering—of persons and of blood units—which together form the "vein-to-vein chain."[6]

After the first serious communal riots of post-Independence India in Jabalpur in 1961, Nehru convened a National Integration Conference at Vigyan Bhavan, New Delhi. Inaugurated by President Dr. S. Radhakrishnan, it was attended by educationalists, scientists, chief ministers, and union ministers, the aim being to formulate methods that would be effective in countering communalism, "casteism," and regional and linguistic separatist movements. Soon after the conference, a National Integration Council was constituted that still sits today.[7] The Ministry of Home Affairs, which has a special division for the promotion of national integration, organizes an annual National Integration Day, and on the death anniversary of Indira Gandhi, it awards the Indira Gandhi Prize for National Integration to public figures thought to have contributed to the nurturance of this ideology.[8]

Nehru's identification of the need to foster national integration reflects the fact that "there is no ideological or cultural guarantee for a nation to hold together" (Khilnani 1997: 207). The idea of an India "united into a single political community" (ibid.: 5), capable of containing immense internal diversity, requires persistent cultural effort in order to be maintained, and the continual emphasis in India on national integration, or alternately "unity in diversity" (anekta me ekta), in its seeking to overcome the potential for national fracture (further partitions, separatist agitations, and so on), continually admits its possibility. The great "Depressed Caste" leader B. R. Ambedkar wrote in the 1940s that "There is no nation of Indians in the real sense of the word, it is to be created. In believing that we are a nation, we are cherishing a great delusion. How can people divided into several thousands of castes be a nation? The sooner we realize that we are not as yet a nation, in the social and psychological sense of the word, the better for us" (1989: 67). Nehru's attempts to foster a sense of national integration, in seeking to counter Ambedkar's vision of division and fissure, implicitly recognized its validity.

The phraseology of national integration is extremely prevalent in Indian public life, and is put to work in diverse situations. The construction of new highways is promoted in government newspaper advertisements as a project of national integration; concert series in New Delhi, made up of performers from the different states of the country, are designed "to promote the cause of national integration." A Class X exam paper from 1997, displayed on the *Times of India* Web site, shows that schoolchildren had to answer the question: "What is meant by National Integration?"[9]

Religious movements also profess to seek to foster national integration. A Radhasoami-run university, for example, delivers courses that seek to "ingrain . . . a sense of national integration" (Juergensmeyer 1991: 162). In his analysis of the Indian comic book series *Amar Chitra Katha*, Hawley shows how the ideology of national integration is read back into the lives of the great sages and saints in Indian history. Kabir, for instance, is billed as "the mystic who tried to bring the Hindus and the Muslims together." The integrative message of these comics stops short of espousing resistance to inequality, instead preaching common origins and "gentle amalgam" (Hawley 1995: 120, 127). In her study of the relationship between Hindu gurus in Rishikesh and the ideology of Hindutva, McKean goes further in viewing "national integration" as a dogma deployed by gurus in order to disguise violent domination by "ruling-class groups" (McKean 1996: 272). Though the somewhat tendentious suggestion would seem to be that because some Hindu nationalist activists valorize national unity and integration, anybody who speaks of these concepts must be a Hindu nationalist, McKean's study is useful in drawing our attention to the strikingly prevalent usage of this terminology among both guru movements and Hindu nationalist organizations. In March 2006, for example, BJP leader L. K. Advani undertook a "National Integration Yatra" (pilgrimage) around India to try to restore his party's flagging fortunes. So Hindutva organizations have long used an assertively counter-Nehruvian version of national integration to project an exclusive Hindu vision of the nation. My approach, however, is to see these redefinitions as challenges to the still widely circulating and revered Nehruvian doctrine rather than, as McKean does, as having usurped it.

In order to make the 1997 exam paper, discussed above, into a revision resource for future examinees, the *Times of India* Web site provides a sample answer in which the definition of national integration is given as "assimilation but not extinction, synthesis but not non-existence, solidarity but not regimentation of the many segments of the people in a territorial sovereignty."[10] In order not only to express but also to help instantiate national integration, a frequent "scenography" is enacted in which people of different states, linguistic regions, religions, or castes (representing "the many segments of the people") are brought together in a single place (representing a "territorial sovereignty") in order that they may interact and thereby foster integration.[11] Such choreographed gatherings or "spatial concentrations" (Marriott 1989: 21) of different communities may be understood to be political acts of composition intended to display and nurture a sense of unity in diversity.[12] The political composition of such gatherings is an explicit aim of the Ministry of Youth Affairs and Sports. Referencing religious fundamentalism, linguistic diversities, and "age-old caste system," the ministry claims that such factors "pose a serious challenge to India's unity and integrity and therefore conscious efforts will have to be made by all concerned to preserve the same." Its scheme for the Promotion of National Integration envisages national integration camps, designed "to provide the youth from different parts of the country and from diverse religious and cultural backgrounds a common platform to interact with each other, know each other's customs and lifestyles, to work together in community welfare projects and in the process make them aware of the underlying unity amidst diversity." A key condition for the ministry's funding of such camps is that "at least 25% of the participants would have to be drawn from a minimum number of five states representing some linguistic and cultural diversity."[13] A news article on one such national integration camp, staged in Chennai, reports that volunteers hailed "from 11 states including Assam, Meghalaya, Maharashtra, Tripura, Arunachal Pradesh, Mizoram, Orissa, Manipur, Sikkim, Kerala, and Tamil Nadu."[14] The scenography of integration thus involves gathering together representatives of India's diverse constituent populations in single spaces.

The scenography stretches back to the early days of independence. For instance, an annual folk dance festival was instituted in New Delhi at the Republic Day celebrations of 1953 which showcased folk dances from across the country (Tarabout 2005: 197). The event was a political act of composition arising out of an early incarnation of congregative thought. As Nehru is reported to have declared: "The idea of several folk dancers from different parts of India coming to Delhi brings home to them and to all of us the richness of our cultural heritage and the unifying bond which holds it together" (cited ibid). Parry (2003: 226) provides a further example in his work on Indian industrial labor, speculating that a regionally heterogeneous migrant labor force at the government steel plant in Bhilai arose from a recruitment policy which reflected "the post-independence ideology of national integration. It was the new India that was being built in Bhilai." It should by now be clear that the recruitment policy was enacting a familiar scenography.

Further, as the Bhilai recruitment policy and the national integration camps attest, and as will further be demonstrated below through examples drawn from blood donation processes, what Kapila (2008: 120) aptly calls the "governmentalization of difference"—state practices of classification and enumeration tied to minority recognition, the granting of entitlements and the state's pluralistic self-image—may evoke not merely fixity and recognition-based fissiparousness, but also promissory narratives of integration and cohesiveness. This is the case because communities need to be distinguished and enumerated in order to be able to be gathered together in microcosmic visions of a national *unitas multiplex*. This, indeed, is the irony of enumeration. Just as Cohn (1987) suggested in his classic work on the census, enumeration *does* politicize identity and involve processes of reification: diversity exists on different levels, and the calling forth of different state and/or religious representatives at national integration camps denies the internal diversity of the represented "community" in order to make a claim about diversity on a different level (that of the nation) (see Greenhouse 1996: 230). At the same time, enumeration is emphatically a condition of the congregative thought at the heart of the ideology of national integration—it is precisely because identities have been defined and made countable that promissory images of a national "holding together" become possible. Enumeration, then, contains dual tendencies toward reification and promissory holdings together.[15]

Omnium Gatherum I: Camps

As places of assembly and convergence, camps are a spatial form that comes almost ready-made for interpretations emphasizing their capacities for promoting national integration. We have seen that the Ministry of Youth Affairs and Sports actively solicits the participation of distinct communities in its national integration camps; the focus now turns to blood donation camps, which can be politically composed in comparable ways.

The Dera Sacha Sauda's spectacular blood donation enactments provide excellent examples of a blood donation camp's ability to "hold together" diverse constituents. The scale of the Dera Sacha Sauda's two record-breaking camps, held in Sirsa and Sri Gurusarmodia village, respectively, required very particular organizational arrangements. Since the quantities of units to be collected would far exceed local requirements, it was necessary for the Sacha Sauda to invite blood bank collection teams from distant regions of the country. Fifty blood banks in total attended the 2004 camp, hailing from the states of Delhi, Haryana, Punjab, Rajasthan, Jammu, Gujarat, and Andhra Pradesh. For these camps, then, Sirsa and Sri Gurusarmodia became points of confluence with not only pilgrims but also blood banks from multiple origins converging in a single center. The corollary, of course, is the taking back of blood collected in singular centers to multiple destinations. A centripetal movement to a center was thus followed by a centrifugal movement away from it in a concertina-style action of compression and decompression. The latter movement creates a sense of Hazoor Maharaj Ji as an indispensable benefactor of the nation, while also resembling something like a royal progress by proxy, the guru marking the nation through distribution of the blood donated in Sirsa, "like some wolf or tiger spreading his scent through his territory, as almost physically part of them" (Geertz 1983: 125).[16] The former movement, conversely, constructs Sirsa as a gathering point of national multiplicity. The local media in Haryana enumerated the states represented at the 2004 camp, describing it as a truly great example of *anekta me ekta* (unity in diversity).[17]

Recalling the 2003 Dera Sacha Sauda camp in which he had taken part, a Delhi blood bank director told me: "16,000 people donated blood. It can definitely lead to national integration. Fifty-two blood banks came from all over India: from Jammu and Kashmir, Rajasthan, Gujarat. . . . So on the one hand, technical experts came from different states. On the other hand, blood from Haryana state went to many states outside." On World Blood Donor Day, 14 June 2004, the Delhi chapter of the Indian Society for Blood Transfusion and Immunohaematology (ISBTI) held a symposium on the theme of "Quality Standards."[18] It included a panel discussion at which a member of the audience asked whether the insurance cards issued to voluntary donors are valid in all Indian states. Since sectors of Delhi are located in the states of Uttar Pradesh and Haryana, respectively, the question was locally pertinent. The panel, comprising blood bank personnel from the corporate, government, and NGO sectors, was unsure of the answer, but one doctor strongly supported the idea:

> This could go a long way in improving voluntary blood collection in India, because in the Western world there's a system of national directories where every donor gets a national number, and that card is valid, honored and accepted anywhere you go across the country.[19] But here there is only fragmentation. There was a camp in December [2003] in Sirsa where people from 50 blood banks came and 15,000 units were donated in one day and blood banks from as far as Ahmedabad and Jammu and Shimla were there. This was a very fine venture for national integration, for practical secularism. Through these thoughts which come through blood donation, I think we can go a long way in improving several things.[20]

Many blood donation camps, of course, are far less heterogeneously composed—camps staged at colleges are attended by the students in residence there; those staged at corporate offices are attended by the professionals who work there, and so on. However, like the national integration camps discussed above, attempts to secure the presence of people from distinct regions or communities are often an integral part of a blood donation camp's planning. At the Nasik *kumbh mela* in 2003, for example, Muslims in the Samajwadi Party organized a blood donation camp.[21] The party's state general secretary Mushir Sayyed declared that the camp was "for the benefit of the millions of pilgrims converging here. . . . We are planning to help anyone with road directions, drinking water, et cetera. The blood camp is to promote national integration."[22] The presence of pilgrims from multiple origins, held together at a single point and donating in concert at a Muslim organized camp, strongly reflects the scenography of integration discussed above.[23] Nasik lies close to the location of the serious communal riots that swept through Gujarat in 2002. The newspaper report is headlined "Secularism in a time of strife," the implicit proposition being that blood donation, performed together by people from diverse origins, for unknown others, helps to counter the divisions of communalism.

Soon after the Gujarat riots a blood donation camp in Kolkata "was inaugurated by the Bengal Chief Minister . . . where 521 people donated their blood to register their support for a country free of communal strife."[24] Similarly, in the city of Allahabad, the Inquilabi Blood Donors Association is reported to stage blood donation camps that "lay particular stress on communal harmony and the fact that blood recognizes no sectarian boundaries." In popular discourse it is "benighted" Allahabad that epitomizes Uttar Pradesh state's "half-closed society." The association's camps, however, "soon acquired the status of a social movement where boys and girls mingled freely."[25]

The anonymity characterizing voluntary blood donation is a further factor that contributes to the perception of it as an act promoting "national integration" and "communal harmony." Although voluntary donation can, when compared with replacement donation, appear abstract and depersonalized, Taussig (1998) argues that where there is facelessness, the face can stand for anyone. Following from this, faceless transfusion recipients can, from the standpoint of donors, stand for any number of possible beneficiaries. Anonymity thus provides an additional mode of enumeration: as I show below, voluntary donors frequently enumerate prospective recipients according to their caste or religious background. This kind of imaginative engagement amounts to an "active not knowing" (Taussig 1999: 7) on the part of donors, and is in line with Smith's (1963: 181) famous definition of the Indian state policy of secularism as ideally involving "active nonpreference" toward the different communities over which it governs.[26] From this angle, the notion of "practical secularism," formulated by the doctor cited above, is apt: donors cannot specify the community to which the recipients of their donations belong. They know their gift may literally be given to anyone; hence, donors' donations result from their enactment of active nonpreference.

The point about anonymous blood donation's mechanical transgression of community boundaries is emphasized in recruitment posters. An Indian Red

Cross slogan reads: "Your blood will be used to treat patients without any distinction of caste, creed, or status." A Kolkata recruitment poster states: "Haru [a
Hindu] donated blood and saved the life of Harun [a Muslim]. Rohim [a Muslim]
has donated to Ram [a Hindu]. A little gift sometimes becomes much bigger
[*asamanya*—rare, incomparable]." Syed Hussain, whom I met at a Youth
Congress camp, told me: "I am a Muslim and I am donating blood. And that goes
to the blood bank. And tomorrow, the patient does not know whose blood it is
they take, and nor do I know for whom I have donated. It may be a Hindu; an
upper-caste man may give to a lower caste; an upper-caste woman may receive
the blood of a lower-caste person. This is for the integration of the people."

Two foci of enumeration have so far been discussed: the blood donation
camp, as a convergence of possibly distinct groups of people, and the anonymity
of voluntary donation, which encourages donors to prospectively enumerate
the possible destinations of their gift. Enumeration, as discussed above, is key to
a fairly standardized scenography of integration. An annual Kolkata blood donation event in which both modes of enumeration were clearly visible provides a
striking example of a blood donation camp as a political act of composition.

The *raksha bandhan* festival, notes Vanita (2002: 157–158), is "widely celebrated in north India when sisters tie a thread (*rakhi*) on their brothers' wrists
to affirm bonds of protection and nurturance. There is a long history of fictive
kin relations being established between women and men, even across Hindu-
Muslim lines, through the tying of the *rakhi*."[27] West Bengal's Association of
Voluntary Blood Donors (AVBD) organizes a donation camp on this day in a central Kolkata museum, which draws inspiration from the festival's association
with fictive kinship and the undoing or healing of religious divisions. The
AVBD's founder, Debabrata Ray, described to me the interesting way in which
the AVBD engages in the political composition of the camp: "We request organizations to attend that represent different languages, religions, and castes. For
each state, also, there are different organizations. We approach the different
caste groups beforehand, though at the camp itself we don't ask their caste."
Having closely observed the persons donating, and examined the names on the
donor questionnaire forms, Debabrata showed me an incomplete list he had made
during the camp delineating the different constituencies he had brought together
in its composition: "Total donors: 265. Women: 45. Muslim: 8 (4 women).
Christian: 33. Jain: 12. Sikh: 1. By language: Tamil: 4. Telegu: 3. Kannada: 2.
Malayalam: 2. Hindi: 26. Oriya: 2. Assamese 1. Bengali: rest. Among Hindus: all
castes." The camp's composition thus corresponded closely to the scenography
of integration witnessed in national integration camps and in the Bhilai steel
plant's recruitment policy, with the actively sought-out representatives of different communities donating side by side.

In addition to the diverse constituencies of donors present at the camp,
donors I spoke with were acutely aware of the diverse constituencies of

recipients to which their donated blood would travel. In its publicity materials, the AVBD refers to the festival's association with sibling bonding, while using the universalistic property of anonymously giving for anyone to take the notion of bonding further—donors would enact active nonpreference in creating bonds of protection for any family member rather than for one family member in particular. As was noted above, rakhis are usually tied by sisters on their brothers for their protection; this is in return for the brother's protective role as regards his sister. Donors at the raksha bandhan camp I attended told me they were expanding the beneficiaries of the festival to include anybody's sister or family member. Their donations were thus absolutely in keeping with the family-oriented nature of the festival, but with "family" understood in a far wider sense: "Today we are protecting other people's sisters if they are in danger. That is the philosophy of this camp. When a little girl tied the rakhi on my hand, I felt I really am doing something to help someone's little sister somewhere."[28] Another donor told me: "What we say here is, donate blood and that blood will be used for protecting *some sister or her family member*" (my emphasis). Donated blood complements or even supplants the rakhi as an agent of protection, with the beneficiaries of protection "centrifuged" to include all families, rather than simply the ones to which specific donors belong.[29] The "centrifuged" festival thus mirrors the centrifuge of the form of donation, from family-replacement donation for a relative to voluntary donation for anyone. Translated into the anonymous structures of voluntary donation, the festival makes protection the result of "active not knowing" on the part of celebrants, this a consequence of voluntary donation's own shunning of preference in being the enactment of a practical form of secularism.

The AVBD's operating of raksha bandhan in order to create indicative continuities between it and voluntary blood donation ideology thus recalls the arguments of chapters 2 and 4 about the alliances that have come to exist between interlocking sets of widening movements: institutional, spiritual, familial, and so on. The case of the raksha bandhan festival presents further evidence that the transition from replacement to voluntary donation does not entail the elimination from this domain of family-based ideational reckoning. Rather, kinship is reconceptualized according to what in this instance is a nationalist logic of m/any. The significant point here is that the process of blood donation "re-familialization" is at the same time one of the family's re-formation (its centrifugation).

Omnium Gatherum II: Blood Banks, Transfusions, and Units of Blood

The camp is thus both a gathering point and the point from which dispersal to many others originates. The "vein-to-vein chain"—the processes through which

blood is extracted, transported, stored, tested, treated, and transfused—consists
of a series of moments of gathering and dispersal. The next gathering point,
after the camp, is the storage of donated blood in the blood bank. As was
observed earlier, the Sathya Sai Baba hospital in Puttaparthi recently lodged a
world record claim for possessing in its blood bank refrigerators the blood of
most nationalities. As the ex-director of the blood bank, informed me: "The
blood bank, the entire hospital is a dream land. It is the only blood bank in the
world where I can safely claim pilgrims from more than 110 countries have voluntarily donated blood." The blood bank thus "holds together" units of blood
donated by the citizens of numerous different countries, creating a vision of
international integration.[30]

Transfusions may in addition be viewed as gathering points. Transfusions
are usually made up of several donated units; a single unit of blood is rarely
transfused. A transfusion is therefore a centering of multiply sourced units,
which are "held together" in a single patient's body. Huyler (2000: 97), in his
account of working as a doctor in a U.S. hospital, vividly shows how transfusions
render the patient a center:

> The ringing phone: "Blood bank."
>
> "This is Dr. Huyler. We need four more units of blood for Maria
> Gonzales."
>
> "OK, we're sending it up. But we're running low. We're going to have
> to send out for it soon."
>
> And so the blood started coming in by air from California and
> Colorado. It arrived cold, a deep icy red, the plastic bags stacked in card-
> board boxes, with labels: Biohazard.
>
> She became the center of something. Airplanes converging, the whis-
> pering voices of consultants. Literature searches, abstracts of scientific
> papers inserted in the chart. The whir of machines, and she bled through
> it all.

Diversely sourced gathering points, as has been demonstrated, are open to
readings that emphasize their integrative properties, and the transfusion is no
exception. Cohen has described the 1977 film *Amar Akbar Anthony* in which
three brothers, separated at birth, have been brought up as Hindu, Muslim, and
Christian, respectively. A woman, who unbeknownst to them is their mother,
requires a transfusion: "In the transfusion scene, three intravenous lines connect the men to the woman, Bharati, whose name ["Indian"] and body figure the
nation. The camera pans showing the three young transfusers in turn with a
temple, mosque or church respectively as backdrop" (Cohen 2001: 15). India
herself is the center into which its constituent religious populations deliver
themselves in an image of transfusion as national integration.

As Cohen is careful to point out, however, that the transfused woman is Hindu ensures that "integration" takes place under a Hindu sign, thus suggesting a vertical interpretation of national integration, with Hinduism the overarching national schema into which "minorities" must obligingly position themselves. This, of course, can be read as a departure from the Nehruvian insistence on the equal status of all religions, and serves as a reminder that "national integration" is a contested category, the egalitarian content of which cannot be taken for granted (McKean 1996; Sheth 1996).

There is a further matter that makes the transfusion image ambiguous from a Nehruvian standpoint. As I mentioned above, the brothers were separated at birth—by birth, that is, they were Hindu, before being brought up separately as Hindu, Christian, and Muslim. There is a sense therefore in which the assembly of "diversely" sourced blood in the patient center is in fact a gathering of the same. This becomes clearer in the light of recent comments made by Hindu nationalist leaders. RSS chief K. S. Sudarshan recently declared that "The blood flowing in the veins of Indian Muslims is the same as Lord Rama and Krishna . . . in a true sense, both Lord Rama and Krishna are ancestors of Indian Muslims."[31] And, recalling Vanaik's (1997: 309) comment that the rhetorical "respect" offered by Hindu nationalist leaders to India's Muslims exists "not because they are Muslims and believe in Islam but because, in a more fundamental sense, they are not Muslims!" the former BJP President Banguru Laxman has similarly asserted that "Muslims are the flesh of our flesh and the blood of our blood but they never got their rightful share in the nation's development nor have they been able to join the national mainstream to play their due role in nation-building," the implication being that if they were not of the same blood then such privileges would not follow.[32]

From this perspective, the transfusion image provides an instance of a gathering of the same: the Christian and the Muslim may have "converted" from Hinduism, but their blood is still Hindu—what is being gathered together is thus Hindu blood. I do not, however, wish to overstate its departure from the Nehruvian model; after all, it has been argued, notably by Benei (2006), that Nehru's integrative message itself operated "under a Hindu sign." And yet, the image does represent a departure from the examples of the Nehruvian nationalist vision presented in this chapter, which engage in active traversals and enumerations of diversity in order to make visible its constituents and acknowledge their presence within the containing nation. The transfusion image is more ambiguous, with gatherings of the same operating not far beneath the more overt narrative of a holding together of difference. The example is helpful in drawing attention to some of the uneasy coexistences and dialogues that exist between vertical and horizontal models of integration.

An additional key "holding together" resides in the unit of donated blood itself. As we have seen, blood component separation is a technological procedure that separates donated blood into its constituent components in order that several people may be treated from one donated unit. The development of this technology in the 1950s revealed that blood, instead of being a single, self-similar substance, is a "holding together" of red cells, platelets, and plasma—all useful in different ways for diverse types of treatment. Plasma can be further subdivided through a procedure called fractionation. Bayer and Feldman (1999: 8) state that "As blood plasma is increasingly subject to transformation by pharmaceutical firms, it is difficult to sustain the symbolic attachments evoked by whole blood." Waldby and Mitchell (2006: 43–44), too, state unequivocally that techniques of blood-splitting dilute the ontological and civic value of donated blood. My experience, however, suggests otherwise; indeed, I show now why micro-technically ordered blood may be particularly *well-suited* to evoking images of a "whole" and integrated nation. As a "heterogeneous collective" (Callon 1998: 30) of different sorts of cells, the single unit of blood, prior to its separation, can be and is understood by donors as a holding together of diversity and thus as a kind of microcosm of "national integration."

Some of the donors I spoke with at camps knew about the division procedures and some did not. However, when I asked both sets of donor what they thought about the separation of their donated blood, a recurring motif—especially among followers of gurus with universalizing orientations like Sathya Sai Baba or the Nirankari master Baba Hardev Singh, and among avowed secularists, followers of Nehru's "universalist version of nationalism" (Jaffrelot 1996: 83)—was the hope that their singularly donated unit would be transfused into three persons from three different communities.

A woman I met at a camp staged by an insurance company in New Delhi, well aware of and enthusiastic about the idea of component therapy, told me: "There is no discrimination, it is non-attachment. I am hopeful my blood will go to three different castes (*jatis*)." A Hindu devotee of Sathya Sai Baba, whom I met at a donation camp organized by devotees in Delhi, declared that he hoped his one donated unit would be split and transfused into a Christian, a Muslim, and a Sikh respectively, in order to show that all people and religions are one. He then pointed to Sai Baba's Sarvadharma symbol, assembled of emblems from the major world religions. The symbol, like the camp, the blood bank, the transfusion, and the unit of blood prior to its division, holds together signs of diverse origins, providing an image of integration. Component therapy is evidently an act of technical decomposition rather than composition, but it reveals that the unit, prior to the separation procedure, is a gathered entity and thus, like the idealized nation, a holding together of the many in the one. In imagining their singularly offered donations as forming the transfusions of several persons belonging to different castes or religions, donors see donation as an integrative action. The one gift's route to m/any serves to reveal m/any's oneness, with the undivided unit, by virtue of the diverse destinations to which, in its divided form, it travels, being construed as India herself, a gathering up and holding together—all of India, as it were, in a unit of blood.

This discussion of the "undivided" unit prior to its separation and that of the raksha bandhan camp has demonstrated the power of anonymity in creating a space for prospective enumeration on the part of donors of their gifts' possible recipients. This anonymity-enabled enumeration makes blood donation into an "extensional field" (Konrad 2005: 49) in which, to recall the exam paper, it is the "many segments of the people" constituting the nation that are extended across. Here we can draw out the implications for conceptualizations of the nation of Konrad's insistence on the inventiveness of anonymity. Konrad's claim is borne out by the data presented in this chapter, with "inventiveness" being located in the idioms of integration employed by donors in thinking about blood donation. Though Konrad distances herself from Titmuss's concern with integration, the substance of donors' creative engagement with anonymity finds a reflection in Titmuss's (1970) argument about the integrative potential of anonymous blood donation.

Anderson (1991: 90) highlights the important place of anonymity in national imaginaries, noting that "no more arresting emblems of the modern culture of nationalism exist than the cenotaphs and tombs of Unknown Soldiers . . . void as these tombs are of identifiable mortal remains or immortal souls, they are nonetheless saturated with ghostly national imaginings." Similarly unidentifiable, transfusion recipients are a medicalized variant of the "unknown soldier," invisible loci of ghostly national imaginings. Adorning the office desk of a Delhi blood bank director is a handmade poster, designed by the child of an employee, depicting a check which reads: "Pay: Unknown Soldier. Amount: one life." It is the impossibility of knowing who recipients will be which means they can be imagined as being anyone at all, and this chapter has shown that anonymity is often the occasion for imaginative traversals of India's "many segments." This book has explored multifarious usages and deployments of the anonymous conditions of voluntary blood donation in India, with a particular focus on spiritual "widenings," and familial centrifugation. The present chapter has identified a further usage of anonymity, drawing attention to its important role in Nehruvian nationalist conceptualization. Konrad employs the term "transilient" in an attempt to conceptualize oblique forms of relationality—in particular anonymized relations of multiplicity and extension (2005: 112). The anonymity of blood donation, as the condition of possibility of donors' prospective traversal of the nation's "many segments," forms the basis of a "national transilience": the enactment of threadlike imaginative extensions across diverse plurality as the folding of different constituencies into a single social field.

As was noted in chapter 3, Mauss famously saw reciprocal gifts as key instruments in the instituting and sustaining of enduring social relations and solidarity. Anonymous and nonreciprocal, voluntary blood donation appears precisely contrary to the Maussian ideal. And yet, we have seen an abundance of integrative narratives in which anonymity not only fails to thwart but actively facilitates imaginings of integration. In her foreword to Mauss's *The Gift*, Douglas (1990) is quite certain that integrative social relations and anonymity are mutually exclusive. Taking issue with Titmuss's (1970) claim that anonymously donated blood is capable of providing, in Simpson's (2004: 855) phrasing, the "invisible stitches [that could] hold society together," Douglas exclaims: "as if there could be an anonymous relationship." While I am not claiming that blood donation contributes to national integration, the fact is that some Indian donors and doctors do construct a nationalist variant upon the Maussian claim—and this for anonymously given gifts. Anonymity provides an imaginative canvas for obliquely conceived relations of multiplicity and extension, thus being a key condition of this nationalist relational reckoning. So the anonymous, nonreciprocal gift of blood that seems so clearly counter to Maussian thinking, actually turns out to conform to it—at least in terms of indigenous analyses. There are relations, plenty of relations, only not as anthropologists have traditionally conceived them.

Conclusion: Counter Currents

I have been at pains throughout to avoid the claim that Nehruvian thought has found an unproblematic refuge in the field of blood donation. Aside from the contested versions of national integration I have outlined, there are some other notable counter currents. Recruiters, for example, sometimes refer to voluntary blood donors as a "minority community" deserving of special privileges such as free medical insurance. Several recruiters even suggested there ought to be a quota of job reservations for donors. A Mumbai donor made the same point to me: "I have donated so many times. A percentage should be given to donors for jobs. There should be more recognition. They are not honored by the government." This is strongly redolent of debates surrounding caste reservations, that is, caste-based compensatory discrimination schemes based on quotas for educational access and public service employment, with different communities struggling for special privileges and access to state resources (Khilnani 1997: 57; S. Bayly 1999: 285). Where Nehruvian "ideas of India" tend to see many community populations feeding seamlessly into the one voluntary donor population that thereby connotes the very unity of the nation, the view described above sees the donor population as a "community" in competition with other caste and religious communities for state windfalls. This amounts to nothing less than the "*jati*-ization" of the donor constituency as a radical countering of Nehru's universalist vision of an integrated nation.[33]

Those broadly Nehruvian doctors who advocate donation as a means to achieve national integration tend to disparage the offering to donors of material incentives such as free insurance or other benefits. Several told me that the giving of clocks, T-shirts, mugs, and food by the Lions and Rotary blood banks can be explained by the fact that both institutions are funded and peopled by a "lot of *agarwals*." The people I am calling "Nehruvian" in outlook have a longstanding predilection for disparaging certain widely recognized forms of what they see as venality and vulgarity—traits stereotypically associated with a money-grubbing *bania*-caste mentality (see Hardiman 1996; Laidlaw 1995: 88–89). Several Mumbai doctors similarly complained to me about the business-minded *khatri* community's influence within the NGOs that collaborate with blood banks to organize camps in the city at which anything from steel plates to kitchen tiles are provided as incentives.[34] Such doctors are reminiscent of the "high-minded Hindu," described by Bailey (1981: 23), "who does what is right because it is right."[35] Blood donation, according to these professionals, like other virtuous activities, should remain "exempted from the process of accounting" (Bailey 1981: 25). Thus, not only is the high-minded doctors' broadly Nehruvian commitment to national integration seen as being under threat from competing Hindutva and reservation-related claims, doctors also seek to protect blood donation from what they perceive as the creeping bania influence that would reinstate crassly self-interested and materialist values into an arena within which, with the banning of paid donation, they are meant to be taboo.

Some doctors, however, do view what they see as the bania-fication of blood solicitation techniques as a necessary evil. This approach could be termed an "impure pragmatics." One Bangalore doctor, for instance, employs a slogan that directs donors' attention to the putative health benefits of donation: "An apple a day keeps the doctor away, but a couple of donations a year keeps the cardiologist at bay." Reflecting on his slogan, the doctor told me: "The primary motivation should be to donate selflessly as a dan, as nishkam seva, not to protect from heart disease. But it is *kali yug* so I feel I can use this for motivational purposes."[36] This impure pragmatics, in which doctors continue to exalt nonreciprocal dan rhetorically while, with regret, recognizing its practical unfeasibility, appears to be gaining some currency—at least in Delhi.

The ideology of voluntary blood donation is thus contested terrain and, as these counter currents demonstrate, Nehruvian thinking by no means dominates the field. But neither can it be dismissed as dead and buried, which has been a tendency in many recent writings on the apparently unstoppable spread of anti-secular Hindutva and other clearly non-Nehruvian ideas and perspectives in contemporary India. This chapter has explored the continuing conceptual power and prevalence of the Nehruvian ideology of national integration, identified a particular scenography according to which images of integration are staged, and focused on the moral significance of anonymity in the formation of what I earlier termed the difference-traversing gift. I suggested that it is not merely from the physical connectivity of blood donation that the ideology of national integration is made physically manifest and potent but also through a powerful combination of anonymity as an imaginative canvas and a series of moments of gathering—of persons, blood units, and separable cells—which together form the "vein-to-vein chain."

The chapter has also focused attention on the important place of enumeration as a component of the aforementioned scenography. What Kapila has shown in a discussion of how the Gaddi pastoral group of Himachal Pradesh went about securing "Scheduled Tribe" status is how the "unifying . . . modernizing nationalist discourse" and "separating technologies of governmentality" go hand in hand; for "in its pursuit of unity, the Indian state has been forced into the recognition of ever more evolved forms of cultural difference" (2008: 129). The point is made in reference to the politics of recognition and redistribution, but it has wider implications. Separation and unification frequently proceed together in other contexts too, for separation produces the entities to be unified (contained). This chapter has argued that the analytical implications of enumeration are not exhausted by existing emphases on fixity and fissiparousness. As a necessary condition of congregative thought, enumeration contains other possibilities too. The examples presented here attest that the scenography of integration relies on separate and separable identities for the promissory visions of a national "holding together" they instantiate.

Such a scenography is well suited to the gathering procedures of blood donation's vein to vein chain which are capable of reproducing it at a variety of scales. The cohesive nation can be encapsulated, via this scenography, in a geographic territory, a camp, a single unit of blood, a transfusion and so on. The existence of this scalar framework—the fact that different parties should wish to replicate the scenography of integration on different planes—suggests that at a time when the Nehruvian worldview is supposedly under threat in all sorts of domains of Indian life, Nehruvian thought continues to possess a powerful and creative presence in the Indian blood donation milieu. Blood procurement technologies of gathering and disbursal provide instantiations of national integration in vivo, its recreation and reassertion demonstrating that it is a project, rather than a given datum, which continues as an ongoing labor in new and unexpected contexts.

8

Conclusion

MARK but this flea, and mark in this,
How little that which thou deny'st me is;
It suck'd me first, and now sucks thee,
And in this flea, our two bloods mingled be;
Thou know'st that this cannot be said
A sin, nor shame, nor loss of maidenhead,
Yet this enjoys before it woo,
And pamper'd swells with one blood made of two,
And this, alas, is more than we would do.

John Donne, "The Flea"

To conclude I begin by reviewing the themes of time-space distanciation and Nehruvian thinking, and demonstrate a significant connection between them. In my discussion of "donor-soldiers" in chapter 6, I noted that blood donation enables Sant Nirankari and Dera Sacha Sauda devotees, from a distance, to play an intimate role in the nation's military affairs. The distanciating function of blood donation, through which simultaneous convergence and separation is achieved between different entities, is vital here. The potentially fraught commitment of the patriotic devotee of soldierly provenance to the values of ahimsa is made experientially practicable by way of this corporeal system of concurrent intimacy and distance. Indeed, one of the most obvious but important facts about blood donation is that, at the point of transfusion, the donor is present in absentia. This is the case in all countries but has particularly significant implications in India. Like money, which, "owing to the abstractness of its form . . . can exercise its effects upon the most remote areas" (Simmel 1991: 504), anonymous voluntary blood donation enables donors to act in various ways at a distance. A further key distanciation function comes into view in an interesting conjunction with what I have been calling Nehruvian thinking.

Consider now the stanza reproduced above from Donne's "The Flea." Swelling "with one blood made of two," the blood of the poet and his lady is "mingled" in the flea but the "donors" themselves are present only in absentia. As Paglia remarks, "The couple have somehow vaulted to procreation without sexual intercourse." With their blood mingling, but at a distance from their own bodies, the flea has become their "weird child" (Paglia 2005), despite the lack of direct sexual contact.

The logic of mixing at one remove conveyed in the poem can, I believe, shed light on Nehruvian thinking and conflicted ideas about caste. Donors and doctors often claim that voluntary blood donation constitutes an active means of transgressing caste distinctions, thereby rendering them irrelevant—biological continuities following blood group rather than caste substance. In broad terms I would call this approach Nehruvian. Throughout my fieldwork, however, I was struck by the fact that many of those who express vigorous anti-caste sentiments nevertheless employ "clean caste" cooks and justify having no contact with blood bank cleaners and city sweepers for reasons of hygiene. One bania acquaintance of mine, for instance, who expressed the hope that his blood would be transfused into recipients of a caste other than his in order to show that "we are all one," declines to eat with the cleaning staff at the school in which he teaches.[1] The donation of blood by those who claim to be anticaste but who nevertheless harbor misgivings about contact with "unclean" caste members appears to allow them to "perform" the anticaste sentiments they profess. What could be more anticaste than mixing one's substance with that of one from any conceivable jati? And yet this is a mixing at one remove from the donor—blood donation enables nonimperiling contact with others, just as the distanciation function of the flea enabled Donne and his lover to vault to procreation with no "loss of maidenhead."

I have briefly discussed issues concerning nonimperilling caste contact in order to show that distanciation can be subject to deployments beyond moral dilemmas about violence. There is a more general point, which is that blood donation opens up new possibilities of connective configuration in enabling donors to form relations at one remove. This study has presented just two examples of this—Nirankari and Sacha Sauda soldiering from a distance and "anticaste" mixing at a distance—though there may well be others that I did not encounter directly during ethnographic research. What seems clear is that the time-space distanciation aspect of blood donation permits a "secret sympathy" between variegated conceptions of violence and caste, enabling certain types of blood giver to adhere to and yet to simultaneously disavow martial commitments and caste distinctions. As Laidlaw (1995: 21) notes, logical consistency is "not something which is necessarily there to be found." Rather, "it takes work to create, reproduce, and maintain it, and it is always partial." In situations of apparently divergent allegiances, blood donation can facilitate partial and provisional experiential solutions, its properties of distanciation, in certain situations, enabling complex accommodations between different aims and imperatives.

The blood bank's mediating role ensures that donors and recipients do not meet and is therefore the guarantor of the anonymity which facilitates time-space distanciation. In making blood donation "work" to produce particular effects, it is most often its anonymity that is operationalized. In chapter 7, I explored the nationalist implications of anonymity, arguing that it offers an imaginative canvas that enables donors to prospectively enumerate and thereby conceptually gather together along "community" lines the gift's possible recipients. Building on Konrad's path-breaking work on anonymity, I proposed the term "national transilience" in order to draw attention to the significance of anonymous relations of extension and multiplicity in processes of nationalist ideation. Chapter 5 demonstrated a further usage of anonymity as a means to portray conspicuous extraction and benefaction as a secret gift. Anonymity also plays a vital role in the "centrifuge" of directional intentionalities required by the formal conceptual logic underpinning the institutional transition from replacement to a voluntary blood donation system in which blood is donated for m/any rather than for singular, known recipients.

This centrifuge of directional intentionalities connects with and helps bring forth other processes of "widening" through what I called centrifugal alliances. As was seen in chapters 2 and 7, concepts of family are one key area of widening (cf. Harriss 2003). In a further example, chapter 4 demonstrated that Nirankari spiritual expansionism finds a key facilitative structure in the centrifugal pathways of voluntary donation which enable devotees' viscous love to travel to m/any. The "feedback" in each of these cases of "active not knowing" is the practical provision of materia medica which brings to fruition the formal systemic transition that is under way. This formal transition requires not only the centrifugation of directional intentionalities but is also heavily dependent on temporal centrifugation: voluntary donation requires not one-time extravagant extractions but "widened out," routinized giving activity.

Chapters 2 and 3 in particular explored questions concerning the morality of widening, with the ideology of voluntary blood donation locating virtue squarely within centrifugal directional intentionalities and the mechanical transgression of community distinctions. It follows that centripetal directional intentionalities, where, for instance, blood is explicitly donated for one community and not another, have attained an ignominious stature of transgression: soon after the extreme sectarian violence that engulfed the state of Gujarat in 2002, a recruiter in urgent need of blood went to a Hindu guru and was provided with 200 donations: "As the camp was finishing [the guru] told me his devotees had requested the blood go only to Hindus. I said, No way! At the same time a Muslim hospital told me they needed blood. I said come and take it. We provided the blood. After 15 days there were 70 Muslim donors at my [Red Cross] blood bank saying that they were ready to reciprocate the help done for them by donating for the Hindus. I said, forget it. I will give the blood to anyone, not

Hindus." Conversely, shortly after the catastrophic "Boxing Day tsunami" struck the coastal regions of south and southeast Asia in December 2004, an eighty-two-year-old widow from Kolkata was reported to have donated to the relief effort "the Rs 2,001 she was going to spend on her late husband's annual *shradh* ceremony."[2] In distributing the resources earmarked for the memorial rites of her dead husband instead to the needy and unknown victims of a natural disaster, she "centrifuged" her offering from one to m/any, causing it to resonate with the transition in modes of giving blood which has been the focus of this study.

And yet, as was argued in chapters 1 and 4, centrifugal movements are frequently structured according to centripetal patterns. To take the example of the Nirankari guru, the two sorts of directional movement interlock in a "to" and "through" model, with gifts singularly (centripetally) aimed at the guru by devotees subsequently being multiply refracted by him toward "humanity." Simultaneously recipient and donor, the guru repersonalizes the gift, even as the formal changeover to a voluntary system seems to depersonalize it. The Nirankari case is a particularly striking example of a wider set of comparable instances in which a specific object is relied upon to facilitate the abstracted gift. In chapter 1, the example was given of a thalassemic child, and death anniversary and birthday donation camps are further cases in which specific personalities constitute the multiply refractive cynosures of donation. The transition to a voluntary system thus reflects Ramanujan's (1989) claim that while modernization in India can be seen as a movement from the context-sensitive toward the context-free, the context-free is prone to become subject to complex processes of recontextualization (Ramanujan 1989: 55, 57).

In addition to these processes of repersonalization, chapters 2 and 7 focused on analogous instances of refamilialization. The complex and paradoxical trajectory of the relation between blood donation and sacrifice presents a comparable picture. Cohen (2001: 18) has explored prevalent public representations of intrafamilial corporeal sacrifice, such as kidney selling to raise dowry funds, as a means of restoring conventional kinship structures and dependencies seen as under threat from "selfish, Western modernity." Replacement blood donation similarly centers on familial obligation and sacrifice—especially for the many relatives who are unconvinced of the safety of blood donation but who nonetheless donate their blood. The policy shift to voluntary donation removes these sacrificial flows from what many see as their natural familial domain, and has also necessitated a set of campaigns designed to counter the widespread association between donation and physical peril. Indeed, chapter 1 discussed Delhi recruiters' attempts to portray donation as a health-enhancing activity through promoting a purificatory, even yogic conception of the activity.

And yet, just as the compelling forces of payment, family, and personal specificity resurface (albeit transfigured) as incubuses within a voluntary mode officially resistant to them, several forms of sacrificial logic retain a powerful presence within the new system. As was seen in chapters 3 and 6, blood dona-tion as sacrifice for the nation or expression of *desh-bhakti* is an established theme in donor solicitation. The "freedom fighter" songs frequently played at corporate and educational donation camps are one such example, as are the camps staged in honor of policemen or soldiers considered to have shed their blood for the nation. These camps share with those held in memory of assassi-nated gurus and politicians a familiar sacrificial template—commemorative blood donation retrospectively bestows on the original death capacities of regeneration, the victim bringing forth new life via the blood donations enacted in his or her memory.

A further distinct but connected dimension of the relation between sacri-fice and blood donation came into focus in chapter 6. For one animal rights organization, the life-giving bloodshed of blood donation is enacted on Kali Puja as the substitutive ennoblement of the life-taking bloodshed of animal sacrifice—a practice closely associated with the worship of this bloodthirsty Bengal goddess. Strongly recalling instances discussed in chapter 3 of blood donation as the substitutive ennoblement of instances of "waste" and "extrava-gance" such as pind-dan and feasting, there is also a sense here in which blood donation joins the lopping of cucumbers and lemons as a consummate reformist practice of nonviolence. But blood donation possesses neither a trans-parent nor a singular relationship with violence and nonviolence. Even in the instance of Kali Puja it cannot but refer to violence in substituting for it. What I drew attention to in chapter 6 is the mediating, double-edged role of blood donation in the subcontinent through which it has become both an exemplary sign of nonviolence and a means of engaging in violent action at one remove (cf. Pocock 1973).

As was mentioned in chapter 3, classical dan is "officially" a surrogate for both asceticism and sacrifice in the Age of Kali (Parry 1994: 190). That human blood is given on Kali Puja brings sacrifice full circle, with human substance substituting for that of the animals substituting for humans. In a comparable move, there is a sense in which Nirankari and Sacha Sauda rakt-dan, which in various ways translates blood donation into ascetic practice, reclaims the ascet-icism which dan is meant to imitate. Attempts to donate blood despite being physically unfit to do so (chapter 4), or to give twice at one camp (chapter 5), or three times on consecutive days (chapter 3) suggest a conception of blood dona-tion as an austerity. Self-denying on one level, it is "enlightened self-interest" on another. Inwardly directed forms of asceticism such as these, where "returns" such as blessings and spiritual advancement are key motivating factors, may be considered "centripetal asceticism." Centripetal asceticism enacted in blood donation contexts endangers transfusion recipients because it propels the med-ically unfit toward donation, who welcome it as an austerity. This brand of asceticism is evidence, in Strathern's (1988: 131–132) words, that "intention and motivation have physiological consequences. The person is vulnerable, so to speak, both to the bodily disposition of others toward him or her and to their wills and desires." What I wish to emphasize here is that centripetal asceticism appears to conflict with another mode of asceticism that I call "donation asceticism." I now take further the arguments of chapter 4 in delineating these contrasting modes of asceticism.

"Donation asceticism" refers to the ways in which the doctrine of voluntary donation as formulated by international arbiters of health policy such as the WHO and the Red Cross makes demands on donors, requiring that they enact self-care as the simultaneous care of the other (the transfusion recipient). This brand of asceticism applies and is responsive to the contemporary globalized blood donation ecumene (S. Bayly 2004b: 321; Hannerz 1999) and is encapsulated in the slogan, "Safe Blood Starts with Me," which, originally formulated by the WHO, has been adopted by various medical authorities and institutions worldwide including those in India. An apparently fairly vapid slogan, possessed neither of dense signification nor particular moral weight, it in fact suggests that donors' conduct and desires must be subjected to "habits of control and self-surveillance" (Laidlaw 1995: 189). Voluntary donors, so reads the subtext, must abstain from actions such as drug use or sexual promiscuity that might lead to the transmission of infection to recipients. Moreover, the two primary functions of the first World Blood Donor Day, held on 14 June 2004, were to thank donors and *to promote healthy lifestyles* among them. The French Voluntary Blood Donors Code of Honor, to which I referred in chapter 4, states: "I declare on my honor:—to remain worthy of being a Voluntary Blood Donor, respecting the rules of morality, good behavior, and solidarity with fellow human beings" (Ray 1990: 69).

This French code recalls the formal vows undertaken by initiate renouncers (see Laidlaw 2005; van der Veer 1988: 118–119), and the doctrine of voluntary donation does indeed make ascetic demands on donors, with asceticism defined here as "a regime of self-imposed but at the same time authoritatively prescribed and ordered bodily disciplines" (Laidlaw 1995: 151). In Alter's (1992: 324) view, "a key symbol of the [classically defined] *sannyasi*'s world renunciation is his mastery of sensual desire." Donor-ascetics must similarly control their desires and pledge—implicitly or explicitly—to enact "responsible" corporeal trusteeship. The following example again recalls the renouncer's vow: when the son of a friend of mine in Delhi turned eighteen he made a pledge (*sankalp*) to donate blood three times a year until the age of seventy, recognizing that it is was his responsibility (*jimmedari*) to live healthily and take precautions to avert the causes of hypertension, diabetes, or any other disqualifying condition that could make him an agent of the transmission of infection. Foucault's (1984: 47) term "gift-obligation" draws attention to the interrelation of freedom and diligence characteristic of the care of the self as found in Epictetus's *Discourses*, but something like the same nuanced interrelation is also a feature of the expectations placed upon voluntary donors. To be a blood donor is to enter a subtle complex of duty and obligation—one is asked to safeguard that part of oneself which may become part of another.

The modes of religious asceticism described by Laidlaw (2005) and van der Veer (1988) differ from donation asceticism in that they are undertaken for the "centripetal" purpose of self-perfection and subsequent freedom from rebirth. Donation asceticism, instead, possesses a centrifugal quality: donors engage in bodily discipline for the protection of the m/any abstract future recipients of their donated blood.[3] This can best be understood in proprietorial terms, since there is a sense in which repeat donors are expected to "renounce" ownership of their bodies and instead enact a futurially oriented "distributed ownership." The term "corporeal trusteeship," employed above, is apt. The trustee administers another's property for a specified purpose. Donation asceticism proposes a corporeal extension of the same idea. Repeat blood donors "administer" their bodies on behalf of hypothetical future recipients (their bodies' "owners"). Additional bodily care and defense is required because as repeat donors, their bodies are no longer *only* their own. Strathern (n.d.) writes that "there are diverse ways in which [people] might be said to 'own' one another." In this instance, the donor's body is "owned" by a quantity of persons equivalent to the sum of its future extractions. Donation asceticism reflects one such previously unacknowledged way in which implicit claims are made by persons on other persons. (Future recipient "owners" remain, of course, abstract and hypothetical, with claims being made on their behalf by proponents of the doctrine of voluntary donation.)

Whereas donation asceticism makes recipients central in opening up the donor's body to their ownership, the fusion between centripetal, or self-oriented, asceticism and blood donation conceptually effaces transfusion recipients, with donation enrolled as an austerity "to improve the condition of [the devotee-donor's] soul" (Laidlaw 1995: 152). The latter brand of asceticism volitionally "conceals" the very recipients the former is designed to protect. The issue of recipient concealment was discussed in chapters 4 and 5. And yet, there need not be a conflict between these modes of asceticism. As was seen in chapter 4, a group of Thai Buddhist monks has configured the relationship between merit, act, and effect in such a way that foregrounds the enactment of responsibility for vulnerable recipients as the very condition of obtaining merit. Such an innovative configuration demonstrates how the safety requirements of blood donation and devotees' concern with merit might be fruitfully reconciled. It could in consequence serve as a kind of ascetic template for devotional orders such as the Dera Sacha Sauda and Sant Nirankaris. What I hope to have shown here is that juxtaposition of fresh ethnographic data from the corporeal donation ecumene with the rich anthropological literature on "classical" asceticism can shed new light on emergent interrelations between biomedicine, asceticism, and responsibility.

A further important dimension of this study has been a focus on the complex intertwinings between blood donation and Nehruvian modes of conceptualization. Chapter 3 considered a photograph of Nehru donating blood, placing it in the context of Nehruvian sacrificial logics. A broadly Nehruvian disparagement of the "bania-fication" of donor solicitation was also discussed, as were depictions of voluntary blood donors as a jati-like minority community. As chapter 7 showed, however, the most striking manifestation of Nehruvian thinking in the blood donation milieu is that which relates to "national integration." Anthropologists have long been somewhat overawed by and seemingly unable to move beyond the rise in extremist Hinduism. The Hindutva phenomenon is, of course, of critical significance but it is not and has never been the only game in town. In a challenge to the prevailing assumption that the only thing that counts politically in India today is the debunking or overriding of Nehruvian ideals of the secular inclusive nation, the present study has rehabilitated Nehruvianism and secularism as important ethnographic subjects. This has been through a focus on national integration, an aspect of Nehruvian secularism that is often overlooked and which has found a key sanctuary in the emergent Indian ideology of voluntary blood donation.

Anthropologists have over recent years learned the important lesson that ethnographic expectations of integration can come "at the expense of vividly imagined ethical life" (Laidlaw 1995: 389). But this of course should not cause them to overlook vividly imagined indigenous analytics of integration. The Nehruvian integrative tool kit consists of a scenography of gathering and spatial concentration and of the anonymous conditions of donation. Both factors enable modes of enumeration that obsessively locate the diverse sources of the gathered entities (whether conceptual, physical, or both). Powerful correlations are thereby set up with the idea of a multiply composed and yet singularly coherent nation.

This study has been particularly concerned with the ways in which practices of enumeration and calculation operate in ways that move between and across categories of the "spiritual" and the ostensibly scientific or utilitarian. As was seen in chapters 2, 3, and 5, the quantification of seva is an important qualitative aspect of devotional practice and more generally of the ways in which donors envisage their giving. Mass camps are a case in point. Such events of conspicuous extraction produce gargantuan numbers for publicity purposes, but on the level of the individual devotee who wishes to donate twice or thrice, numbers are in an intimate relation with sacrifice and merit. If in such instances the three months meant to elapse between donations acts as a bar to grand extractive gestures capable of building up merit, chapter 2 showed how

Hinduism's existing calculative repertoire can interact with new blood bank technology to produce a possible solution. This novel conjunction is seen to generate meritorious multiplications not through the giving of more but through the treatment of donated blood in order to increase its destinations. What results is the technological production of merit.

To further demonstrate Indian blood donors' propensity to treat numbers not as stable objects but as protean conceptual material, I briefly refer to blood bank director Dr. Bhatia's virtuoso reflections concerning apheresis, a special form of component therapy in which only one component of donors' blood is removed, the "leftover" portion being transfused into them even as they donate. Since this allows more to be taken of a specific component than is obtainable from conventional donations, recipients in need of only one component can avoid having to have a multiply sourced and therefore riskier transfusion. As Bhatia puts it: "the apheresis donor can donate platelets every 48 hours because platelets get regenerated within 48 hours in the body. So every 48 hours you can donate your platelets, we say subject to a maximum of 24 times in a year." Apheresis thus enables donors to donate with increased frequency. As was seen in chapter 2, conventional component therapy enables three or four recipients to receive blood deriving from a single donation. Bhatia combines the two arithmetical models of component separation and apheresis to produce an arresting figure of massively expanded gift destinations: "You donate your platelets 24 times per year, so you help or save 24 lives through the apheresis system, plus you donate your blood four times a year—and each of these units gets separated into at least three components; thereby you are helping another 12 lives. So the total you can save is 36 lives in one year. If you donate for about 40 years from 18–60 years of age, 1,200–1,500 people will be saved during the lifespan of a healthy, active, regular voluntary donor." The figure prior to component separation and apheresis for a lifetime of lifesaving was a comparatively paltry 168.

Consider now a recruitment poster sponsored by the Canara Bank Social Banking Cell, widely displayed before the advent of the new arithmetic of component therapy, which contains the text: "Between the ages of 18–60 you can save 168 lives. How many lives have you saved so far?" The analogy here between saving money and lives suggests possible interrelations between banks of money, merit, and blood. Since units of blood may at the same time be units of merit (see chapter 2), one can "save up" the lives one has saved in the karma bank and also make withdrawals.[4] As a female teacher told me, "*simran* [remembering God] is like a bank (*kosh*). You are storing something. You store your good deeds and your simran and you can cash it any time. When you need money you go to the bank, so when you are suffering too much you say to God, Oh help me, and He will say, this person never forgot me, so how can I let him down now?" At a recruitment event staged before Delhi schoolchildren, this overlapping of varieties of bank was made explicit in a song adapted by a medical student from the film *Mukadar ka Sikander* (The Luck of the Winner):

> Do a great contribution of rakt-dan and earn punya.
> The whole life we work hard to fill our banks with money,
> But if we devote our deeds to *punya-karma* [meritorious action]
> We can fill up our banks with good deeds.

So Bhatia's numerical emphasis draws attention to the quantitative basis of much seva activity and the related calculability of spiritual credit, but his personal donation theology goes even further. As was seen in chapter 3, Bhatia recently addressed a large gathering of students of the yoga guru Swami Ramdev at which a donation camp had been organized: "You people will probably not think that what Swami Ji is telling you about *pranayam* [a yogic breathing technique] and meditative posture is like a single act of blood donation, but just do blood donation and you will automatically go into those states. Do it more regularly, do it more regularly, still more regularly, get into apheresis, get apheresis done every 48 hours. Maybe another technique comes up tomorrow where every five minutes you can give something—who knows? Science might develop something where everyday you can give blood and this will be *satat dyan* [a continuous meditation]." In this prospective regime of total donation, meditation is medicalized, machinic, and unending.

But why should Ramdev's students reach yogic and meditative states through blood donation? The answer lies in a "metacorrespondence" (Alter 2004: 78) between yoga and blood donation which centers on oneness and the universal. "Meditation," says Bhatia, "is the method of communicating with the creator. It is a mode to realize the oneness of everything. Blood donation is equal to meditation in this manner: your donated blood goes into many patients." The high-frequency donation enabled by apheresis and the concurrent distribution to numerous recipients enabled by component therapy radically multiplies the extensional reach of donors, and it is this which generates a sense for Bhatia of a cosmic, universal connectivity and therefore of a kind of technological samadhi. Samadhi, the telos of yoga in which the individual self is united with the universal Self, similarly dissolves oppositions of subject and object, observer and observed (Alter 2004: 95, 100). Further, the narrowing of the interval between donations enabled by apheresis leads Bhatia to envisage no intervals at all, with donation assuming a state of uninterrupted continuousness—this being a further key attribute of samadhi.[5] A "reflective practitioner" (Schön 2002), Bhatia's theorizing of a cosmic yoga achievable through continuous donation and the multiplication of recipients concerns envisaged states of being rather than actual practices. This study too has unabashedly had as much to do with ways of thinking about blood donation as with actual donation activity.

What Bhatia describes are potential spiritual effects consequent on the increased "technicity" of blood. In a related manner, chapter 2 portrayed component separation as a kind of technological supplement to auspiciousness, while chapter 7 noted how the divisibility of singular blood units can be imagined according to nationalist templates of "unity in diversity." "Technicity" is an analytic term developed by Waldby and Mitchell in their recent work on biological exchange. Their focus is on "the intersection of the material qualities of tissues—their location and function in the body, their durability, their immunological specificity—with the kinds of technology available to procure, potentiate, store and distribute them." The "complex technical ordering" of tissues in order to make them more prolific amounts, they say, to a kind of husbandry (Waldby and Mitchell 2006: 32–33). The authors' focus on technicity is apt and a significant contribution, even if the argumentation is somewhat empirically sparse. The present study complements that of Waldby and Mitchell in providing ethnographic specificity concerning the engagements of real people with the husbandry of tissues, demonstrating that the "biotechnical leverage" of such tissues can produce prolific effects for imaginings of spirit and the nation as well as markets. To paraphrase Waldby and Mitchell (ibid.: 30), this study has shown how the human body's productivity is sutured into *and plays a transformative role in relation to* religions of productivity and productive national imaginings.

In addition to questions concerning multiple units of blood and merit, multiplicity also arose as a methodological issue: I conducted fieldwork in multiple settings among multiple communities; camps are composed of multiple collaborators and multiple meanings about blood donation are constantly being generated. The donation camp in particular is frequently the locus of extremely interesting juxtapositions; to paraphrase Pinney (2006), individuals who outside the camp might not inhabit the same terrain are here brought within a common epistemological space. A critical part of the theoretical aim of this study has thus been to provide a vocabulary that acknowledges that there exist multiple understandings of blood donation but which at the same time recognizes the bridge of common thought and action which bestows some semblance of order on this plurality. Blood donation is the thing ("boundary object") which "sits in the middle" of a set of heterogeneous participants ("communities of practice"). The object that unites these diverse constituencies is also that about which they have signally contrasting ideas. "Rationalist" doctors participate in camps cheek by jowl with devotee-donors adamant that their viscous love-imbued blood will foster the expansion of their order. Of course, excessive collection and attempts to donate by the medically unfit cause consternation among doctors, but the production of "bad meanings" is a risk built into solicitation techniques that actively customize donation for appropriation and resignification by extremely diverse communities of practice.

This returns us to the interoperability of north Indian devotional orders and campaigns to promote voluntary donation, the subject of chapters 4–6. I used "interoperability" to describe the ways in which these phenomena interlock and bring each other to fruition. However, the focus has also been on the frequent problematic divergences at the heart of the relationship: what has resulted, perhaps, is disjunctive synthesis. Nevertheless, in working through each other, significant quantities of blood are provided to blood banks for transfusion, while for devotional orders, the collaboration with biomedicine makes available to them a wellspring of new and surprising devotional possibilities from which to shape their religious lives.

What voluntary blood donation procedures offer devotional movements is a harnessable centrifugal directionality and an apparently unambiguous engagement with social utility. Utility-valorizing orders ("religions of utility") such as the Sant Nirankaris and the Dera Sacha Sauda are committed to spiritual operations that possess a complex but discernible manifestation in a utility irreducible to valueless instrumentality. There do exist, however, ambiguities and counteradaptive tendencies: as was seen in chapter 5, for example, doctors claim the Dera Sacha Sauda smothers utility in its quantitative embrace. But the fact that this movement employs utility as a means to sanction its mode of spectacular religiosity in fact says something about utility's elevated stature; that is, the power of "utility" is actually demonstrated as a circulating store of virtue in its being employed to sanctify or at least facilitate its own oppositional force.

Chapter 3 explored the exaptation of the gift, arguing that culturally and historically transmitted forms and structures are in the process of being extended into "fresh involvements" (Crease 1997: 222) with utility. The logic of parasiting is not one of erasure but of insinuation and augmentation. Modes of classical giving reemerge in the forms extended from them. The process is almost one of revelation: recruiters and other interpretive entrepreneurs revisit the "medley" of ancient and extant cultural forms, revealing them to be not only congruent with but active catalysts of utility. Of course, "utility" is a contested category and any definition of it must be provisional. But that provided by Bataille (1985) which sees utility as a signifier of conservation and production is helpfully lucid and resonates with blood donation in several important ways. I would point here in particular to the depictions discussed in chapter 2 of donated blood as an indispensable force of familial conservatism, and to the discussion in chapter 6 of donating blood as a Vishnuite project to help preserve and sustain a populace in imminent danger of calamitous harm.

All this is evidence that utility is far from being a mere abstraction devoid of ethical content and divorced from context. Some of the more dramatic manifestations of virtuous utility are provided by the gurus who induct their devotees into its purview. Building on the "to" and "through" model of gift repersonalization presented in chapters 1 and 4, chapter 6 attempted to locate more precisely the role played by gurus in Indian blood donation activity and also more widely in Indian society, arguing for an understanding of gurus as gateway figures through which their devotees pass into an osmotically produced modernity. Through the operations performed on identifiably modernist tenets such as utility by the gurus who advance them, such tenets come to be saturated with spiritual significance and amenable to incorporation within diverse sorts of donation theology. Biomedical utility is not just biomedical utility—it is the sum of its interactions with other phenomena: yoga, ayurveda, devotional religion, and different sorts of guru are some of its most significant constitutive elements in its Indian manifestation. The guru as gateway compellingly demonstrates how interaction between religious practice and medical utility may result not in the disenchantment of religion but in the sacralization of utility.

In a noteworthy recent contribution to the study of "sects" in India, Shah (2006) calls for an approach to such religious configurations that would place them in the context of their role in society as a whole rather than more narrowly in "Indian religion." My focus here on the seva activities of religious movements in the sant tradition would appear to be in line with such an approach, especially since the devotional orders documented here are in the vanguard of the wider phenomenon of the "making social" of the gift—and what is the making social of their seva activities in order that they come to serve m/any if not a widening out and a movement beyond themselves? This study has delineated the contours of a very particular orientation toward "society" and "humanity" on the part of north Indian sant devotees which attains its dynamism by virtue of a "to" and "through" movement toward and beyond the key intermediary agent and devotional cynosure—the multiply refractive guru.

As a kind of afterthought and pointer for future enquiry, Shah alludes in the final parts of his article to important processes of change under way in the array of Hindu sects. Here lies part of the value of the present study. In attempting to describe and account for the place of devotional movements in Indian blood donation settings and also more widely in contemporary life, I have explored their multiple engagements with utility and ultimately their transmutation into religions of utility. While the main focus of Shah's article lies elsewhere, on the relationship between sects, renunciation, and caste, Shah (2006: 244) does briefly refer to the contribution of sects to "modern, secular, developmental activities" such as relief work after major disasters, the setting up of hospitals and colleges, and so on. Chapters 3–6 of the present study, however, provided ample evidence that so far as north Indian sant movements are concerned, the donation of blood is hardly a secular activity (though it may buttress "secularism"; see chapter 7). Shah is, though, broadly correct in seeing the pursuit of such development activities as bringing sects into a closer relationship with the state. More accurate, however, would be an understanding that saw the former as substituting for rather than cooperating with the latter. According to Rao

(2003), economic liberalization (she calls it "neoliberalism") in India has created a situation where "the state must continue to assert a protective relationship to its largely poor population while withdrawing from its welfare role in
practice." If this argument were to be accepted—and I believe there are grounds
for doing so—then an interesting conclusion would follow. If devotional networks such as the Dera Sacha Sauda and Sant Nirankaris can legitimately be
understood as providing services that prior to liberalization would have
emanated from state authorities, then one unintended consequence of economic liberalization, it could be argued, is the religious dynamism and efflorescent biospiritual medical creativity formed in interaction with biomedical and
other developmental projects that presently marks north Indian "religious
society."

This biospiritual medical creativity—and by creativity I mean striking
processes of "carrying forward" in which actors "apply everything that has been
culturally and historically transmitted to [them] and . . . wind up acting originally and with fresh involvements" (Crease 1997: 222)—is a "dispersed creativity"
(Leach 2004) that occurs at several different levels and locales. As was seen in
chapter 6, gurus enact this creativity in shaping various sorts of donation theology, and recruiters too engage in creative acts of customization. But donors as
well provide some of the most remarkable instances: donation as a mode of capture or physical austerity, component separation as a technological means of
merit production, and so on. This all seems to suggest that biomedicine in its
north Indian manifestation is much less a terrain of loss and "cognitive enslave-
ments" (S. Bayly 2004b: 340) than a storehouse of manipulable conceptual
material ripe for spiritual expropriation.

But "creativity" is a term much in vogue and requires caution. Osborne
(2003: 508, 510) complains that it has become a central doctrine of contemporary global culture, a kind of moral imperative and a form of capital in its own
right. The Hindu tradition in India has frequently been described by anthropologists as creative and protean (for example, Babb 1986: 1), and Mazzarella (2003:
282) argues that this presumption is mobilized to justify the imposition of all
kinds of social and economic change in India, with Hinduism's famed versatility
pulled into service as a "prophylactic" against all potentially debilitating social
transformation. Pinney (2006) too argues persuasively against what he sees as
an anthropological affinity with creative reformulation, "heroic man (and his
"culture") [always] break[ing] free from the determinations of technology."

Several points follow from this. First, whatever the predilections of anthropology at large, much of the existing literature on corporeal donation is highly
deterministic, and the multiple parasitings, extensions, and instances of
biospiritual creativity that characterize the Indian involvement with blood
donation thus present a significant challenge to it. Second, while I am largely
sympathetic to Pinney's argument, what is in essence a theoretical rejoinder

should not blind ethnographers to real cases of creative change. Third, it must be stated emphatically that an acknowledgment of creativity does not preclude due recognition of disciplinary or deterministic processes. Dr. Bhatia's linking of yoga and blood donation before an audience of Swami Ramdev's yoga students may have been instrumentally grounded as a means to bolster donations, but that does not mean it wasn't creative. His pressing of yoga into a fresh involvement with blood donation was both highly innovative and the very means of medical utility's instrumental advancement.

Finally, my study has at no stage naively celebrated the instances of creativity it has documented. This book has delineated the deployability of gurus' captive voluntary devotees and recognized that on one level biospiritual medical creativity is indeed a political economy of innovation designed to make Indians bioavailable for extractive purposes. While many examples have been presented of conscientious recruiters eager not only to persuade people to give blood but also to persuade them to give it in the right way, this study has also been unequivocal in acknowledging that many recruiters consider gurus' devotees convenient donor banks. According to some of them at least, the activation of these donor banks is a shortcut method of acquiring blood where "from the master of discipline [the guru] to him who is subjected to it [the devotee] the relation is one of signalization: it is a question not of understanding the injunction but of perceiving the signal and reacting to it immediately" (Foucault 1977: 166).

And yet to state that recruiters simply appropriate gurus' devotee bases, with devotees becoming mere "inscription surfaces" (Kittler cited in Pinney 2006) of medical utility, would be to eviscerate devotees' own experiences and the ways in which they and their gurus employ biomedical procedures as a rich corpus of conceptual substance from which to shape their religious lives. I have sought to keep in view both the deployability of devotees and the nuances of their devotional experience, to recover a space of the biospiritual within the biopolitical, and thereby to treat with due weight and sensitivity the manifold, and yes, highly creative and compelling donation theologies that have arisen around blood donation in India.

NOTES

Chapter 1. Introduction

1. Anonymity is a key feature of voluntary systems of corporeal donation. The normative practice of not telling the recipient about the donor or the donor about the recipient is a means of avoiding indebtedness (Fox and Swazey 1992: 37).

2. The family replacement system is not unique to India. Part of the blood supply in the United States was until recently reliant on this mode of collection; the same system currently prevails in Sri Lanka (Simpson 2004: 850) and in many other countries. Most medical opinion is now strongly opposed both to paid and to replacement donation. Paying donors is said to provide an incentive to conceal disqualifying factors such as HIV/AIDS (Brooks 2004: 282). Replacement donation is said to pressurize patients' relatives unduly, pushing many to seek so-called professional donors to donate in their stead, and threatening those who cannot arrange for this kind of donation with denial of life-saving treatment.

3. The *National Guidebook on Blood Donor Motivation* (2003), published by the government, estimates India's blood need as 8 million units per annum. The constant stream of new, blood-requiring treatment techniques causes this figure to increase year by year. The total annual collection figure, says the *Guidebook*, is 4 million units, with roughly 2 million of these being voluntary donations and 2 million replacement (ibid.: 203). The gap between demand and supply is extremely serious and results in many preventable deaths; however, these are not as many as the figures may suggest— there are several established alternatives to transfusion, and doctors are reported to overprescribe blood (Bray and Prabhakar 2002: 477).

4. Founder of Jainism. See Laidlaw (1995) for an account of annual celebrations of his birth. See Glossary for basic background on all these groups.

5. I define "utility" provisionally here in a classical sense as the state of being productive, conservative, useful, or beneficial. "Social utility" refers to that which is socially useful; "medical utility"—a term I employ throughout the book—comes under this definition. These are only provisional definitions—this is extremely contested analytical terrain which I explore in depth in chapter 3. The Sanskrit term for "useful" is *upyogi*; more colloquially, the word *fayademand* is often used.

6. See, for example, Ohnuki-Tierney (1994) and Lock (2003). Simpson (2004: 841) too has noted that utility is often framed in opposition to "intrinsic value" in such studies. I term "corporeal donation" all willed transfers of bodily substance for medical or research purposes, including blood, cadavers, kidneys, eyes, ova, and many other body-derived substances.

7. It could be argued that these spiritual orders and movements are not in themselves religions. However, devotional orders in the north Indian sant tradition often see themselves as wholly new religious dispensations (see Babb 1986; Juergensmeyer 1991). In addition, Indianist scholars frequently wrestle with definitions of Hinduism: that is, is it one religion or a conglomeration? (see Gellner 2004). These points I hope lend legitimacy to my use of the term "religions of utility."

8. I see this usage of "interoperability" as preferable to the more conventional vocabulary used by anthropologists, that is, "interdependency" or "mutual constitution," the latter being a term often used to indicate the way in which seemingly separate phenomena can work with or against each other to transform and in a sense create one another. While "interdependency" is less problematic than "mutual constitution" because it offers more precision in conveying a sense of the reciprocal reliance that can develop when one thing (in this case medical blood donation initiatives) connects with or makes contact with another (the activities of devotional orders), what I point to particularly in my use of "interoperability" is the practical nature of the set of interactive operations involved when so-called separate systems may come to interlock and work through each other. This, I emphasize, can involve disjuncture as well as fruitful combination.

9. The Sant Nirankari Mission is distinct from the Nirankari reform movement founded by Baba Dayal (1783–1855) in order to address creeping "deformities" within Sikhism. The difference is elaborated in chapter 4. The Radhasoami movement, it should be noted, has intermittently collected its devotees' blood since the 1960s. I am grateful to Chris Crookes for making me aware of this.

10. Though the words *sant* and *saint* are extremely close in meaning, there is apparently no etymological connection between them (Juergensmeyer 1991: 22). Some Nirankari devotees claim the Mission has 20 million adherents, far more than the 4 or 5 million Radhasoami initiates (see Juergensmeyer 1991: 236–238), but the Nirankari figure is unofficial and probably unreliable. The Mission is, however, a very substantial organization, with a presence throughout India and the world, so the lack of scholarly work on it is certainly curious. The Dera Sacha Sauda claims to possess more than 2 million devotees.

11. *Satsang* means literally "association of the good." Sant and bhakti movements are "congregational religion[s]" (Lorenzen 1995: 24).

12. I am influenced here by Miller's (1998) determination to avoid the sociological obviations that result from treating the consumer-subjects of late capitalism as simply enacting a script laid down for them.

13. "Biospiritual" is my term for describing situations in which there is either reliance on spirit to facilitate biological aims/goals or reliance on biological facts or techniques to facilitate spiritual goals.

14. Cohen (2004: 166) proposes a set of three connected terms: to be "operable" is to be a "bioavailable" body, extracted from as a kind of countergift to the state. "Supplementable" persons are those able to receive, "from the sovereign state," parts of others' bodies.

15. Other key anthropological works on blood donation include Weston (2001, United States), Cohen (2001, India), Erwin (2006, China), and Dalsgaard (2007, Denmark). I have previously written on memorial blood donation events in India (Copeman

2004), and on temporal and affective aspects of giving blood (Copeman 2005). See also Rabinow (1999, France), Valentine (2005), Healy (2006), and Waldby and Mitchell (2006).

16. I am most grateful to Joseph Alter (personal communication) for the term "mechanical transgression."

17. *Guanxi* refers to social networks, consisting of identifiable persons, which are created and sustained by the exchange of gifts and favors.

18. In the United States most whole blood donations are nonremunerated, while the donation of specific blood components—a more time-consuming process for donors—is usually paid for (Vicziany 2001: 387; see also Starr 2002 on the American situation). The United Kingdom's system is wholly nonremunerated. The same is true for Denmark; though see Dalsgaard (2007) on the hidden returns which he sees as greasing the system.

19. Seventeen of these were run by the state or central government, two by NGOs, fifteen were attached to private hospitals, and seven were private "stand-alone."

20. The transmutation of "altruism" into hefty profits for recipient institutions is a feature of numerous corporeal economies. Hayden (2007: 730) has noted how "altruistically" given tissue, blood, or gene samples in the United States and Europe can cause disquiet among ethicists, for "such gifts may well enable quite a lot of profit for those on the receiving end of such transactions." Or as Waldby and Mitchell (2006: 24) put it, the norm of altruism in corporeal giving "has simply rendered the body an open source of free biological material for commercial use." Familiar with the charge against them, blood banks, both government and commercial, protest that the fee they demand of recipients is merely a "processing charge" which barely covers the costs of testing, storing, and matching donated blood. Such protests usually fall on deaf ears, especially when the blood bank in question is a commercial one.

21. Doctors tend to be Anglophone, middle- and upper-middle-class, and "clean caste" Hindus. However, Muslim, Christian, and Dalit doctors are by no means unheard of. The social background of donor recruiters overlaps with that of doctors, though is somewhat more diverse. Many blood banks cannot afford to employ recruiters. The two blood banks with which I was most closely associated in Delhi do, however, employ them. Though both are female, I do not think that this represents a wider linkage between women and recruitment activity. The social profile of the many doctors with whom I interacted largely matches that described by Madan (1980) in his earlier study of Delhi medics, despite the intervening years. In his survey of doctors and medical academics at New Delhi's prestigious All India Institute of Medical Sciences (AIIMS), the location of two of the blood banks with which I had contact, Madan found that nearly all the doctors had had "elite" school and college educations (1980: 61) and that 87 percent were Hindus, the rest being Christians and Sikhs. Eighty-six percent of his respondents were "clean" caste (ibid., 50–51). Madan encountered no Muslim medics, though the Muslim community constitutes nearly 11 percent of the population of India. Similarly, during the fifteen months of fieldwork on which this study is based, I met only two Muslim doctors, at government hospitals in Mumbai and Kolkata, respectively. Madan (ibid.) claims that this absence is related to Muslims' "lower general educational levels and socioeconomic conditions."

22. Doctors report that Muslims are extremely reluctant to donate blood. As a religious minority, the low donation figures reported in surveys (e.g., Ray, Singh, and

Banerjee 2005) partly reflect the lower proportion of Muslims in the population at large. There is, however, some substance to doctors' reports. Camps are staged at Delhi's Muslim Jama Milia University, but other than that, I heard of very little Muslim involvement in blood donation. There is, I suggest, a fine line between stereotypes of the reluctant Muslim and the reality. One doctor told me of the tactics he employs in order to persuade Muslim relatives of the patients admitted to his hospital to provide replacement donations: "I tell them quietly that Muslims are very bad people. He'll say 'No.' I say, 'I tell you, they're bad—they don't donate blood.' He'll say, 'No, they'll do it. I'll show you.' So, out of vengeance they'll donate. It's the only way." Though I collected much data on this thorny issue, the devotional focus of this study does not permit a full consideration here of the relation between Islam and blood donation.

23. This is a controversial practice because it appears to reintroduce "payment" as a feature of a supposedly nonremunerated system. I do not have space to fully consider these debates in this study, but provide a brief discussion in chapter 7.

24. A similar situation pertained in the days following the 11 September 2001 attacks on the United States. The Congress staged a blood donation event at which senators and representatives gave blood. Each of them was presented with a videotape depicting their blood donations for showing to their constituents (Starr 2002). See chapter 5 on the documentation of mass camps, and Copeman (2004: 140–141).

25. *Outlook*, 22 October 2001.

26. Although this is indicative of the educated class's disparagement of ignorant or poor people's "superstition," it is in fact a very general fear—I quickly discovered that even many blood bank staff are frightened of blood donation. Arnold (1993) records the acute anxieties harbored by many nineteenth-century Indians about the extractive aspects of Western medicine as practiced by their colonial masters.

27. Chapter 4 provides a fuller discussion of blood donation and socioeconomic status. On widespread Indian anxieties about blood quality and quantum, see Marriott (1959: 59), Minocha (1996: 91–92), and Osella and Osella (1996: 43).

28. Message from Chief Medical Officer of Lok Nayak Hospital, souvenir publication, *Jai Hind* (NGO), 2003; http://www.bloodbanksdelhi.com/content/FAQ.htm.

29. *Rakta-Kranti* souvenir, April 2004.

30. The phrase is employed by Alter (2004: 200) in reference to auto-urine therapy as a practice of "self-containment and self-sufficiency."

31. *Dosa* is "force in the body or mind responsible for illness; also trouble" (Langford 2002: 274). The *Concise Oxford Dictionary of Current English* (1976) defines an "armamentarium" as the resources available to someone engaged in a task, or a set of medical equipment or drugs.

32. Red cells live for 120 days. Dr. Debasish Gupta of the National AIDS Control Organization (NACO) informed me that "In your circulation you have plenty of red cells, millions and millions. Of these cells, some are one day old, some are 10 days old, some are 20 days old, some are 110 days old, some may be 119 days old. So when you are donating blood you are donating a mixture of differently aged red cells."

33. See Reddy (2007: 434–435) on invocations of dan among Indians in Houston who were asked to donate tissue samples for genetic research purposes.

34. This is because of the medical policy axiom that offering donors incentives increases the likelihood that they will conceal risk factors that, if revealed, would disqualify them from donating.

35. Although replacement donations given by relatives are rarely actually transfused into their sick family members, such donations are nevertheless in essence given "for" them in order to facilitate their treatment.

36. This move outward from the family finds a parallel in the business world. Harriss (2003) has recently demonstrated that Indian family businesses are seeking to widen their "circles of trust" in order to adjust to economic change.

37. Ramanujan (1989: 57) points to the way in which the English language has acquired markedly Sanskritic characteristics in its Indian usage.

38. Dr. P. Srinivasan, director of Jeevan blood bank, Chennai, quoted in *The Hindu*, 31 July 2001.

39. See Dominique Lapierre's famous Kolkata-based epic, *The City of Joy* (1999), for a semi-fictional account of the desperation and squalor that characterizes the life of a "professional" blood donor.

40. During an interview with the director of a government blood bank, I witnessed exactly this. A BJP member of the Delhi Legislative Assembly (MLA) telephoned my interviewee to request the release of blood, without replacement or cost, to an acquaintance in his constituency. The director complied, reasoning to me that the BJP, after all, organizes blood donation camps from time to time.

41. Newspapers regularly report on Delhiites' purported indifference to one another. One article, consisting of snapshot interviews with Delhiites bemoaning their city, was memorably headlined: "Capital Shame: Filth, Boorish Behaviour" (*Times of India*, 12 December 2003). When changes are carried out on the world that make it conform better to particular descriptions of it, a "principle of convergence" is enacted, according to Bowker and Star (1999).

Chapter 2. Generative Generosity

1. Platelets are disk-like structures that are the foundation of clots (Starr 1998: 211). Plasma is the colorless coagulable part of blood in which the fat globules float (*OED*)— usually frozen after extraction and centrifuge, it becomes known as Fresh Frozen Plasma (FFP). Red cells contain hemoglobin that helps carry oxygen from the lungs to other parts of the body. Red cells also collect carbon dioxide waste, moving it to the lungs for expulsion (Ray 2003).

2. Interview with Dr. N. K. Bhatia, director of Rotary Blood Bank, Delhi, 2004. In my experience, government blood banks are less likely to possess the technology than private or NGO blood banks, though the biggest government hospitals in Delhi do practice separation techniques.

3. Compare to Scheper-Hughes's (1996) article "Theft of Life," in which theft of life derives not from irrational prescription but from illicit extraction.

4. This is important for the same reason that dividing blood is important—the single unit transfusion, like the "whole" unit, is a figure of censure, an "irrational" waste of precious substance. For if one can give a unit of blood with no resulting physical

harm, say modernizing doctors, then what possible benefit could occur from transfusion of the same quantity?

5. In anthropological writings on Hinduism's apparatuses of return, blessings (*ashirvad*), merit (*punya*), and fruits (*phal*) are related but differentiated concepts—all are "benefits" that can be secured by donation (*dan ka labh*). Punya is merit that results from ethically good actions. For the donors I had dealings with, blood donation, roughly speaking, may result in both punya and blessings, with the benefits of blessings likely to bear fruit in this life rather than the next. The blessings that donors can expect to receive from transfusion recipients are continually stressed by blood bank donor recruiters—"Give blood, get blessings," as one Indian Red Cross slogan puts it. Blessings may predominate, but punya also—which is likely to come not from recipients but from a higher authority or impersonal spiritual mechanism—is a feature of poetry of solicitation and also of donors' own expectations. One recruitment poster, for instance, declares, *Rakt-dan punya ka kaam* (Blood donation is the work of a good deed). In my experience, phal (fruits) can stand for both punya (merit) and ashirvad (blessings). The point I wish to emphasize is that, though different words, and formally different concepts, ashirvad, phal, and punya often appeared to me during fieldwork mixed together and difficult to distinguish. For example, a devotee of the Dera Sacha Sauda (see chapter 5), who when I met him had recently narrowly survived a car crash, told me on one occasion that he had been saved through the punya of his guru and *manav seva* (service of the guru and humanity), and on another that it was simply the guru's blessings (*ashirvad*) that had saved him.

6. The Indian Web site http://www.bloodsavers.com emphasizes the ease with which donors can save not only one but several lives: "Saving the world isn't easy. Saving a life is. Donating one pint of blood can save up to three lives. Maybe even someone you know."

7. "Such volunteers are also eligible for the benefit of ten (10) Grace Marks Under Section 0.229-A of the University Act. Preference is given in Public Service Commission to a candidate who is holding such certificate for two years of service in NSS and for attending the Y.F.S.D (i.e., Youth for Sustainable Development) camp. The motto of NSS is "Not Me, But You." It stands for the following two ideals, "(i) to forget and surrender the self and (ii) to render selfless service to the entire nation" (http://www.karmayog.com/ngos/nss.htm).

8. I am grateful to Amrit Srinivasan for drawing my attention to these differentials. Social service schemes are featured at all levels of the Indian education system. See Reddy (2007: 437) on the obligation to perform Socially Useful Productive Work (SUPW) at school. See also chapter 5 on protests staged by trainee medics against a new requirement that they spend a year conducting social service in rural areas. On the National Service Scheme (NSS), see http://yas.nic.in/yasroot/schemes/nss.htm.

9. The phrase is Zaloom's (2003: 263); she uses it to refer to factors influencing decision making among Chicago finance traders.

10. Lohri, celebrated annually on the 13 or 14 of January, is the Punjabi version of the famous Makar Sankranti and Pongal festivals of northern and southern India, respectively.

11. This all recalls Ramanujan's argument (1989), discussed in chapter 1, that India is a predominantly "context-sensitive" society. See Heim (2004: 117, 126) on the foregrounding of time, place, and calculability in regard to the giving of dan in the Dharmashastras.

12. See http://www.umich.edu/~urecord/9899/Mar15_99/7.htm.

13. Developed by Debabrata Ray, founder of the Association of Voluntary Blood Donors (AVBD).

14. On the revered category of the secret gift (*gupt-dan*), see Laidlaw (1995), Mayer (1981), and chapter 5 below.

15. As has been observed in other contexts, notably that of the nation and its kin or blood-based appeals, idealized expansion of family ties becomes a basis for many forms of modern civic-mindedness (see, for example, Stafford 1992).

Chapter 3.   The Reform of the Gift

1. Corsín Jiménez (2007) has documented the way in which "utility" has acted as a proxy for "society" in Western economic theory since the beginning of the twentieth century.

2. "In everyday life, ideology is at work, especially in the apparently innocent reference to pure utility" (Žižek 1999: 90).

3. Though, as Parry (1986: 463) makes clear, dan is far from being the only kind of gift in India. Many gifts, not governed by the laws of *danadharma*, are indeed reciprocally structured (ibid.: 460). In such cases, says Parry, there is little evidence of the transfer of spirit. Chapter 4 considers this matter in some detail.

4. Mayer (1981) too has described socially active asceticism as eschewing the conventional association between ascetic practices and merit making. I take issue with this view below.

5. Analyses of classical dan have emphasized the importance of the worthiness of recipients. The "worthy vessel" (recipient) is extremely reluctant to accept the gift (Parry 1986: 460). Laidlaw (2000) analyses *supatra-dan*—a gift to a worthy recipient—from lay to renouncer Jains. Worthiness remains an element of the reformed gift, but the recipient is worthy not by virtue of status but by virtue of need.

6. I mean that they are epiphenomenal from the point of view of the actor pursuing his self-interest ("Private Vice").

7. Swami Vivekananda (1863–1902), a "sage-polemicist" (S. Bayly 1999: 150) and giant figure in twentieth-century Hinduism, taught that "one should see "man as god," and that "true worship consist[s] in work for social ends" (Hansen 1999: 70).

8. Though see Bornstein's (2006; forthcoming) work on interrelations between philanthropic giving, receipts, trust, and notions of dan in Delhi. Kent (2004) and Reddy (2007) describe translations and extensions of dan concepts in the Indian diaspora.

9. http://www.sachasauda.com/satsangs/English2.htm.

10. Ibid. See Vidal (2000) on the ambiguous role of intermediaries in other Indian contexts.

11. *Rupana Times*, 11 October 2004. Pagri ceremonies are held for the passing of the deceased male's turban to the new head of the family, ideally the deceased's eldest son.

12. *Taze*, 13 October 2004. The term *gaddinashin* generally refers to the occupier of the usually hereditary seat of custodianship of a Muslim shrine. The designation, however, is also used in Sikhism, in this case in reference to a nonhereditary guru.

13. The gift of a cow to a Brahmin and pind-dan (balls of grains or rice offered to the dead) are not the same thing, though both may be performed in mortuary ceremonies (see Parry 1994: xxiv, 173). It is possible that their conflation here may be an error on the part of my informant.

14. The rasam pagri events at which blood was donated, Dr. Banerwal told me, were conducted mainly by Jats—commonly "non-servile cultivating people" (S. Bayly 1999: 37).

15. Pind-dan, as described by Parry (1994: 191), consists of balls of rice or grains given by mourners to mediating Brahmins in order to make merit for the deceased and mitigate their sufferings. I referred above to Sacha Sauda devotees' depictions of pind-dan as an offering of exemplary wastefulness. Banerwal's mentioning of the peace of the departed, when juxtaposed with Parry's exposition of pind-dan, suggests that blood donation may have been given as, or in place of, pind-dan as its nonwasteful substitutive ennoblement.

16. I heard several other accounts, however, of marriages extended-to-utility. I was told, for instance, that at his son's marriage, a Delhi Rotarian demanded monetary donations to Delhi's Rotary blood bank instead of gifts to the couple. In Calcutta I met Swarup Das, a volunteer in the AVBD, whose wedding had been preceded by a blood donation ceremony. Being a regular donor, he had postponed the event to a date on which he would be able to donate. He and his wife have additionally organized donation camps on each of their wedding anniversaries (and they named their son Sonitasroti, which in Bengali means "flow of blood"). Cohen too (1999: 161) heard of a Delhi couple "who insisted all their wedding guests sign up to donate something [i.e., parts of their body]." Watt (2005: 81) notes that in the early years of the twentieth century there was a spate of weddings in which invitees were encouraged to make monetary donations to nationalist educational initiatives instead of to the couple. Marriages have for several hundred years been a key target of Indian social reformist activity. These examples attest to the Indian marriage's continuing status as critical reformist target, now for the inculcation of virtuous utility.

17. *Times of India*, 12 February 2002; *Times of India*, 7 February 2002.

18. *The Hindu*, 19 January 2001.

19. A renowned yoga instructor, he has gained national prominence over the past ten years with broadcasts watched by over a million viewers throughout India on the private Aastha TV channel. He also presides over huge "yoga camps" staged in Indian cities, attended by up to 75,000 students.

20. The *pranayama* breathing techniques taught by Swami Ramdev are advertised as benefiting the practitioner's "heart, lungs, brains, depression, migraine, paralysis, neural system, obesity, constipation, gastric, cholesterol, allergic problems, asthma, snoring, concentration, and even cancer and AIDS," to name but a few conditions (http://research.iiit.ac.in/~smr/knowyoga/tiki-index.php?page=pranayama).

21. On donation as self-purifying, see chapter 1. This is a further example of the metamorphosis of blood donation into bloodletting.

22. http://timesofindia.indiatimes.com/articleshow/958057.cms. See Copeman (forthcoming) for a full account.

23. *Deccan Herald*, 26 December 2004.

24. Quoted by NDTV television correspondent, 12 December 2004.

25. The first part of this sentence paraphrases Laidlaw (2005).

26. "In Bangalore and Delhi I was told stories of a kind of donation madness: a man desperate to give away any organ he could; a couple who insisted all their wedding guests sign up to donate something" (Cohen 1999: 161).

27. http://www.time.com/time/asia50/c_people.html.

28. http://164.100.24.208.Is/Ismember/biodata.asp?mpsno=184.

29. "The Delhi Police organized a blood donation camp to commemorate the courage of the five police personnel who were killed while preventing heavily armed Pakistani militants from entering the Parliament House complex on December 13 last year" (*Hindustan Times*, 14 December 2003).

30. *The Tribune*, 25 September 2006.

31. Commenting on letters written by French soldiers to their loved ones during the First World War which envisage their bloodshed as a kind of gift to the nation, Koenigsberg (2004) writes that such images evoke "a blood transfusion where the life-sustaining substance of an individual body passes into the collective body, functioning to keep it alive." See chapters 4 and 6 for more on convertibility between blood sacrifice and blood donation.

32. See Copeman (2006) for a fuller account of the samiti's activities. Myths surrounding Dadhichi are analyzed by Babb (2004). See also Heim (2004: 138) on bloody gifts of the body (*deh-dan*) as discussed in Hindu and Buddhist sacred texts, and Reddy (2007) on Indians in Houston looking to mythical examples of bodily gift-giving as templates of a kind for their own giving of blood for genetic research.

33. Simpson has documented a comparable move in Sri Lanka by medical authorities to install the Buddha, as he appeared in a previous birth, as an eye donor, and thus to mobilize Buddhists in the region to act as their master had done. As Simpson (2004: 840) comments, "stepping into a biogenetic future rich in technological possibility also involves an engagement with the past."

34. "Conjunctive structure" paraphrases Sahlins's (1981) "structure of the conjuncture."

Chapter 4.   Devotion and Donation

1. On the sant tradition and bhakti movements in north India, see Lele (1981), Schomer and McLeod (1987), and Lorenzen (1995). Though the Sant Nirankaris are briefly mentioned in Madan (1997) and McKean (1996), there are no substantial existing scholarly treatments of the movement.

2. This is sold cheaply in Nirankari Colony in Delhi, the location of the Mission's headquarters. Originally in Hindi, much of it has been translated into English, and it is on these translations that I draw.

3. Dr. Bharat Singh, director of the Delhi State Blood Transfusion Council, informed me that roughly 350,000 units of blood are collected in the capital each year. Eighty percent of this is replacement donation, 20 percent voluntary. Therefore approximately 70,000 voluntary donations are collected. The Mission claims to collect 20,000 units of blood annually, which therefore represents 28.6 percent of the 70,000 voluntary donations overall.

4. At donation camps, as in blood banks, medical professionals perform a series of tests on devotees' hemoglobin, weight, blood pressure, and so on in order to ascertain prospective donors' eligibility to donate. As Brooks (2004: 282) notes, "While the donor offers the gift of blood, the blood service is the arbiter of its suitability."

5. Devotees use the language of bhakti devotion for key elements of donation practice—notably the employment of the term *prashad* for postdonation snacks, this being the term for the sweets, flowers, and other sanctified "leavings" imparted to devotees in token of the God's or guru's divine favor in a wide range of Indian religious contexts (see Fuller 1992: 85).

6. Devotees I met claimed a following of 20 million, but I emphasize that this is an unofficial figure.

7. These exchanges took place in the context of extreme tensions surrounding the growing Sikh separatist militancy of the late 1970s and 1980s. See Grewal (1990: chapter 10) for an account of this period.

8. I am making an ethnographic rather than a political point here. I am not seeking to debunk or challenge the necessity of these medical tests.

9. An example of the specifically guru-centered orientation of devotees' seva was provided at a Nirankari donation camp I attended in Haryana. One *bhajan* (devotional song) sung by women donors as they were bled referred to their souls' marriage to their guru, and asked him for strength so that they would be able to endure giving this gift *to him*. Another bhajan, sung by the same women, went: "Great father, great soul, every bit (*kan-kan*) of us belongs to you; please accept our offering (*dan*)."

10. The Nath Sampradaya is a master-disciple initiatory tradition, made up of different guru lineages, and largely associated with Shaivism. See White (1996) for further details of the Nath tradition.

11. The guru makes a similar claim about devotees' purity of intention, declaring that "while the world has the tendency to forget what it receives, the saints [devotees] forget what they give" (http://www.nirankari.com/archive/reports/2003_04_20_bdcamp.htm).

12. See Juergensmeyer (1991: 142) on Radhasoami devotees needing to be restrained from giving too large a proportion of their salaries to their guru. See also chapter 5, which documents attempts by Dera Sacha Sauda devotees to give more than one unit of blood at a time.

13. Vessey's (2002) observation that "The body does not always collaborate with our plans" finds strong support in these stories of disqualification.

14. The Association of Voluntary Blood Donors stages a Parliament of Motivators conference, the title of which consciously recalls Vivekananda's address to the Parliament of Religions in Chicago (1893), in Kolkata every five years in order to share best practices in donor recruitment techniques.

15. Osella and Osella (1996: 41) similarly draw attention to a strong correlation between physical and moral states in Kerala.

16. Warrier (2003a: 277) records Mata Amritanandamayi's comparable aim "to alleviate suffering and infuse love into the modern world."

17. http://www.nirankari.org.

18. Sermons delivered by Jain renouncers are considered *gyan-dan* (gifts of knowledge) (Laidlaw 1995: 297), while gifts of learning are known more commonly as *vidya-dan* (Watt 2005: 71). Devotees' understanding that their *gyan* (knowledge) is reified in their donated blood resonates with the Jain case, even if the context of transmission differs. See also Copeman (2006) on cadaver donation as gifts of learning to trainee doctors.

19. As Sharma (1987: 276) has noted, the transfer between persons of karma "violates the doctrine to the extent that one is supposed to be the legatee of one's own deeds and not of others."

20. Though this devotee explicitly attributes "corporeal capture" to the satguru's strategizing, I heard no official endorsements of these views.

21. As these examples indicate, devotees' descriptions of the effects of their gifts on recipients are frequently rendered in a cellular or genetic idiom: Nirankari blood donations work upon recipients' nerves, genes, and cells; the spirit of the gift is expounded through a lay scientific dialect of biospiritual capture and loving control.

22. See also Arnold (1993: 143) on concerns among nineteenth-century Indians that colonial vaccination projects were an instrument to force their conversion to Christianity.

23. Parry (1999: 137–138) and S. Bayly (1999: 314) also note that caste boundaries can be maintained through restrictions in flows of substance.

24. A paraphrasing of Rafael (2003: 415).

25. Though see Gregory's (forthcoming) essay "The Auspicious Gift in Middle India."

26. This citation is drawn from a posting by Laurie Maund made on 11 November 2005 to an e-group called "SEA-AIDS," hosted by http://www.healthdev.org/eforums. Its title is "Living Blood Bank: How Thai Buddhist Monks Are Helping Their Communities Prevent HIV." Laurie Maund works on the project she describes.

Chapter 5. Blood Donation in the Zone of Religious Spectacles

1. Guinness World Records (2004).

2. There is a large discrepancy between the number of donors attracted to the events and the number of units actually collected. Many devotees, subsequent to their registration, are found to be ineligible for medical reasons. See chapter 4 on the high prevalence of medical disqualification among the devotees of guru-led movements.

3. See Glossary for background on the Limbdi Ajramar Jain community and on the other organizations listed in this section.

4. http://coca-colaindia.com/limca_book_of_records/default.asp.

5. *The Hindu*, 22 May 2005.

6. *Times of India*, 7 October 2004. See chapter 1 on the gender ratio of voluntary blood donors. Roughly 200 units were donated at the Lord Ayyappa camp, more than a third of which were provided by women. This is a higher than usual proportion, but is hardly unique. Migrants from Kerala, a state in which women are commonly regarded to share a more equal status with men than elsewhere in India, the camp organizers hoped to highlight the "enlightened" nature of persons hailing from there.

   I return in chapter 7 to the Puttarparthi blood bank. Though there is an epidemic of claims, many are clearly for categories of record that do not exist (e.g., the Ayyappa and Sathya Sai Baba claims). I know of at least three further attempts made by Indian organizations to break the record for most units of blood collected in a single day: a Gujarat cultural group tried and failed to achieve the record in 2002 (http://www.ahmedabad.com/news/2k2/oct/21argcrowd.htm); the Tamil Nadu State Aids Control Society claimed to have broken the record in 2003, though there is no record of this (http://www.ananova.com/news/story/sm_413841.html?menu=); and a Surat blood donation society collected 8,008 donations in 1999, intriguingly from only 8,000 donors (http://www.prideofindia.net).

7. The present study, along with Mines's (1994) and others', seriously calls into question Michaels's (2004: 7) recent claim that the Hindu "identificatory habitus" is marked by an absence of competition and recognition of individual achievement.

8. *The Guardian*, 22 June 2007.

9. Ibid.

10. See also Godelier (1999: 77), who notes that the Kwakiutl word *p'asa* means "to give but to flatten at the same time, by crushing the name of a rival, of the receiver."

11. Such statements recall Gandhi's (1949: 385) complaint about the Indian "popular attitude" of "partiality for exciting work, dislike for quiet constructive effort."

12. He is also called Hazoor Maharaj Ji in the movement's literature, and Pita Ji (father) by his devotees.

13. Cf. Laidlaw (1995: 245) on the Jain idol as an "assemblage of excellences, in which abstract ideas are given bodily form."

14. The Dera Sacha Sauda is not unique in pursuing commercial ventures. See Juergensmeyer (1991: 159) on the Radhasoami movement's "enlightened" industrial undertakings. Parry (1989: 85) has argued that antipathy to money often goes hand in hand with an ideology of autarky, which is exactly the case with the Dera Sacha Sauda.

    The provision of this level of care for pilgrims runs counter to most anthropological accounts that emphasize the hardships and austerities of pilgrimage (e.g., Osella and Osella 2003; Daniel 1984). In fact, the Sacha Sauda site recalls McKean's (1996: 4) depiction of "amusement park–like" ashrams in Rishikesh which she sees as venues for "the production and consumption of fetish-like commodities."

15. http://www.sachasauda.com/satsangs/English2.htm.

16. McKean (1996), like the Sacha Sauda guru, excoriates Indian gurus for their exploitation of credulous devotees. However, though the Sirsa guru sets himself up in opposition to these other nefarious masters, he has unfortunately joined them in opprobrium. In a 2003 news article headlined "Godman under a Cloud," the Sacha Sauda is said to be under police investigation after the murder—reportedly committed by devotees—of a journalist who had published allegations that the guru had sexually exploited several female ascetics (*sadhvi*s) (*Frontline*, 1 March 2003). A letter, copies of which were sent by one of these sadhvis to the prime minister, union home minister, the Central Bureau of Investigation (CBI), and the Haryana chief minister, alleges that the guru threatened to kill her if she disclosed his activities, and also that he regularly boasts of his political influence in Haryana and Punjab. With headlines like these, and a continuing police investigation into its activities, the Sacha Sauda's large-scale, highly visible adoption of "virtuous" activities such as blood donation may at least in part be an attempt to create a media presence capable of obscuring or

hiding from view a different set of damaging stories that are threatening to define its public image.

17. Unlike the Nirankari Mission, whose previous three gurus have been installed through descent, Dera Sacha Sauda gurus choose their successors.

18. http://www.derasachasauda.org.

19. Since its inception in 1875, the Arya Samaj has been particularly active in pursuing campaigns against idolatry, caste, and popular ritual traditions (Hansen 1999: 71).

20. The assumption is logical but problematic in the Indian context, in which many doctors are said to administer transfusions as a "tonic" rather than on the basis of need. An everyday example of the encoding of utility in gifts occurs when passersby give food instead of money to beggars in order to forestall their spending of the money given to them on drugs or alcohol.

21. *Dhan Dhan Satguru Tera Hi Aasra, The Truth*. DSS Video CD Vol. 1 (Dera Sacha Sauda n.d.c.). Cf. the classic view that "the cow is seen as an embodiment of Laxsmi. She is also a maternal figure associated with nourishment and nurture. Eating her flesh is therefore suggestive of matricide" (Babb 2004: 233n).

22. http://www.sachasauda.com/satsangs/English2.htm.

23. These phrases are contained in a Sathya Sai Baba calendar, given to blood donors at a Delhi camp organized by the Sathya Sai Baba Seva Samiti.

24. *Kirti-dan* is not a term I heard during fieldwork, but suspicion as regards public giving and earning fame through acts of largesse is extremely widespread. The principles informing kirti-dan were thus very much evident in my primary field sites, if not the formal category itself.

25. *Dhan Dhan Satguru Tera Hi Aasra, The Truth.*

26. See Babb (1986: 176–77) for a discussion of problems arising from application of the "tendentious" Western concept of miracles in non-Western contexts. In India, notes Babb, there is nothing particularly "remarkable in the idea that human beings can cultivate extraordinary powers." At the same time, "scientific rationalism is very much part of the Indian scene."

27. Participatory and yet not so in terms of attribution. What devotees see as evidence of the guru's miraculousness—his wonderful gifts to humanity—are at the same time their gift to him. These "miraculous" constructions and donations were, after all, carried out for free (if one for a moment discounts blessings) by devotees as guru seva, and it is the guru who is credited with the miracles that *they* perform. Though objectively miracles of participation, such "miracles" are performed multiply but attributed singularly. Partaking of the miracles for which they praise their guru, devotees are awestruck by their own ability to be mobilized. The singular attribution of multiply performed feats is not an exclusively Dera Sacha Sauda phenomenon—it is shared by other guru-led movements in India. As discussed in chapter 3, devotees of the south Indian guru Mata Amritanandamayi give her credit for happenings as mundane as having enough petrol in a car to get home. In addition, writes Warrier (2003a: 256), the Mata's devotees view the enlargement and spread of the movement she heads as evidence of her miraculous powers, whereas it is in fact "the perseverance of the devotees and disciples themselves that has made this institution building possible in the first place." Thus, rather like Dera Sacha Sauda devotees, followers of the

Mata are responsible for the "miracles" they attribute to her. Such singular ascription ought to qualify any sense of the democratizing of the miraculous by way of its newly multiple generation. Instead, miracles' multiple performance is ideologically denied by both the movement's literature and by devotees themselves. Participation is expected as "spiritual duty," but what occurs, in fact, is devotees' simultaneous enrolment and erasure.

28. Juergensmeyer (1991: 82) notes that accounts of miracles performed by Radhasoami masters, such as the multiplying of food, are reminiscent of those attributed to Jesus. When this data is taken together with my own, I think it becomes clear that Jesus has assumed the status of miraculous exemplar for reform-minded Hindus. Furthermore, the example of Christ is often used by these groups in order to demonstrate the importance of living spiritual masters: just as God came to earth in the human form of Christ 2,000 years ago, runs the argument, so he now takes the form of this or that guru.

29. *Navan Jamana*, 12 October 2004.

30. This, of course, contravenes all official guidelines. See chapter 4 on blood donation as an austerity.

31. Although the Nirankari guru does attend the annual Human Unity Day (*manav ekta divas*) camp where he observes his wife donate (the guru himself reportedly can no longer donate due to diabetes), he does not attend the smaller-scale camps staged throughout the summer months.

32. Juergensmeyer sees the importance attached to darshan as a significant driver of the annual eye treatment camps staged by the Radhasoamis. The high value for devotees of experiencing the darshan of their guru means that blindness is looked upon by the movement with particular pity. The blind suffer "an enormous weight of bad karma, and as a result some within Radhasoami have thought it impossible for the blind to achieve a high degree of spiritual achievement" (1995: 81). Juergensmeyer does not say it directly, but the strong implication is that Radhasoami eye operations give not only sight back to the patients but also the opportunity for spiritual advancement.

33. After the Dera Sacha Sauda gained renown as a result of its record-breaking activities, several entrepreneurial blood banks in Delhi contacted the movement's local branches and compiled lists of devotees who they could contact when in need of blood.

34. Sometimes a rabbit and sometimes a deer accompany the guru on his public excursions. Several devotees said the movement had rescued them from being slaughtered, and that they accompany the spiritual master as a reminder to devotees about the importance of vegetarianism. See Hibbets (1999) on Indian gifts of protection, which include saving animals from slaughter.

35. http://www.sify.com/news/fullstory.php?id=14454113.

36. *Times of India*, 21 May 2007. Though in many ways like a strike, a *bandh* is frequently forcible rather than voluntary. The word itself means "closed." Responses to the controversy were highly politicized, with the Congress—which has been the beneficiary of Sacha Sauda electoral support—defending the order, and the BJP, which is in an alliance with the Akali Dal, heavily criticizing it.

37. *The Hindu*, 30 May 2007.

38. *Times of India*, 21 May 2007.

39. http://rtv.rtrlondon.co.uk/2007–05–21/37340eb3.html.

40. Most frequently in West Bengal, according to the *Economic Times* (18 December 2006), where the average number of bandhs per year is 40–50.

41. *The Hindu*, 31 January 2005.

42. http://www.rediff.com/news/2003/jul/30diary.htm.

43. *The Hindu*, 13 June 2007.

44. *Indian Express*, 26 October 1999. See also http://www.oasiswebsite.com. *Dharna* usually refers to a hunger protest, classically performed by a creditor at the door of a debtor in order to exert moral pressure for repayment. Though officially proscribed during British rule, protestors still frequently characterize their protests as dharnas.

45. The phenomenon is not entirely restricted to India. http://bloodforpeace.com is a U.S. Web site protesting against the U.S.-led war in Iraq. Its designers' aim was to find "a patriotic and constructive way to show our outrage at the loss of life." The U.S. public was enjoined to "make this the most successful and *productive* war protest in American history!!" (my emphasis). The contrast, of course, is with the blood shed by U.S. soldiers: "Our beloved troops are shedding their own blood every single day because of extremely poor decision making in Washington." Blood donation, here, is not patriotism by other means, but patriotism by the same means that the soldiers endure, loss of blood.

46. http://www.ndtvblogs.com/views/viewblogs.asp?gl_guid=&blogname=sami& q_userid=12887.

47. Ibid. A crore is 10 million.

48. Devotees' "calm" and "silent" giving of their blood as a method of protest led to newspaper declarations that the Dera Sacha Sauda action was an attempt at *gandhigiri* (e.g., see http://sify.com/news/fullstory.php?id=14454113, http://www.ibnlive.com/news/ dera-takes-to-gandhigiri-as-sikh-clergy-talks-tough/40955–3.html ["Dera Takes to Gandhigiri"]). The term *gandhigiri* (loosely, action/actions characteristic of Gandhi) was popularized by the 2006 Bollywood film *Lage Raho Munna Bhai* (Rajkumar Hirani) which has been credited with reviving interest in Gandhi throughout the country. The main protagonist in the film protests through the delivery of bouquets of flowers to the "oppressor" he seeks to challenge, and there has apparently been a spate of "flower protests" in the wake of the film. As Ghosh and Babu (2006) put it, "Gandhi, the man, was once the message. In the India of the post-liberalization brand, *gandhigiri* is the message."

49. See, in this respect, Cohen (2004) on Vajpayee and *hijras*.

50. *The Hindu*, 30 November 2007.

51. He was referring to Scheduled Castes/Schedules Tribes/Other Backward Classes. See http://www.savebrandindia.org.

Chapter 6.   Utility Saints and Donor-Soldiers

1. Indians are by no means unique in connecting blood donation and war-flavored patriotism. See Starr (2002) on patriotic donation in the United States and Rabinow (1999) for the French variant. The National Blood Service Web site for England and North

Wales, colored red, white, and blue, asks people to "do their bit for the nation" (https://secure.blood.co.uk/index.html).

2. Admittedly a very small proportion, but I did meet several Muslim Nirankari devotees and one Christian Sacha Sauda devotee.

3. Bhakti Parav is, as far as I am aware, a specifically Nirankari day of devotion.

4. *Indian Express*, 19 June 1999.

5. Vegetarianism is central to most Indians' ideas about what constitutes nonviolence (see Babb 2004: 21).

6. See Laidlaw (1995: 104) on the popularity of Hindu nationalist political organizations among Jaipur Jains.

7. http://www.animalcrusaders.org/ex_editorial.html. See Samanta (1994) for a recent ethnographic account of bloody sacrifice to Kali.

8. Shah (2006: 211) lists a variety of titles: acharya, baba, guru, mahant, maharaj, sadhu, sant, sanyasi, and swami.

9. "Osmotically" is from "osmosis," "the tendency of the solvent of a less concentrated solution of dissolved molecules to pass through a semi-permeable membrane into a more concentrated solution," or "diffusion through any membrane or porous barrier, as in dialysis" (*Collins Concise Dictionary of the English Language* [1988]).

10. Heidegger ([1953] 1993) uses this term in reference to modern technology.

11. Titmuss (1970) discusses the U.S. case, and http://www.aegis.com/news/ips/2001/IPO10903.html the Indian one.

12. The phrase "tournaments of blood value" is adapted from Appadurai (1986: 21).

13. During the annual Ganpati festivities, idols of Ganesh—often coated with toxic chemicals—are submerged in rivers and seas. Vermiculture refers to the use of worms as an environmentally friendly method of converting organic waste into valuable organic manure.

14. See also Roscoe (1988), Lindstrom (1984), and Empson (2006) on millenarian and prophetic ideas. Mumbai's most notable recent catastrophic events have been the large-scale sectarian violence of 1992, followed by a series of simultaneous bomb blasts, said to have been instigated by the Mumbai underworld, also in 1992; the serious flooding of 2005; and the bomb blasts on the Mumbai Suburban Railway in July 2006.

15. See Starr (2002) and Waldby and Mitchell (2006: Introduction) on the acute symbolism that surrounded acts of blood donation in the days following 11 September. The Indian government is reported to have offered to send blood for the victims, "even though its supplies are neither adequate nor safe" (Starr 2002).

16. The Beslan school siege and massacre took place in Beslan, North Ossetia, in September 2004. Chechen separatist militants killed 344 civilians, including 186 schoolchildren, and injured many hundreds more. See Stewart and Harding (1999: 291) on catastrophe as media spectacle.

17. Founded by prophetic visionary Dada Lekhraj in the 1930s, the Brahma Kumaris (Daughters of Brahma) prepare themselves for a period of calamities and a subsequent heavenly world in which there will be perfect gender equality. Particularly active in urban north India, the movement claims in excess of 100,000 devotees and

has internationalized rapidly with branches in Britain, Australia, and the United States. Its headquarters lie at Mt. Abu, Rajasthan. See Babb (1986: chapters 4–6).

18. Devotees claim a following of 100,000. The Trust has branches throughout Maharashtra but has yet to become a pan-Indian phenomenon.

19. Many seemed not to be aware of the perishability of blood: refrigerated red cells expire after thirty days, platelets after six days. Only frozen plasma lasts indefinitely.

20. "Theology of ultimacy" is after Barkun's (1998: 459) definition of millennialized politics, where politics has "cease[d] to be an instrument for the incremental adjustment of conflicting interests, [becoming] instead a 'politics of ultimacy' where ultimate issues are at stake in a once-and-for-all confrontation."

21. Ingold (2006: 15) gives the example of the movement of the sun through rather than across the sky.

22. A yagna is a popular fire offering ritual. *Maha-yagna* means "great offering."

Chapter 7.   The Nehruvian Gift

1. Recent essays by Peabody (2001) and Guha (2003) have been more nuanced in their approach to the question of enumeration, presenting evidence of both precolonial modes of community enumeration and of the active role played by communities themselves in formulating self-descriptions. The present argument, I hope, complements those of Peabody and Guha in demonstrating that analysis of the telling aspects of enumerative processes in the subcontinent is by no means exhausted by those studies that, as Guha (2003: 162) puts it, focus upon "the warm, fuzzy continuum of premodern collective life [being] suddenly and arbitrarily cut up by colonial modernity."

2. *The Times* (London), 13 July 2006.

3. http://in.christiantoday.com/template/news_view.htm?code=gen&id=53.

4. A central figure in the history of blood donation and transfusion, Karl Landsteiner discovered blood groups in 1900, thereby increasing the safety of transfusion and enabling it to become a major component of modern medical treatment.

5. *Frontline*, 2 August 2002.

6. Though I contrast the Nehruvian and Hindutva variants of national integration, Benei (2006) argues that Nehru's conceptualization of the nation was unwittingly "Hindu." While Benei may be correct that the two variants represent the different extremes of a continuum, I maintain that there remain important qualitative differences between them.

7. See Brass (1990: chapters 5–7) and Husain (1996) on political moves to foster "national integration" in post-Independence India.

8. The irony here is the pivotal role Indira Gandhi played in undoing the efforts of her father in promoting national integration. In the years preceding the so-called Emergency of 1975–1977, the Congress's populist goals "had come to be expressed in terms which covertly signaled the importance of *jati* and *varna* classifications to anyone who could be thought of as wronged or deprived" (S. Bayly 1999: 285; see Khilnani 1997: chapter 1). This led to sometimes violent competition between different caste groups in order to secure the state windfalls promised by Indira Gandhi.

9.   http://learning.indiatimes.com/test_papers/papers/social_%20science/1997/
     setIa9_aI5.htm

10. Ibid.

11. A term originating in theater, "scenography" refers to the work of constructing,
     adapting, transforming, and filling a dramatic space. Edwards and Osborne (2005)
     use the term in relation to suicide, and its "staging" in various contexts.

12. The phrase "unity in diversity" (*anekta me ekta*), "one of the most oft-repeated state-
     sponsored slogans" (Kapila 2008: 120), is often uttered in the same breath as
     "national integration." The notion of political composition I take from Mosse (2004:
     647), who, drawing on Latour (2000), notes that "actors in development are con-
     stantly engaged in creating order and unity through political acts of composition."

13. http://yas.nic.in/yasroot/schemes/integration/integration.htm.

14. *The Hindu*, 3 December 2005.

15. The term "holding together" is Hirsch's (1995), used in relation to ritual among the
     Fuyuge of the Papuan highlands.

16. I do not have space for a full consideration of the kingly aspects of the Dera Sacha
     Sauda guruship, though it is a rich and interesting subject. The term "fictive king-
     ship" (after "fictive kinship") was coined by Juergensmeyer (1991: 166) in reference to
     the Beas branch of Radhasoami gurus. Beas, the Punjab headquarters of the organiza-
     tion, has the appearance of a "magical kingdom," or a "spiritual court"; several of the
     Beas masters have been members of the caste from which Punjab's princes were
     drawn; and their honorific title, "Maharaj," of course, directly equates them with roy-
     alty. As mentioned above in chapter 5, the full title of the Sirsa master is Guru
     Maharaj Gurmeet Ram Rahim Singh Ji, and the literature generated by the organiza-
     tion refers to his kin as members of the "Holy Royal Family."

17. For example: *Navan Jamana*, 12 October 2004.

18. World Blood Donor Day was begun in 2004 for the global promotion of voluntary
     blood donation, and is promoted by the Red Cross and WHO.

19. He is partly correct in that in most Western countries people can indeed receive blood
     at any government-run hospital capable of providing it and do not have to have given
     previously in order to receive it without charge.

20. I return below to this doctor's interesting concept of "practical secularism."

21. The kumbh mela is a massive Hindu convocation which takes place four times in
     every twelve years. Rotating between Prayag, Haridwar, Ujjain, and Nasik, these are
     the locations where, in the vedic period, four drops of *amrita* (the nectar of immor-
     tality) are said to have fallen to the ground during a battle between gods and demons
     for its possession. Attended by millions, including thousands of sadhus, its center-
     piece is a ritual bathing at the banks of the rivers in each location.

22. *Times of India*, 28 July 2003.

23. The Dera Sacha Sauda camps also consist of pilgrim donors. Medical pilgrimages are
     commonplace in a wide variety of global contexts (e.g., Lourdes); the difference in the
     case of the Sacha Sauda is that, though pilgrims do often themselves get treated at the
     Sirsa clinics, they also provide blood for the treatment of others.

24. *Ganashakti Newsmagazine*, 18 March 2002.

25. *Outlook*, 22 October 2001. The reputation of Uttar Pradesh state, along with that of Bihar, is blighted by its poor record on women's rights, communal tensions, and criminal activity. The leading figure in the association, Shahid Askari, faced initial opposition to his camps, with residents of the city chasing him through the streets, calling him *raktu*—one who draws blood.

26. Though the state has indeed subjected the practices of different religious communities to regulation, it is supposed to do so in a balanced and equal manner (Hansen 1999: 53). Of course, controversial debates surround the question of whether this ideology is adequately put into practice.

27. See Freed and Freed (1998: 250–256) for a colorful description of *raksha bandhan* as celebrated in a north Indian village.

28. Schoolgirls from a central Kolkata Catholic school tied lovely rakhis of fresh flowers onto the wrists of donors. Having engaged in a brotherly act of protection, donors were provided with rakhis by these schoolgirl "sisters."

29. Hibbets (1999) provides a fascinating account of the Indic gift of protection (*abhayadana*), as elaborated in medieval texts. It may be possible that the protective gift of blood is considered by some donors a variant of abhayadana.

30. The blood bank's location at a pilgrimage centre creates a parallel with the Dera Sacha Sauda camps, which are also points at which extractable pilgrims converge. The kumbh mela camp provides another example of pilgrims as a medical resource.

31. *Times of India*, 19 October 2000. Bryant (2002: 521–523) has found similar attitudes among Greek Cypriots, some of whom express the view that "Turkish Cypriots are Greeks 'by blood,' but that they had converted to Islam in the early years of Ottoman rule. Or as one young professional expressed it to me, 'Even if my brother goes astray [i.e. becomes a Muslim], he's still my brother.'"

32. *The Week*, 10 September 2000.

33. While it could be argued that reservations form part of a Nehruvian concern with social justice—and therefore that my distinction between Nehruvian thought and reservations is illegitimate—Nehru himself saw only an extremely limited application for reservation schemes, with caste "slated to wither away through a process of modernization" (Rao 2003). One anti-reservation commentator recently quoted with approval Nehru's view that "these external props, as I might call them, the reservation of seats, and the rest—may possibly be helpful occasionally, but they produce a false sense of political relation, a false sense of strength, and, ultimately therefore, they are not nearly so important as real educational, cultural and economic advance which gives them inner strength to face any difficulty or opponent" (*Indian Express*, 7 April 2006).

34. *Agarwal*, *khatri*, and *bania* usually denote people of merchant-trader background of middling clean-caste status, often of vaishya varna.

35. As was noted in chapter 1, very many though by no means all doctors are high-caste Hindus. In a seeming irony, some of the doctors who complain of the bania influence in donor solicitation are themselves banias. As Laidlaw (1995: 88) has shown, however, "bania" is often understood as much as an attitude or mentality as a caste into which one may be born. It is therefore not unreasonable or surprising for bania doctors to complain of new "bania"-style modes of recruitment.

36. This is an example of the longstanding Indian tradition of making explicit references to kali yug as a way of explaining or justifying practices apparently at variance with standard Hindu ethics or morality.

Chapter 8. Conclusion

1. This situation resembles that reported by Säävälä (2003: 237–238) for Hyderabad. While most Hyderabad urbanites rhetorically deemphasize the significance of caste, caste anxieties and distinctions continue to be of vital importance in various overt and covert ways.

2. *Sunday Express*, 9 January 2005.

3. Though I readily acknowledge that this "centrifugal" aspect is implicit in some varieties of Indian asceticism: Laidlaw (2005), for example, notes that austerities undertaken by Jain renouncers, full of volitional complexity, though not directed toward purposes outside of the self, can and do have "radiating effects," possibly removing the sins and faults of those around them.

4. See Mathur (1991: 66) on karma as a form of "divine accountancy."

5. "*Yoga* results in the nonconditioned state of *samadhi* or of *sahaja*, in the perfect spontaneity of the *jivan-mukta*, the man 'liberated in this life.' From one point of view, we may say that the *jivan-mukta* has abolished time and history" (Eliade 1990: 339–340).

GLOSSARY OF GURUS AND ORGANIZATIONS

All India Institute of Medical Sciences (AIIMS). Prestigious government-funded but independently functioning hospital and research center, established in 1956 and located in New Delhi. Has two attached blood banks.

Aniruddha Bapu. Mumbai-based guru espousing millenarian theology. Has set up Academy of Disaster Management.

Art of Living. An internationally taught yoga course centered on breathing techniques, designed by south Indian guru Shri Shri Ravi Shankar. Devotees conduct blood donation camps and other seva activities throughout India.

Arya Samaj. A socioreligious organization, has engaged in Hindu "reformist" activity since its inception in 1875 by Swami Dayananda, pursuing campaigns against idolatry and caste. Its teachings "exalt rationality, restraint and austerity. The movement is radically monotheistic, abhorring priestly authority and elaborate ritual. Its experience of Hinduism is action-centered, soldierlike, and explicitly masculinized" (S. Bayly 2004a: 130).

Association of Voluntary Blood Donors, West Bengal (AVBDWB). Vanguard voluntary movement for the promotion of nonremunerated blood donation in West Bengal. Extremely successful, it has spawned imitator organizations in other states such as Kerala and Tamil Nadu.

Bharatiya Janata Party (BJP). Indian People's Party; a Hindu nationalist party founded in 1980. Ousted from power in 2004, it considers the Rashtriya Swayamsevak Sangh (q.v.) a moral authority.

Brahma Kumaris. "Daughters of Brahma"; founded in the 1930s. Particularly active in urban north India, possessing in excess of 100,000 devotees. Promulgates a millenarian theology.

Congress Party. Also known as Indian National Congress; founded 1885, political organization at forefront of struggle for Indian Independence. Heads the present government.

Dera Sacha Sauda. "True deal"; also known as Sacha Sauda. Devotional order founded in 1948, located in Sirsa, Haryana. In the sant tradition, it claims more than a million devotees. Holds Guinness world record for largest-ever blood donation camp (2004).

Dev Sangha. Small West Bengal community centering on worship of the goddess Haimavati, an amalgamation of Brahma, Vishnu, Shiva, and Durga.

Divine Life Society. Religious movement founded in 1936 by Swami Sivananda emphasizing universality of Hindu thought and practice. Has links with the Vishwa Hindu Parishad (q.v.).

Indian Society of Blood Transfusion and Immunohaematology (ISBTI). Professional organization and health pressure group with members deriving from blood banking, transfusion medicine, and donor recruitment. Established 1972.

International Society of Blood Transfusion (ISBT). Founded in 1935, a scientific society bringing together professionals involved in transfusion medicine from more than eighty-five countries.

International Federation of Red Cross and Red Crescent Societies. World's largest humanitarian organization with over a 185 member national societies. Holds the seven fundamental principles of: humanity, impartiality, neutrality, independence, voluntary service, unity, and universality.

Limbdi Ajramar Jain Community. Followers of eighteenth-century Jain guru, Acharyashri Ajramarji Maharaj Saheb. Organized a series of spectacular fasts and blood donation events in 2003 on the 250th birth anniversary of Ajramar, also the year of Lord Mahavir's 2600th birth anniversary.

Mata Amritanandamayi Mission. Established by Kerala guru Mata Amritanandamayi in 1981 to undertake charitable works that include the donation of blood. The Mata (mother) is believed by her devotees to be an incarnation of the goddess Devi (see Warrier 2003a).

Narendra Maharaj. Maharashtrian guru whose followers regularly donate blood.

National AIDS Control Organization (NACO). Government body that oversees and coordinates all AIDS-related public policy areas in India. Actively seeks to foster voluntary blood donation.

Radhasoami. Spiritual movement in the sant tradition, founded in 1861 by Swami Shiv Dayal, who was succeeded by other spiritual masters. There are now more than twenty lineages in the Radhasoami family tree, the three largest being based in Dayalbagh, near Agra; Beas, in the Punjab; and Delhi (Juergensmeyer 1991: 4–5). Both the Beas and Agra branches enjoin devotees to seek God-Realization through a living spiritual master.

Rashtriya Swayamsevak Sangh (RSS). "Association of National Volunteers"; a militant, highly disciplined Hindu nationalist organization. Treated as a moral authority by other Hindutva groups.

Red Cross Blood Bank, Delhi. Busiest blood bank in the capital, and one of the oldest, it collects mainly replacement donations, despite most days conducting voluntary camps.

Rotary Blood Bank, Delhi. Opened in 2002; this NGO-run blood bank was the first in the capital to accept only voluntary blood donations and not to demand replacement.

Safe Blood. Small Delhi NGO that maintains lists of donors and conducts school visits to publicize voluntary blood donation. Founded by a hematologist who practices in Delhi's Apollo Hospital.

Sant Nirankari Mission/Mandal. Large Delhi-based devotional movement in the sant tradition, founded in 1929. Claims millions of devotees.

Sathya Sai Baba. Charismatic "godman" based in Andhra Pradesh, south India, with large international following. Devotees conduct a range of seva activities, including blood donation. See Babb's (1986) excellent study of his Indian devotees.

Sawan Kirpal Ruhani Mission. Delhi-based offshoot of the Radhasoamis (q.v.).

Shiv Sena. Nativist political party based in Maharashtra espousing a particularly virulent and Islamaphobic brand of Hindutva.

Swami Ramdev. Nationally prominent yoga instructor and guru who showcases his techniques on television and at huge "yoga camps" in metropolitan settings.

Vishwa Hindu Parishad (VHP). "World Hindu Council"; founded in 1964. Pursues a staunchly Hindutva-based agenda.

World Health Organization (WHO). United Nations special agency for health, established in 1948. Governed by 192 member states through the World Health Assembly.

Youth Congress. Youth wing of Congress Party (q.v.). Was, under Indira Gandhi's son Sanjay in the 1970s, a "delinquent boys' club" (Khilnani 1997: 47). Now conducts social service activities and campaigns for the Party.

REFERENCES

Web sites last accessed in February 2008.

Abrahams, Ray. 1991. "Plus ça change, plus c'est la meme chose?" *Australian Journal of Anthropology* 1, 2–3: 131–146.

Adas, Michael. 1981. "From Avoidance to Confrontation: Peasant Protest in Precolonial and Colonial Southeast Asia." *Comparative Studies in Society and History* 23, 2: 217–247.

Addlakha, Renu. 2001. "State Legitimacy and Social Suffering in a Modern Epidemic: A Case Study of Dengue Hemorrhagic Fever in Delhi." *Contributions to Indian Sociology* 35, 2: 151–179.

Allen, Tim. 1989. "Violence and Moral Knowledge: Observing Social Trauma in Sudan and Uganda." *Cambridge Anthropology* 13, 1: 45–65.

Alter, Joseph. 1992a. "The *Sannyasi* and the Indian Wrestler: The Anatomy of a Relationship." *American Ethnologist* 19, 2: 317–336.

———. 1992b. *The Wrestler's Body: Identity and Ideology in North India.* Berkeley: University of California Press.

———. 1994. "Celibacy, Sexuality, and the Transformation of Gender into Nationalism in North India." *Journal of Asian Studies* 53, 1: 45–66.

———. 1999. "Heaps of Health, Metaphysical Fitness: Ayurveda and the Ontology of Good Health in Medical Anthropology." *Current Anthropology* 40 Supplement: 43–66.

———. 2000. *Gandhi's Body: Sex, Diet, and the Politics of Nationalism.* Philadelphia: University of Pennsylvania Press.

———. 2004. *Yoga in Modern India: The Body between Science and Philosophy.* Princeton: Princeton University Press.

Ambedkar, B. R. 1989. *Thoughts of Ambedkar.* Vol. 1, ed. L. R. Bailey. Jalandhar: Bheem Patrika Publications.

Anagnost, Ann. 2006. "Strange Circulations: The Blood Economy in Rural China." *Economy and Society* 35, 4: 509–529.

Anderson, Benedict. 1991. *Imagined Communities.* London: Verso.

Anidjar, Gil. 2002. "A Note on 'Faith and Knowledge.' " In *Jacques Derrida: Acts of Religion*, ed. Gil Anidjar, 40–41. New York: Routledge.

Appadurai, Arjun. 1981. "Gastro-Politics in Hindu South Asia." *American Ethnologist* 8: 494–511.

———. 1986. "Introduction: Commodities and the Politics of Value." In *The Social Life of Things: Commodities in Cultural Perspective*, ed. Arjun Appadurai, 3–63. Cambridge: Cambridge University Press.

———. 1990. "Topographies of the Self: Praise and Emotion in India." In *Language and the Politics of Emotion*, ed. C. Lutz and L. Abu-Lughod, 92–112. Cambridge: Cambridge University Press.

Arias, Ernesto G., and Gerhard Fischer. 2000. "Boundary Objects: Their Role in Articulating the Task in Hand and Making Information Relevant to It." Boulder: University of Colorado, Center for Lifelong Learning and Design and Institute of Cognitive Science, Department of Computer Science, and College of Architecture and Planning. Available at http://cs.colorado.edu/~gerhard/papers/icsc2000.pdf.

Arnold, David. 1993. *Colonizing the Body: State Medicine and Epidemic Disease in Nineteenth-Century India*. Berkeley: University of California Press.

Babb, Lawrence A. 1986. *Redemptive Encounters: Three Modern Styles in the Hindu Tradition*. Berkeley: University of California Press.

———. 2004. *Alchemies of Violence: Myths of Identity and the Life of Trade in Western India*. Delhi: Sage.

Badrinath, Chaturvedi. 1993. *Dharma, India, and the World Order: Twenty-one Essays*. Edinburgh: Saint Andrew Press.

Bailey, F. G. 1981. "Spiritual Merit and Morality." In *Culture and Morality: Essays in Honour of Christoph von Furer-Haimendorf*, ed. Adrian C. Mayer, 23–41. Delhi: Oxford University Press.

Bailey, James Wood. 1997. *Utilitarianism, Institutions, and Justice*. Oxford: Oxford University Press.

Barkun, M. 1998. "Politics and Apocalypticism." In *Apocalypticism in the Modern Period and the Contemporary Age*. Vol. 3, *The Encyclopaedia of Apocalypticism*, ed. S. J. Stein, 442–460. New York: Continuum.

Barthes, Roland. [1959] 2000. "Tacitus and the Funerary Baroque." In *A Roland Barthes Reader*, ed. Susan Sontag, 162–166. London: Vintage.

Bataille, Georges. 1985. "The Notion of Expenditure." In *Visions of Excess*, ed. and trans. Alan Stoekl, 116–129. Minneapolis: University of Minneapolis Press.

Bayer, Ronald, and Eric A. Feldman. 1999. "Introduction: Understanding the Blood Feuds." In *Blood Feuds: AIDS, Blood, and the Politics of Medical Disaster*, ed. Eric A. Feldman and Ronald Bayer, 1–16. Oxford: Oxford University Press.

Bayly, C. A. 1986. "The Origins of Swadeshi (Home Industry): Cloth and Indian Society, 1700–1930." In *The Social Life of Things*, ed. Arjun Appadurai, 285–321. Cambridge: Cambridge University Press.

———. 1988. *Indian Society and the Making of the British Empire*. Cambridge: Cambridge University Press.

Bayly, Susan. 1989. *Saints, Goddesses and Kings: Muslims and Christians in South Indian Society, 1700–1900*. Cambridge: Cambridge University Press.

———. 1999. *Caste, Society and Politics in India from the Eighteenth Century to the Modern Age*. Cambridge: Cambridge University Press.

———. 2004a. "Conceptualizing from Within: Divergent Religious Modes from Asian Modernist Perspectives." In *Ritual and Memory: Toward a Comparative Anthropology of Religion*, ed. James Laidlaw and Harvey Whitehouse, 111–134. Walnut Creek, Calif.: Altamira Press.

———. 2004b. "Vietnamese Intellectuals in Revolutionary and Postcolonial Times." *Critique of Anthropology* 24, 3: 320–344.

Beckerlegge, Gwilym. 2003. "Saffron and *Seva*: The Rashtriya Swayamsevak Sangh's Appropriation of Swami Vivekananda." In *Hinduism in Public and Private: Reform, Hindutva, Gender and Sampraday*, ed. Antony Copley, 31–65. Delhi: Oxford University Press.

Benei, Veronique. 2006. "Languages, Bodies, Emotions: Schooling Regional/National Citizens in Western India." Lecture given at Cambridge University.

Berger, John. 1974. *The Look of Things*. New York: Viking Press.

Bergman, Gregory. 2006. *Isms.* Avon, Mass.: Adams Media.

Bhabha, Homi K. 1984. "Of Mimicry and Man: The Ambivalence of Colonial Discourse" *October* 28, Spring: 125–133.

Bharadwaj, Aditya. 2003. "Why Adoption Is Not an Option in India: The Visibility of Infertility, the Secrecy of Donor Insemination, and Other Cultural Complexities." *Social Science and Medicine* 56, 9: 1867–1880.

———. 2007. "Biosociality and Bio-Crossings: Encounters with Assisted Conception and Embryonic Stem Cells in India." In *Genetics, Biosociality and the Social Sciences: Making Biologies and Identities*, ed. S. Gibbon and C. Novas, 98–116. London: Routledge.

———. 2008. "Assisted Life: The Neoliberal Moral Economy of Embryonic Stem Cells in India." In *Reproductive Technologies in Non-western Settings*, ed. Marcia Inhorn and Daphna Birenbaum-Carmeli. Oxford: Berghahn.

Bharucha, Zarin. 2000. "Blood Services in India." *Transfusion International* 79: 12–13.

Boas, Franz. 1966. *Kwakiutl Ethnography*, ed. H. Lodere. Chicago: University of Chicago Press.

Bornstein, Erica. 2003. *The Spirit of Development: Protestant NGOs, Morality, and Economics in Zimbabwe*. Stanford: Stanford University Press.

———. 2006. "No Return: A Brief Typology of Philanthropy and the Sacred in New Delhi." In *The Practice of Altruism: Caring and Religion in Comparative Perspective*, ed. Ruben L. F. Habito and Keishin Inaba, 165–179. Newcastle: Cambridge Scholars Press.

———. Forthcoming (2009). "Sacred Philanthropy: Between Impulse and Obligation." *Contributions to Indian Sociology*.

Bowker, Geoffrey C., and Susan Leigh Star. 1999. *Sorting Things Out: Classification and Its Consequences*. London: MIT Press.

Boyer, Pascal. 1999. "Human Cognition and Cultural Evolution." In *Anthropological Theory Today*, ed. Henrietta Moore, 206–233. Cambridge: Polity Press.

Brass, Paul. 1990. *The Politics of India since Independence*. Cambridge: Cambridge University Press.

Bray, Tim. 2001. "The Rational Use of Blood in India: Intervention to Promote Good Transfusion Practice." Ph.D. Thesis, London School of Hygiene and Tropical Medicine.

Bray, Tim, and K. Prabhakar. 2002. "Blood Policy and Transfusion Practice—India." *Tropical Medicine and International Health* 7, 6: 477.

Bray, Tim., P. Salil, H. A. Weiss, and J.D.H. Porter. 2003. "Transfusion Medicine in India: A Survey of Current Practice." *Transfusion Medicine* 13, 1: 17–24.

Brooks, J. P. 2004. "The Rights of Blood Recipients Should Supersede Any Asserted Rights of Blood Donors." *Vox Sanguinis* 87, 4: 280–286.

Bryant, Rebecca. 2002. "The Purity of Spirit and the Power of Blood: A Comparative Perspective on Nation, Gender, and Kinship in Cyprus." *Journal of the Royal Anthropological Institute* 8, 3: 509–530.

Callon, Michel. 1998. "Introduction: The Embeddedness of Economic Markets in Economics." In *Laws of the Markets*, ed. Michel Callon, 1–59. Oxford: Blackwell.

Caputo, John D. 1987. *Radical Hermeneutics: Repetition, Deconstruction, and the Hermeneutic Project*. Bloomington: Indiana University Press.

Chakrabarty, Dipesh. 2007. " 'In the Name of Politics': Democracy and the Power of the Multitude in India." *Public Culture*. 19, 1: 35–58.

Chatterjee, Partha. 1996. "The Manifold Uses of Jati." In *Region, Religion, Caste, Gender and Culture in Contemporary India*. Vol. 3, ed. T. V. Sathyamurthy, 281–292. Delhi: Oxford University Press.

Cohen, Lawrence. 1998. *No Aging in India: Modernity, Senility and the Family*. Delhi: Oxford University Press.

——. 1999. "Where It Hurts: Indian Material for an Ethics of Organ Transplantation." *Daedalus* 128, 4: 135–165.

——. 2001. "The Other Kidney: Biopolitics beyond Recognition." *Body & Society* 7, 2–3: 9–29.

——. 2004. "Operability: Surgery at the Margin of the State." In *Anthropology in the Margins of the State*, ed. Veena Das and Deborah Poole, 165–190. Santa Fe: School of American Research Press.

——. 2007. "Committed to Death." Paper presented at 106th American Anthropological Association Annual Meeting, Washington, DC.

Cohn, B. S. 1987. "The Census, Social Structure, and Objectification in South Asia." In *An Anthropologist among the Historians and Other Essays*, 224–254. Delhi: Oxford University Press.

Coleman, Simon. 2004. "The Charismatic Gift." *Journal of the Royal Anthropological Institute* 10, 2: 421–442.

Connerton, Paul. 1989. *How Societies Remember*. Cambridge: Cambridge University Press.

Copeman, Jacob. 2004. " 'Blood Will Have Blood': A Study in Indian Political Ritual." *Social Analysis* 48, 3: 126–148.

——. 2005. "Veinglory: Exploring Processes of Blood Transfer between Persons." *Journal of the Royal Anthropological Institute* 11, 3: 465–485.

——. 2006. "Cadaver Donation as Ascetic Practice in India." *Social Analysis* 50, 1: 103–126.

——. Forthcoming. "Extractive Endings: Death, *Dan*, and Virtuous Utility in India." In *The Politics of the Gift*, ed. Nikolai Ssorin-Chaikov. Oxford: Berghahn.

Copley, Antony. 1997. *Religions in Conflict: Ideology, Cultural Contact, and Conversion in Late Colonial India*. Delhi: Oxford University Press.

Corbin, John. 1986. "Insurrections in Spain: Casas Viejas 1933 and Madrid 1981." In *The Anthropology of Violence*, ed. D. Riches, 28–49. Oxford: Blackwell.

Corsín Jiménez, Alberto. 2005. "Changing Scales and the Scales of Change: Ethnography and Political Economy in Antofagasta, Chile." *Critique of Anthropology* 25, 2: 157–176.

——. 2007. "Introduction: Well-being's Re-proportioning of Social Thought." In *Culture and Well-Being: Anthropological Approaches to Freedom and Political Ethics*, ed. Alberto Corsín Jiménez. London: Pluto Press.

Crease, Robert P. 1997. "Responsive Order: the Phenomenology of Dramatic and Scientific Performance." In *Creativity in Performance*, ed. R. K. Sawyer, 213–225. London: Ablex.

Cunningham, Andrew, and Bridie Andrews. 1997. "Introduction: Western Medicine as Contested Knowledge." In *Western Medicine as Contested Knowledge*, ed. Andrew Cunningham and Bridie Andrews, 1–23. Manchester: Manchester University Press.

Dalsgaard, Steffan. 2007. " 'I Do It for the Chocolate': An Anthropological Study of Blood Donation in Denmark." *Distinktion* 14: 101–117.

Daniel, E. Valentine. 1984. *Fluid Signs: Being a Person the Tamil Way*. Berkeley: University of California Press.

Daniel, Sheryl B. 1983. "The Tool Box Approach of the Tamil to the Issues of Moral Responsibility and Human Destiny." In *Karma: An Anthropological Inquiry,* ed. Charles F. Keyes and E. Valentine Daniel, 27–62. Berkeley: University of California Press.

Das, Veena. 1983. "Language of Sacrifice." *Man* 18, 3: 445–462.

——. 2004. "The Signature of the State: The Paradox of Illegibility." In *Anthropology in the Margins of the State*, ed. Veena Das and Deborah Poole, 225–252. Santa Fe: School of American Research Press.

Derrida, Jacques. 1992. *Given Time: 1. Counterfeit Money*. Chicago: University of Chicago Press.

———. 1995. *The Gift of Death*. Chicago: University of Chicago Press.

———. 1998. "Faith and Knowledge: The Two Sources of 'Religion' at the Limits of Reason Alone." In *Religion*, ed. Jacques Derrida and Gianni Vatimo, 1–78. Stanford: Stanford University Press.

Donne, John. 1937. *The Love Poems of John Donne*. London: Chatto and Windus.

Douglas, Mary. 1990. "No Free Gifts." Foreword to Marcel Mauss, *The Gift: The Form and Reason for Exchange in Archaic Societies*, trans. W. D. Halls, vii–xviii. London: Routledge.

Dumont, Louis. 1966. *Homo Hierarchicus: An Essay on the Caste System*. Chicago: University of Chicago Press.

Eco, Umberto. 1997. *Kant and the Platypus: Essays on Language and Cognition*. London: Secker and Warburg.

Edwards, Catharine, and Thomas Osborne. 2005. "Scenographies of Suicide: an Introduction." *Economy and Society* 34, 2: 173–177.

Eliade, Mircea. 1990. *Yoga: Immortality and Freedom*. Princeton: Princeton University Press.

Empson, Rebecca. 2006. "Reproducing People and Prophecy in Mongolia." *Cambridge Anthropology* 25, 3: 52–60.

English, James F. 2005. *The Economy of Prestige: Prizes, Awards, and the Circulation of Cultural Value*. Cambridge: Harvard University Press.

Erwin, Kathleen. 2006. "The Circulatory System: Blood Procurement, AIDS, and the Social Body in China." *Medical Anthropology Quarterly* 20, 2: 139–159.

Favero, Paolo. 2005. *India Dreams: Cultural Identity among Young Middle Class Men in New Delhi*. Stockholm: Stockholm Studies in Social Anthropology.

Foucault, Michel. 1977. *Discipline and Punish: The Birth of the Prison*. London: Penguin.

———. 1984. *The History of Sexuality*. Vol. 3, *The Care of the Self*. London: Penguin.

———. 1994. "On the Government of the Living." In *Ethics: Subjectivity and Truth. Essential Works of Foucault 1954–1984*, ed. Paul Rabinow, 81–85. London: Penguin.

Fox, Renee C., and Judith P. Swazey. 1992. *Spare Parts: Organ Replacement in American Society*. Oxford: Oxford University Press.

Fox, Richard G. 1985. *Lions of the Punjab: Culture in the Making*. Berkeley: University of California Press.

Freed, Stanley A., and Ruth S. Freed. 1998. *Hindu Festivals in a North Indian Village*. Seattle: Anthropological Papers of the American Museum of Natural History.

Froerer, Peggy. 2006. "Emphasizing Others: The Emergence of Hindu Nationalism in a Central Indian Tribal Community." *Journal of the Royal Anthropological Institute* 12, 1: 39–59.

Fuller, C. J. 1992. *The Camphor Flame: Popular Hinduism and Society in India*. Princeton: Princeton University Press.

Gandhi, Mohandas K. 1949. *An Autobiography: The Story of My Experiments with Truth*. London: Phoenix Press.

———. 1961. *Non-Violent Resistance (Satyagraha)*, ed. Bharatan Kumarappa. New York: Schocken Books.

Geertz, Clifford. 1983. "Centers, Kings, and Charisma: Reflections on the Symbolics of Power." In *Local Knowledge: Further Essays in Interpretive Anthropology*, 121–146. New York: Basic Books.

———. 2000. "The Pinch of Destiny: Religion as Experience, Meaning, Identity, Power." In *Available Light: Anthropological Reflections on Philosophical Topics*, 167–186. Princeton: Princeton University Press.

Gell, Alfred. 1992. *The Anthropology of Time: Cultural Constructions of Temporal Maps and Images*. Oxford: Berg.

———. 1998. *Art and Agency: An Anthropological Theory*. Oxford: Clarendon Press.

Gellner, David. 2004. "Hinduism. None, One or Many?" *Social Anthropology* 12, 3: 367–371.

Ghosh, Arunabha, and Tapan Babu. 2006. "Lage Raho Munna Bhai: Unraveling Brand Gandhigiri." *Economic and Political Weekly* 41, 51: 5225–5228.

Giddens, Anthony. 1990. *The Consequences of Modernity*. Stanford: Stanford University Press.

Godelier, Maurice. 1999. *The Enigma of the Gift*. Cambridge: Polity Press.

Gold, Ann Grodzins. 1988. *Fruitful Journeys: The Ways of Rajasthani Pilgrims*. Berkeley: University of California Press.

Gold, Daniel. 1987. *The Lord as Guru: Hindi Sants in the North Indian Tradition*. Oxford: Oxford University Press.

———. 1992. "What the Merchant-Guru Sold: Social and Literary Types in Hindi Devotional Verse." *Journal of the American Oriental Society* 112, 1: 22–35.

Gordon, Eliza. J. 2000. "Preventing Waste: A Ritual Analysis of Candidate Selection for Kidney Transplantation." *Anthropology and Medicine* 7, 3: 351–371.

Greenblatt, Stephen J. 1996. "Resonance and Wonder." In *Modern Literary Theory: A Reader* 3rd ed., ed. Philip Rice and Patricia Waugh, 268–288. London: Arnold.

Greenhouse, Carol J. 1996. *A Moment's Notice: Time Politics across Cultures*. Ithaca: Cornell University Press.

Gregory, C. A. Forthcoming (2009). "The Auspicious Gift in Middle India." *Contributions to Indian Sociology*.

Grewal, J. S. 1990. *The Sikhs of the Punjab*. Cambridge: Cambridge University Press.

Guha, Sumit. 2003. "The Politics of Identity and Enumeration in India c. 1600–1990." *Comparative Studies in Society and History* 45, 1: 148–167.

Guinness World Records. 2004. *Guinness Book of World Records, 2005*. London: Guinness.

Halliburton, Murphy. 2002. "Rethinking Anthropological Studies of the Body: *Manas* and *Bodham* in Kerala." *American Anthropologist* 104, 4: 1123–1134.

Handelman, Don. 1990. *Models and Mirrors: Towards an Anthropology of Public Events*. Cambridge: Cambridge University Press.

Hannerz, Ulf. 1999. "Notes on the Global Ecumene." In *The Anthropology of Globalization: A Reader*, ed. Jonathan Xavier Inda and Renato Rosaldo, 37–45. Oxford: Blackwell.

Hansen, Thomas Blom. 1999. *The Saffron Wave: Democracy and Hindu Nationalism in Modern India*. Delhi: Oxford University Press.

———. 2001. *Wages of Violence: Naming and Identity in Postcolonial Bombay*. Princeton: Princeton University Press.

Hanson, Stephen. 1997. *Time and Revolution: Marxism and the Design of Soviet Institutions*. Chapel Hill: University of North Carolina Press.

Hardiman, David. 1996. *Feeding the Baniya: Peasants and Usurers in Western India*. Delhi: Oxford University Press.

Harriss, John. 2003. 'Widening the Radius of Trust': Ethnographic Explorations of Trust and Indian Business." *Journal of the Royal Anthropological Institute* 9, 4: 755–773.

Hart, Keith. 2005. *The Hit Man's Dilemma: Or, Business, Personal and Impersonal*. Chicago: Prickly Paradigm Press.

Hawley, John Stratton. 1995. "The Saints Subdued: Domestic Virtue and National Integration in *Amar Chitra Katha*." In *Media and the Transformation of Religion in South Asia*, ed. Lawrence A. Babb and Susan S. Wadley, 107–134. Philadelphia: University of Pennsylvania Press.

Hayden, Cori. 2007. "Taking as Giving: Bioscience, Exchange, and the Politics of Benefit-Sharing." *Social Studies of Science* 37, 5: 729–758.

Haynes, Douglas. 1987. "From Tribute to Philanthropy: The Politics of Gift Giving in a West Indian City." *Journal of Asian Studies* 46, 2: 339–360.

———. 1991. "From Avoidance to Confrontation? A Contestatory History of Merchant-State Relations in Surat, 1600–1924." In *Contesting Power: Resistance and Everyday Social Relations in South Asia*, ed. Douglas Haynes and Gyan Prakash, 239–289. Berkeley: University of California Press.

Haynes, Douglas, and Gyan Prakash. 1991. "Introduction: The Entanglement of Power and Resistance." In *Contesting Power: Resistance and Everyday Social Relations in South Asia*, ed. Douglas Haynes and Gyan Prakash, 1–23. Berkeley: University of California Press.

Healy, Kieran. 2006. *Last Best Gifts: Altruism and the Market for Human Organs*. Chicago: University of Chicago Press.

Heidegger, Martin. [1953] 1993. "The Question Concerning Technology." In *Martin Heidegger: Basic Writings*, ed. David Farrell Krell, 307–342. London: Routledge.

Heim, Maria. 2004. *Theories of the Gift in South Asia: Hindu, Buddhist, and Jain Reflections on "Dana."* London: Routledge.

Hellman, Eva. 1996. "Dynamic Hinduism: Towards a New Hindu Nation." In *Questioning the Secular State*, ed. D. Westerlund, 237–258. London: Hurst.

Heuze, Gerard. 1992. "Shiv Sena and 'National' Hinduism." *Economic and Political Weekly* 27, 40–41: 2189–2195 and 2253–2263.

Hibbets, Maria. 1999. "Saving Them from Yourself: An Inquiry into the South Asian Gift of Fearlessness." *Journal of Religious Ethics* 27, 3: 437–462.

Hirsch, Eric. 1995. "The 'Holding Together' of Ritual: Ancestrality and Achievement in the Papuan Highlands." In *Cosmos and Society in Oceania*, ed. D. de Coppet and A. Iteanu, 213–233. Oxford: Berg.

Hobsbawn, E. J. 1959. *Primitive Rebels: Studies in Archaic Forms of Social Movement in the Nineteenth and Twentieth Centuries*. Manchester: Manchester University Press.

Hogan, David E., and Julio Rafael Lairet. 2007. "Triage." In *Disaster Medicine*, ed. David E. Hogan and Jonathan L. Burstein, 12–39. Philadelphia: Wolters Kluwer-Lippincott Williams and Wilkins.

Holtorf, Christian. 2001. "My Blood for Thee." In *Blood: Art, Power, Politics and Pathology*, ed. James D. Bradburne, 21–31. London: Prestel.

Hopkins, Washburn. 1901. "On the Hindu Custom of Dying to Redress a Grievance." *Journal of the American Oriental Society* 21: 146–159.

Husain, M. G., ed. 1996. *Ethnic Diversity and National Integration*. Delhi: Manak Publications.

Huyler, Frank. 2000. *The Blood of Strangers: True Stories from the Emergency Room*. London: Fourth Estate.

Ingold, Tim. 1997. "Eight Themes in the Anthropology of Technology." *Social Analysis* 41, 1: 106–138.

———. 2006. "Rethinking the Animate, Re-Animating Thought." *Ethnos* 71, 1: 9–20.

Institute of Electrical and Electronics Engineers. 1990. *IEEE Standard Computer Dictionary: A Compilation of IEEE Standard Computer Glossaries*. New York: IEEE.

Jackson, Michael. 2002. "Biotechnology and the Critique of Globalization." *Ethnos* 67, 2: 141–154.

Jaffrelot, Christophe. 1996. *The Hindu Nationalist Movement and Indian Politics: 1925 to the 1990s*. Delhi: Penguin.

Jones, Kenneth W. 1976. *Arya Dharm: Hindu Consciousness in Nineteenth-Century Punjab*. Berkeley: University of California Press.

Joralemon, Donald. 1995. "Organ Wars: The Battle for Body Parts." *Medical Anthropology Quarterly* 9, 3: 335–356.

Juergensmeyer, Mark. 1991. *Radhasoami Reality: The Logic of a Modern Faith*. Princeton: Princeton University Press.

———. 1995. "The Social Significance of Radhasoami." In *Bhakti Religion in North India: Community Identity and Political Action*, ed. David N. Lorenzen, 67–93. Albany: State University of New York Press.

Kakar, Sudhir. 1984. *Shamans, Mystics and Doctors: A Psychological Inquiry into India and Its Healing Traditions*. London: Unwin.

Kapferer, Bruce. 1997. *Feast of the Sorcerer: Practices of Consciousness and Power*. Chicago: Chicago University Press.

Kapila, Kriti. 2008. "The Measure of a Tribe: The Cultural Politics of Constitutional Reclassification in North India." *Journal of the Royal Anthropological Institute* 14, 1: 117–134.

Kaviraj, Sudipta. 1989. "On the Construction of Colonial Power: Structure, Discourse, Hegemony." Nehru Memorial Museum and Library: Delhi (mimeographed).

Kent, Alexandra. 2004. "Divinity, Miracles and Charity in the Sathya Sai Baba Movement of Malaysia." *Ethnos* 69, 1: 43–62.

Khare, R. S. 1984. *The Untouchable as Himself: Ideology, Identity, and Pragmatism among the Lucknow Chamars*. Cambridge: Cambridge University Press.

Khilnani, Sunil. 1997. *The Idea of India*. Delhi: Penguin.

Koenigsberg, Richard. 2004. "As the Soldier Dies So the Nation Comes Alive: The Sacrificial Meaning of Warfare." Available at http://home.earthlink.net/~libraryofsocialscience/as_the_soldier.htm.

Konrad, Monica. 1998. "Ova Donation and Symbols of Substance: Some Variations on the Theme of Sex, Gender and the Partible Person. *Journal of the Royal Anthropological Institute* 4, 4: 643–667.

———. 2005. *Nameless Relations: Anonymity, Melanesia, and Reproductive Gift Exchange between British Ova Donors and Recipients*. Oxford: Berghahn.

Laidlaw, James. 1995. *Riches and Renunciation: Religion, Economy, and Society among the Jains*. Oxford. Clarendon Press.

———. 1996. "The Uses and Abuses of Theology: Comments on Jonathan Parry's *Death in Banaras*." *South Asia Research* 16, 1: 31–44.

———. 2000. "A Free Gift Makes No Friends." *Journal of the Royal Anthropological Institute* 6, 4: 617–634.

———. 2002. "For an Anthropology of Ethics and Freedom." *Journal of the Royal Anthropological Institute* 8, 2: 311–332.

———. 2004. "Embedded Modes of Religiosity in Indic Renouncer Religions." In *Ritual and Memory: Toward a Comparative Anthropology of Religion*, ed. James Laidlaw and Harvey Whitehouse, 89–109. Walnut Creek, Calif.: Altamira Press.

———. 2005. "A Life Worth Leaving: Fasting to Death as Telos of a Jain Religious Life." *Economy and Society* 34, 2: 178–199.

———. 2007. "The Intension and Extension of Well-Being: Transformation in Diaspora Jain Understandings of Non-Violence." In *Culture and Well-Being: Anthropological Approaches to Freedom and Political Ethics*, ed. Alberto Corsín Jiménez, 156–179. London: Pluto Press.

Lal, Vinay. 2002. "Indians and the Guinness Book of Records: The Political and Cultural Contours of a National Obsession." In *Of Cricket, Gandhi, and Guinness: Essays in Indian History and Culture*. Calcutta: Seagull Books.

Lambert, Helen. 2000. "Sentiment and Substance in North Indian Forms of Relatedness." In *Cultures of Relatedness*, ed. Janet Carsten, 73–89. Cambridge: Cambridge University Press.

Langford, Jean. 2002. *Fluent Bodies: Ayurvedic Remedies for Postcolonial Imbalance*. Durham: Duke University Press.

Lapierre, Dominique. 1999. *The City of Joy*. Delhi: Full Circle.

Laqueur, Thomas. 1999. "Pint for Pint." *London Review of Books*, 14 October: 3–7.

Latour, Bruno. 2000. "When Things Strike Back: A Possible Contribution of Science Studies." *British Journal of Sociology* 5, 1: 105–123.

Leach, James. 2004. "A Dispersed Creativity, Or, Persons and Their Boundaries: Some Broader Issues Involved in the Ownership of Intellectual Property." *Cambridge Anthropology* 24, 1: 21–27.

Leder, Drew. 1990. *The Absent Body*. Chicago: University of Chicago Press.

Lele, Jayant, ed. 1981. *Tradition and Modernity in Bhakti Movements*. Leiden: E. J. Brill.

Lewin, M. 1985. *The Making of the Soviet System: Essays in the Social History of Interwar Russia*. London: Methuen.

Lindstrom, Lamont. 1984. "Doctor, Lawyer, Wiseman, Priest: Big-Men and Knowledge in Melanesia." *Man* 19, 2: 291–309.

Lipner, Julius J. 1989. "The Classical Hindu View on Abortion and the Moral Status of the Unborn." In *Hindu Ethics*, ed. H. G. Coward, J. J. Lipner, and K. K. Young, 41–69. Albany: State University of New York Press.

Lock, Margaret. 2000. "The Quest for Human Organs and the Violence of Zeal." In *Violence and Subjectivity*, ed. Veena Das, M. Ramphele and Arthur Kleinman, 271–295. Berkeley: University of California Press.

———. 2002. *Twice Dead: Organ Transplants and the Reinvention of Death*. Berkeley: University of California Press.

———. 2003. "On Making up the Good-as-Dead in a Utilitarian World." In *Rethinking Life and Death: Toward an Anthropology of the Biosciences*, ed. Margaret Lock and Sarah Franklin, 165–192. Santa Fe: School of American Research.

———. 2007. "Alienation of Body Parts and the Biopolitics of Immortalized Cell Lines." In *Beyond the Body Proper: Reading the Anthropology of Material Life*, ed. Margaret Lock and Judith Farquhar, 567–583. Durham: Duke University Press.

Lorenzen, David N. 1995. "Introduction: The Historical Vicissitudes of Bhakti Religion." In *Bhakti Religion in North India: Community Identity and Political Action*, ed. David N. Lorenzen, 1–32. Albany: State University of New York Press.

Macfarlane, Alan. 1997. "On Creative and Analytical Methods." Available at http://www.alanmacfarlane.com/TEXTS/holmes.pdf.

MacIntyre, Alastair. 1981. *After Virtue: A Study in Moral Theory*. London: Duckworth.

Madan, T. N. 1980. "Doctors at the All India Institute of Medical Sciences." In *Doctors and Society: Three Asian Case Studies*, ed. T. N. Madan, 11–112. Ghaziabad: Vikas.

———. 1987. *Non-Renunciation: Themes and Interpretations of Indian Culture*. Delhi: Oxford University Press.

———. 1991. "Introduction." In *Religion in India*, ed. T. N. Madan, 1–25. Delhi: Oxford University Press.

———. 1997. *Modern Myths, Locked Minds: Secularism and Fundamentalism in India*. Delhi: Oxford University Press.

Mahmood, Cynthia Keppley. 1997. *Fighting for Faith and Nation: Dialogues with Sikh Militants*. Philadelphia: University of Pennsylvania Press.

Malleson, G. B. 1987. "Was There a Conspiracy?" In *India in 1857—The Revolt against Foreign Rule*, ed. A. Embree. Delhi: Chanakya Publications.

Marcus, G. E. 2002. "Beyond Malinowski and after *Writing Culture*: On the Future of Cultural Anthropology and the Predicament of Ethnography." *Australian Journal of Anthropology* 13, 2: 191–199.

Marriott, McKim. 1959. "Western Medicine in a Village of Northern India." In *Health, Culture, and Community*, ed. B. D. Paul, 239–268. New York: Russell Sage Foundation.

———. 1989. "Constructing an Indian Ethnosociology." *Contributions to Indian Sociology* 23, 1: 1–39.

Mathur, K. S. 1991. "Hindu Values of Life: Karma and Dharma." In *Religion in India*, ed. T. N. Madan, 63–77. Delhi: Oxford University Press.

Mauss, Marcel. 1990. *The Gift: The Form and Reason for Exchange in Archaic Societies*, trans. W. D. Halls. London: Routledge.

Mayer, Adrian C. 1981. "Public Service and Individual Merit in a Town of Central India." In *Culture and Morality: Essays in Honor of Christoph von Furer-Haimendorf*, ed. Adrian C. Mayer, 153–173. Delhi: Oxford University Press.

Mazzarella, William. 2002. "Cindy at the Taj: Cultural Enclosure and Corporate Potentateship in an Era of Globalization." In *Everyday Life in South Asia*, ed. Diane Mines and Sarah Lamb, 387–399. Bloomington: Indiana University Press.

———. 2003. *Shovelling Smoke: Advertising and Globalization in Contemporary India*. London: Duke University Press.

McKean, Lise. 1996. *Divine Enterprise: Gurus and the Hindu Nationalist Movement*. Chicago: University of Chicago Press.

McLeod, W. H. 1996. *The Evolution of the Sikh Community: Five Essays*. Delhi: Oxford University Press.

———. 1999. *Sikhs and Sikhism*. Delhi: Oxford University Press.

McSherry, Corynne. 2001. *Who Owns Academic Work? Battling for Control of Intellectual Property*. Cambridge: Harvard University Press.

Mehta, B. C. 2000. *Iron Deficiency Disease in India*. Mumbai: Dr J. C. Patel Medical Research Foundation.

Michaels, Axel. 2004. *Hinduism: Past and Present*. Princeton: Princeton University Press.

Miller, Daniel. 1998. *A Theory of Shopping*. Cambridge: Polity Press.

Mines, Diane P. 2005. *Fierce Gods: Inequality, Ritual, and the Politics of Dignity in a South Indian Village*. Bloomington: Indiana University Press.

Mines, Mattison. 1994. *Public Faces, Private Voices: Community and Individuality in South India*. Berkeley: University of California Press.

Minocha, Aneeta. 1996. *Perceptions and Interactions in a Medical Setting: A Sociological Study of a Women's Hospital*. Delhi: Hindustan Publishing Corporation.

Miyazaki, Hirokazu. 2005. "From Sugar Cane to 'Swords': Hope and the Extensibility of the Gift in Fiji." *Journal of the Royal Anthropological Institute* 11, 2: 277–295.

Mosse, David. 2004. "Is Good Policy Unimplementable? Reflections on the Ethnography of Aid Policy and Practice." *Development and Change* 35, 4: 639–671.

Nandy, Ashis. 1970. "The Culture of Indian Politics: A Stock Taking." *Journal of Asian Studies* 30, 1: 57–79.

Nanu, A. 2004. "What Ails the Indian Blood Transfusion Service?" Lecture given at the 19th National Conference of the Indian Society of Blood Transfusion and Immunohaematology, Chennai.

Nanu, A., S. P. Sharma, K. Chatterjee, and P. Jyoti. 1997. "Markers for Transfusion-Transmissible Infections in North Indian Voluntary and Replacement Blood Donors: Prevalence and Trends 1989–1996." *Vox Sanguinis* 73, 2: 70–73.

National Blood Policy. 2002. In *The Blood Banker's Legal Handbook*, compiled by M. L. Sarin, 44–53. Chandigarh: Sarin Memorial Legal Aid Foundation.

Oberoi, Harjot Singh. 1994. *The Construction of Religious Boundaries: Culture, Identity, and Diversity in the Sikh Tradition*. Oxford: Oxford University Press.

Ohnuki-Tierney, Emiko. 1994. "Brain Death and Organ Transplantation: Cultural Bases of Medical Technology." *Current Anthropology* 35, 3: 233–254.

Osborne, Thomas. 2003. "Against 'Creativity': A Philistine Rant." *Economy and Society* 32, 4: 507–525.

———. 2005. " 'Fascinated Dispossession': Suicide and the Aesthetics of Freedom." *Economy and Society* 34, 2: 280–294.

Osella, Filippo, and Caroline Osella. 1996. "Articulation of Physical and Social Bodies in Kerala." *Contributions to Indian Sociology* 30, 1: 37–68.

———. 2003. " 'Ayyappan Saranam': Masculinity and the Sabarimala Pilgrimage in Kerala." *Journal of the Royal Anthropological Institute* 9, 4: 729–754.

Paglia, Camille. 2005. *Break, Blow, Burn.* New York: Pantheon Books.

Panikkar, K. N. 1999. "Introduction: Defining the Nation as Hindu." In *The Concerned Indian's Guide to Communalism*, ed. K. N. Panikkar, vii–xxxv. Delhi: Viking.

Parry, Jonathan. 1980. "Ghosts, Greed and Sin: The Occupational Identity of the Benares Funeral Priests." *Man* 15, 1: 88–111.

———. 1986. "*The Gift*, the Indian Gift, and the 'Indian Gift.' " *Man* 21, 3: 453–473.

———. 1989. "On the Moral Perils of Exchange." In *Money and the Morality of Exchange*, ed. Jonathan Parry and Maurice Bloch, 64–93. Cambridge: Cambridge University Press.

———. 1994. *Death in Banaras.* Cambridge: Cambridge University Press.

———. 1999. "Two Cheers for Reservation: The Satnamis and the Steel Plant." In *Institutions and Inequalities: Essays in Honour of Andrei Beteille*, ed. Ramachandra Guha and Jonathan Parry, 128–169. Delhi: Oxford University Press.

———. 2000. " 'The Crisis of Corruption' and 'The Idea of India': A Worm's Eye View." In *The Morals of Legitimacy*, ed. I. Pardo. Oxford: Berghahn.

———. 2003. "Nehru's Dream and the Village 'Waiting Room': Long-Distance Labour Migrants to a Central Indian Steel Town." *Contributions to Indian Sociology* 37, 1–2: 217–249.

———. n.d. "The Sacrifices of Modernity in a Soviet-Built Steel Town in Central India." Unpublished manuscript.

Peabody, Norbert. 2001. "Cents, Sense, Census: Human Inventories in Late Precolonial and Early Colonial India." *Comparative Studies in Society and History* 43, 3: 819–50.

Pinch, William. 1997. "Subaltern Sadhus? Political Ascetics in Indian Myth, Memory, and History." Available at http://www.virginia.edu/soasia/symsem/kisan/papers/sadhus.html.

Pinney, Christopher. 2005. "Things Happen: Or, From Which Moment Does That Object Come?" In *Materiality*, ed. Daniel Miller, 256–272. Durham: Duke University Press.

———. 2006. "Technomaterialist Photography." Lecture given at Cambridge University.

Pocock, David F. 1973. *Mind, Body and Wealth: A Study of Belief and Practice in an Indian Village.* Oxford: Blackwell.

Poovey, Mary. 1998. *A History of the Modern Fact: Problems of Knowledge in the Science of Wealth and Society.* Chicago: University of Chicago Press.

Prabhananda, Swami. 1991. *The Ramakrishna Movement.* Calcutta: Ramakrishna Mission Institute of Culture.

Rabinow, Paul. 1994. "Introduction. The History of Systems of Thought." In *Ethics: Subjectivity, and Truth: Essential Works of Foucault, 1954–1984*, ed. Paul Rabinow, xi–xlii. London: Penguin.

———. 1999. *French DNA: Trouble in Purgatory.* Chicago: University of Chicago Press.

Rafael, Vincent. 2003. "The Cell Phone and the Crowd: Messianic Politics in the Contemporary Philippines." *Public Culture* 15, 3: 399–425.

Raheja, Gloria Goodwin. 1988. *The Poison in the Gift: Ritual, Prestation, and the Dominant Caste in a North Indian Village.* Chicago: University of Chicago Press.

Rajagopal, Arvind. 2001. *Politics after Television: Hindu Nationalism and the Reshaping of the Public in India*. Cambridge: Cambridge University Press.

Ramanujan, A. K. 1989. "Is There an Indian Way of Thinking? An Informal Essay." *Contributions to Indian Sociology* 23, 1: 41–58.

Rao, Anupama. 2003. "Indian Feminism and the Patriarchy of Caste." *Himal South Asian* Available at www.himalmag.com/2003/february/analysis_1.htm.

Ray, Debabrata. 1990. *National Guide Book on Blood Donor Motivation*. Delhi: Directorate General of Health Services, Ministry of Health and Family Welfare, Government of India.

———. 2003. *National Guidebook on Blood Donor Motivation*. Delhi: National AIDS Control Organisation.

Ray, Sougat, Zile Singh, and A. Banerjee. 2005. "Psychosocial Variables of Voluntary Blood Donors at Blood Bank of a Medical College." *Medical Journal Armed Forces India* 61, 2: 130–132.

Reddy, Deepa. 2007. "Good Gifts for the Common Good: Blood and Bioethics in the Market of Genetic Research." *Cultural Anthropology* 22, 3: 429–472.

———. Forthcoming (2009). "Citizens in the Commons: Blood and Genetics in the Making of the Civic." *Contributions to Indian Sociology*.

Reisz, Emma. 2004. " 'Provident' Political Economy in Indian Forests." In *Worlds of Political Economy: Knowledge and Power in the Nineteenth and Twentieth Centuries*, ed. Frank Trentmann and Martin Daunton, 115–135. London: Palgrave-Macmillan.

Roberts, Michael. 2006. "Pragmatic Action and Enchanted Worlds: A Black Tiger Rite of Commemoration." *Social Analysis* 50, 1: 73–102.

Robinson, Rowena, and Sathianathan Clarke, eds. 2003. *Religious Conversion in India: Modes, Motivations, and Meanings*. Delhi: Oxford University Press.

Roscoe, Paul B. 1988. "The Far Side of Hurun: The Management of Melanesian Millenarian Movements." *American Ethnologist* 15, 3: 515–529.

Rosin, R. Thomas. 2000. "Wind, Traffic and Dust: The Recycling of Wastes." *Contributions to Indian Sociology* 34, 3: 361–408.

———. n.d. "The Street as Public Commons: A Cross-Cultural Comparative Framework for Studying Waste and Traffic in India." Lecture given at the 7th Annual Conference of the International Association for the Study of Common Property, June 10–14, 1998, Vancouver, Canada. Available at http://www.indiana.edu/~iaspc/Drafts/rosin.pdf.

Säävälä, Minna. 2001. "Low Caste but Middle Class: Some Religious Strategies for Middle-Class Identification in Hyderabad." *Contributions to Indian Sociology* 35, 3: 293–318.

———. 2003. "Auspicious Hindu Houses. The New Middle Classes in Hyderabad, India." *Social Anthropology* 11, 2: 231–247.

Sahlins, Marshall D. 1972. "The Spirit of the Gift." In *Stone Age Economics*. Chicago: Aldine.

———. 1981. *Historical Metaphors and Mythical Realities: Structure in the Early History of the Sandwich Islands*. Ann Arbor: University of Michigan Press.

Samanta, Suchitra. 1994. "The Self-Animal and Divine Digestion: Goat Sacrifice to the Goddess Kali in Bengal." *Journal of Asian Studies* 53, 3: 779–803.

Sarkar, Tanika. 2001. *Hindu Wife, Hindu Nation: Community, Religion, and Cultural Nationalism*. London: Hurst.

Schaller, Joseph. 1995. "Sanskritization, Caste Uplift, and Social Dissidence in the Sant Ravidas Panth." In *Bhakti Religion in North India: Community Identity and Political Action*, ed. David N. Lorenzen, 94–119. Albany: State University of New York Press.

Scheper-Hughes, Nancy. 1996. "Theft of Life: The Globalization of Organ Stealing Rumours." *Anthropology Today* 12, 3: 3–11.

———. 2004. "Parts Unknown: Undercover Ethnography of the Organs-Trafficking Underworld." *Ethnography* 5, 1: 29–73.

Schomer, Karine, and W. H. McLeod. 1987. *The Sants: Studies in a Devotional Tradition of India.* Delhi: Motilal Banarsidass.

Schön, Donald. [1983] 2002. *The Reflective Practitioner: How Professionals Think in Action.* Aldershot: Ashgate.

Segal, D.A. and R. Handler. 1992. "How European is Nationalism?" *Social Analysis* 32: 1–15.

Sen, Amiya P. 2003. *Social and Religious Reform: The Hindus of British India.* Delhi: Oxford University Press.

Shah, A. M. 2006. "Sects and Hindu Social Structure." *Contributions to Indian Sociology* 40, 2: 209–248.

Shao, Jing. 2006. "Fluid Labor and Blood Money: The Economy of HIV/AIDS in Rural Central China." *Cultural Anthropology* 21, 4: 535–569.

Sharma, Arvind. 1987. "The Social Implications of Karma." In *The Dimensions of Karma,* ed. S. S. Rama Rao Pappu, 267–291. Delhi: Chanakya Publications.

———. 1998. *The Concept of Universal Religion in Modern Hindu Thought.* Basingstoke: Macmillan.

Sheth, D. L. 1996. "Changing Terms of Elite Discourse: The Case of Reservation for 'Other Backward Classes.'" In *Region, Religion, Caste, Gender and Culture in Contemporary India.* Vol. 3., ed. T. V. Sathyamurthy, 314–333. Delhi: Oxford University Press.

Simmel, Georg. [1907] 1991. *The Philosophy of Money,* trans. T. Bottomore and D. Frisby. London: Routledge.

Simpson, Bob. 2004. "Impossible Gifts: Bodies, Buddhism and Bioethics in Contemporary Sri Lanka." *Journal of the Royal Anthropological Institute* 10, 4: 839–859.

Singer, Milton. 1972. *When a Great Tradition Modernizes.* London: Pall Mall Press.

Singh, Bir, R. M. Pandey, N. D'Souza, A. Anushyanthan, V. Krishna, V. Gupta, M. M. Chaudhary, S. Ganeshan, S. Jha, S. Uppal, V. Mehrara, R. D. Deepchand, Y. Singh, K. M. Hsia, S. Bhushan, V. Anand, and A. K. Singh. 2002. "Knowledge, Attitudes, and Socio-Demographic Factors Differentiating Blood Donors from Non-Donors in an Urban Slum of Delhi." *Indian Journal of Community Medicine* 27, 3. http://www.indemedica.com/journals.php?journalid=7&issueid=41&articleid=519&action=article.

Smith, Adam. [1776] 1976. *An Inquiry into the Nature and Causes of the Wealth of Nations,* ed. Peter Cannan. Chicago: University of Chicago Press.

Smith, Donald E. 1963. *India as a Secular State.* Princeton: Princeton University Press.

Smith, Brian K. 1989. *Reflections on Resemblance, Ritual, and Religion.* Oxford: Oxford University Press.

Snodgrass, Jeffrey G. 2001. "Beware of Charitable Souls: Contagion, Roguish Ghosts and the Poison(s) of Hindu Alms." *Journal of the Royal Anthropological Institute* 7, 4: 687–704.

Spodek, Howard. 1971. "On the Origins of Gandhi's Political Methodology: The Heritage of Kathiawad and Gujarat." *Journal of Asian Studies* 30, 2: 361–372.

Srinivas, M. N. 1965. *Religion and Society among the Coorgs of South India.* Bombay: Asia.

Ssorin-Chaikov, Nikolai. 2006. "On Heterochrony: Birthday Gifts to Stalin, 1949." *Journal of the Royal Anthropological Institute* 12, 2: 355–375.

Ssorin-Chaikov, Nikolai, and Olga Sosnina. 2004. "The Faculty of Useless Things: Gifts to Soviet Leaders." In *Personality Cults in Stalinism / Personenkulte im Stalinismus,* ed. K. Heller and J. Plamper, 277–300. Göttingen: Vandenhoeck and Ruprecht.

Stafford, Charles. 1992. "Good Sons and Virtuous Mothers: Kinship and Chinese Nationalism in Taiwan." *Man* 27, 2: 363–378.

Star, Susan Leigh. 1989. "The Structure of Ill-Structured Solutions: Boundary Objects and Heterogeneous Distributed Problem Solving." In *Distributed Artificial Intelligence.* Vol. 2., ed. L. Gasser and M. Huhns, 37–54. London: Pitman.

Starr, Douglas. 1998. *Blood: An Epic History of Medicine and Commerce*. London: Warner Books.

———. 2002. "Bad Blood: The 9/11 Blood Donation Disaster." *New Republic* 227, 5: 13–16.

Stewart, Kathleen, and Susan Harding. 1999. "Bad Endings: American Apocalypsis." *Annual Review of Anthropology* 28: 285–310.

Strathern, Andrew. 1971. *The Rope of Moka: Big-Men and Ceremonial Exchange in Mount Hagen, New Guinea*. Cambridge: Cambridge University Press.

Strathern, Marilyn. 1988. *The Gender of the Gift: Problems with Women and Problems with Society in Melanesia*. London: University of California Press.

———. 1993. "Entangled Objects: Detached Metaphors." *Social Analysis* 34, 4: 88–101.

———. 1997a. "A Return to the Native." *Social Analysis* 41, 1: 15–27.

———. 1997b. "Double Standards." In *The Ethnography of Moralities*, ed. Signe Howell, 127–151. London: Routledge.

———, ed. 2000. *Audit Cultures: Anthropological Studies in Accountability, Ethics, and the Academy*. London: Routledge.

———. 2005a. "Robust Knowledge and Fragile Futures." In *Global Assemblages: Technology, Politics, and Ethics as Anthropological Problems*, ed. Aihwa Ong and Stephen J. Collier, 464–481. Oxford: Blackwell.

———. 2005b. *Kinship, Law and the Unexpected: Relatives Are Always a Surprise*. Cambridge: Cambridge University Press.

———. 2006. "Useful Knowledge." *Proceedings of the British Academy* 139: 73–109. (Isaiah Berlin Lecture).

———. n.d. (Draft). "Divided Origins and the Arithmetic of Ownership." Final version in *Kinship, Law and the Unexpected: Relatives Are Always a Surprise*, 135–161. Cambridge: Cambridge University Press.

Tagore, Rabindranath. 1912. *Gitanjali*. London: Chiswick Press.

Tarabout, Gilles. 2006. "Malabar Gods, Nation-Building and World Culture: On Perceptions of the Local and the Global." In *Globalizing India: Perspectives from Below*, ed. Jackie Assayag and Chris Fuller, 185–209. London: Anthem Press.

Tarlo, Emma. 1996 *Clothing Matters: Dress and Identity in India*. London: Hurst.

———. 2003. *Unsettling Memories: Narratives of India's "Emergency."* Delhi: Permanent Black.

Taussig, Michael. 1998. "Crossing the Face." In *Border Fetishisms: Material Objects in Unstable Spaces*, ed. Patricia Spyer, 224–243. London: Routledge.

———. 1999. *Defacement: Public Secrecy and the Labour of the Negative*. Stanford: Stanford University Press.

Titmuss, Richard M. 1970. *The Gift Relationship: From Human Blood to Social Policy*. London: LSE Books.

Uberoi, J.P.S. 1996. *Religion, Civil Society and the State: A Study of Sikhism*. Delhi: Oxford University Press.

Valentine, Kylie. 2005. "Citizenship, Identity, Blood Donation." *Body & Society* 11, 2: 113–128.

van der Veer, Peter. 1988. *Gods on Earth: The Management of Religious Experience and Identity in a North Indian Pilgrimage Centre*. London: Athlone.

———, ed. 1996. *Conversion to Modernities: The Globalization of Christianity*. New York: Routledge.

Vanaik, Achin. 1997. *The Furies of Indian Communalism: Religion, Modernity, and Secularization*. London: Verso.

Vanita, Ruth. 2002. "*Dosti* and *Tamanna*: Male-Male Love, Difference, and Normativity in Hindi Cinema." In *Everyday Life in South Asia*, ed. Diane Mines and Sarah Lamb, 146–158. Bloomington: Indiana University Press.

Varma, Pavan K. 1998. *The Great Indian Middle Classes*. Delhi: Penguin.

Vaudeville, Charlotte. 1974. *Kabir*. Vol. I. Oxford: Clarendon Press.

Vessey, David. 2002. "The Polysemy of Otherness: On Ricoeur's *Oneself as Another*." In *Ipseity and Alterity: Interdisciplinary Approaches to Intersubjectivity*, ed. Shaun Gallagher and Stephen Watson. Rouen: Presses Universitaires de Rouen.

Vicziany, Marika. 2001. "HIV/AIDS in Maharashtra: Blood, Money, Blood Banks, and Technology Transfer." *Contemporary South Asia* 10, 3: 381–414.

Vidal, Denis. 2000. "Markets and Intermediaries: An Enquiry about the Principles of Market Economy in the Grain Market of Delhi." In *Delhi: Urban Space and Human Destinies*, ed. Veronique Dupont, Emma Tarlo and Denis Vidal, 125–142. Delhi: Manohar.

———. 2006 (Draft). "*Darshan*." Available at http://www.soas.ac.uk/scasfile/keywords/denisvidal-darshan.pdf.

Vidal, Denis, Emma Tarlo, and Veronique Dupont. 2000. "The Alchemy of an Unloved City." In *Delhi: Urban Space and Human Destinies*, ed. Veronique Dupont, Emma Tarlo, and Denis Vidal, 15–28. Delhi: Manohar.

Vidal, Denis, Gilles Tarabout, and Eric Meyer, eds. 2003a. *Violence / Non-Violence: Some Hindu Perspectives*. Delhi: Manohar; Centre de Sciences Humaines.

———. 2003b. "On the Concepts of Violence and Non-Violence in Hinduism and Indian Society." In *Violence / Non-Violence: Some Hindu Perspectives*, ed. Denis Vidal, Gilles Tarabout, and Eric Meyer, 11–26. Delhi: Manohar; Centre de Sciences Humaines.

Vidal, Gore. 1997. *Myra Breckinridge / Myron*. London: Penguin.

Wagner, Roy. 1981. *The Invention of Culture*. Chicago: Chicago University Press.

Waldby, Catherine. 2000. *The Visible Human Project: Informatic Bodies and Posthuman Medicine*. London: Routledge.

———. 2002. "Stem Cells, Tissue Cultures, and the Production of Biovalue." *Health: An Interdisciplinary Journal for the Social Study of Health, Illness and Medicine* 6, 3: 305–323.

Waldby, Catherine, and Robert Mitchell. 2006. *Tissue Economies: Blood, Organs, and Cell Lines in Late Capitalism*. Durham: Duke University Press.

Warrier, Maya. 2003a. "The *Seva* Ethic and the Spirit of Institution Building in the Mata Amritanandamayi Mission." In *Hinduism in Public and Private: Reform, Hindutva, Gender and Sampraday*, ed. Antony Copley, 254–289. Delhi: Oxford University Press.

———. 2003b. "Processes of Secularization in Contemporary India: Guru Faith in the Mata Amritanandamayi Mission." *Modern Asian Studies* 37, 1: 213–253.

Watt, Carey Anthony. 2005. *Serving the Nation: Cultures of Service, Association, and Citizenship*. Delhi: Oxford University Press.

Weber, Max. 1958. *Religion of India: The Sociology of Hinduism and Buddhism*, trans. Hans H. Gerth. Glencoe, Ill.: Free Press.

Weiner, James. 1995. "Allegro and Introduction." *Social Analysis* 38, September: 5–17.

Wenger, Etienne. 1998. *Communities of Practice: Learning, Meaning, and Identity*. Cambridge: Cambridge University Press.

Weston, Kath. 2001. "Kinship, Controversy, and the Sharing of Substance: The Race/Class Politics of Blood Transfusion." In *Relative Values: Reconfiguring Kinship Studies*, ed. Sarah Franklin and Susan McKinnon, 147–174. Durham and London: Duke University Press.

White, David Gordon. 1996. *The Alchemical Body: Siddha Traditions in Medieval India*. Chicago: University of Chicago Press.

White, Luise. 2000. *Speaking with Vampires: Rumor and History in Colonial Africa*. Berkeley: University of California Press.

Whitehouse, Harvey. 2000. *Arguments and Icons: Divergent Modes of Religiosity*. Oxford: Oxford University Press.

———. 2004. "Toward a Comparative Anthropology of Religion." In *Ritual and Memory: Toward a Comparative Anthropology of Religion*, ed. Harvey Whitehouse and James Laidlaw, 187–205. Walnut Creek, Calif.: Altamira Press.

Wolfe, A. 1989. *Whose Keeper? Social Science and Moral Obligation*. Berkeley: University of California Press.

Yang, Mayfair Mei-Hui. 2000. "Putting Global Capitalism in Its Place: Economic Hybridity, Bataille, and Ritual Expenditure." *Current Anthropology* 41, 4: 477–509.

Zaloom, Caitlin. 2003. "Ambiguous Numbers: Trading Technologies and Interpretation in Financial Markets." *American Ethnologist* 30, 2: 258–272.

Žižek, Slavoj. 1999. "Fantasy as a Political Category." In *The Žižek Reader*, ed. Elizabeth Wright and Edmond Wright, 87–101. Oxford: Blackwell.

ANIRUDDHA BAPU LITERATURE

Kadu, Kantilalsinh ed. n.d. *Nirbhid Lekh*. Panvel: Matruchhaya Printers.

Sadguru Shree Upasana Trust. 2002. *Textbook of Disaster Management*. Mumbai: Sadguru Shree Upasana Trust.

DERA SACHA SAUDA LITERATURE

Dera Sacha Sauda. n.d.a. *Believe-Me-Not: Simply Incredible!!* Sirsa: Dera Sacha Sauda (HR).

———. n.d.b. *A Saga of Welfare Work for the Sea of Humanity: Shah Satnam Ji Green "S" Welfare Force Society, Dera Sacha Sauda, Sirsa*. Sirsa: Dera Sacha Sauda (HR).

———. n.d.c. *Dhan Dhan Satguru Tera Hi Aasra, The Truth*. Vol. I. DSS Video CD.

SANT NIRANKARI MISSION LITERATURE

Sagar, Kirpa. 1994. *Understanding the Sant Nirankari Mission*. Delhi: Sant Nirankari Mandal.

Sant Niranakri Mandal. 2003. *Sant Nirankari Mission: An Introduction*. Delhi: Sant Nirankari Mandal.

Singh, Amrik. n.d. *The Matchless Mission*. Delhi: Parkashan Vibhag.

Social Welfare Vibhag. n.d (Leaflet). *Religion Essentially Means God-Realization and Love for Every Human Being*. Delhi: Social Welfare Vibhag.

NEWSPAPERS AND OTHER SERIAL PUBLICATIONS

The Deccan Herald (Bangalore)
The Economic Times
Frontline (Chennai)
Ganashakti Newsmagazine (Kolkata)
The Guardian (London)
The Hindu (Chennai)
Hindustan Times (Delhi)
The Independent (London)
The Indian Express (Mumbai)
Navan Jamana
Outlook (Delhi)

Rupana Times
Sacha Kahoon (Sirsa)
The Sunday Express (Mumbai)
Taze
The Times (London)
The Times of India
The Week (Cochin)

INDEX

Adi Granth. *See* Guru Granth Sahib
AIDS. *See* HIV
Allahabad, 20, 159
Alter, Joseph, 23, 26, 90, 128, 130, 137, 146, 174, 187n16, 188n30
"alternating disequilibrium," 105, 107–108, 111. *See also* camps: competitive nature of; world records
altruism, 2, 28, 47–48, 85, 103, 107, 187n20
Ambedkar, B. R., 154–155
Amritanandamayi, Mata, 3, 84, 87, 121, 139–140, 143, 194n16, 197n27
Anagnost, Ann, 10
Anderson, Benedict, 165
Anidjar, Gil, 103
anniversaries. *See under* camps
anonymity: and "active nonpreference," 159, 161, 171; and dan, 10, 27, 115, 130, 133; and enumeration, 30, 153, 159–160, 165, 171; and facelessness, 159; as a feature of voluntary blood donation, 2, 27–32, 37, 159, 171, 185n1; and nationalism, 10, 148, 151, 153, 165–166, 171, 176; and normalization of the difference-traversing gift, 153, 166; and philanthropy, 30, 140; spiritual connotations of, 10, 49, 69, 80, 95, 100, 115, 121, 148; theory of, 10–11, 95, 151, 153, 159, 165–166; and time-space distanciation, 131, 133, 138, 148, 169, 171; and universalism, 80, 100, 151, 161; and Unknown Soldiers, 165; and violence, 132
Appadurai, Arjun, 126, 200n12
Arnold, David, 188n26
asceticism, 5, 9, 35, 56–58, 70, 88, 91, 94, 103, 117, 127–129, 135–136, 173–176, 191n4, 196n16, 204n3. *See also* "donation asceticism"
Association of Voluntary Blood Donors, West Bengal (AVBD), 16–17, 35, 70, 78, 146, 160–161, 191n13, 192n16, 194n14. *See also* Ray, Debabrata
ayurveda, 24–26, 87, 181, 188n31

Babb, Lawrence A., 7, 77, 120, 144, 193n32, 197n26, 201n17
Babu, Tapan, 199n48
Bailey, F. G., 167

Banaras, 22, 28, 42, 54
banias, 167, 170, 176, 203n34
Bapu, Aniruddha, 3, 139, 143–146, 148
Barkun, M., 201n20
Bataille, Georges, 52–53, 180
Bayer, Ronald, 164
Bayly, Susan, 22, 56, 99, 195n23
Beckerlegge, Gwilym, 56
Benei, Veronique, 163, 201n6
Bhabha, Homi, K., 67
bhakti (devotional worship), 5–8, 74, 77–80, 83–88, 114, 134–136, 143–144, 173, 176, 186n11, 193n1, 194n5, 200n3
Bharadwaj, Aditya, 37
Bharatiya Janata Party (BJP), 70, 155, 163, 189n40, 198n36. *See also* Hindutva
bioavailability, 9, 133, 183, 186n14
biomedicine, 3, 20, 23, 26, 28, 77, 89, 91–92, 97–98, 103, 111, 132, 147–148, 176, 180–183
biomorality, 101
biopolitics, 9, 183
biosociality, 37
biospirituality, 9, 132, 147, 182–183, 186n13, 195n21
biotechnology. *See* technology
blessings, 1, 7, 41–42, 45–46, 49, 58, 62–63, 74, 78, 82, 85, 87–93, 96–97, 101–103. *See also* karma; merit
blood banks, 1–2, 4, 10–20, 22–23, 32–34, 39, 41, 43, 59–61, 65, 78–79, 89, 91, 100, 103–104, 107, 120–121, 152, 158, 162, 167, 170–171, 187n20, 189n2, 192n16, 203n30; as a sacred setting, 69, 72–76
blood component separation, 29, 37–40, 42, 46, 48, 163–164, 179, 189n2; apheresis mode of, 177–178; and merit/auspiciousness, 41–43, 45–46, 49, 177–179, 182; and nationalism, 164–165, 168, 179; and meditation/ yoga, 178
blood donation: family-replacement, 2, 10–13, 27–34, 37, 48, 85, 89, 99, 111, 140, 159, 161, 171–172, 185n2, 185n3, 188n22, 189n35, 193n3; paid, 2, 13, 27, 32–33, 83, 89–90, 93, 151, 167, 185n2, 187n18, 189n39; voluntary (nonremunerated), 1–4, 8, 10–16, 18, 19–21, 25, 27–35, 37, 46–49, 69, 72, 76, 78, 83–85, 89–90, 93, 95, 99–101, 104, 111–112, 130, 132–134, 140–141, 147–148, 151–154, 158–161,

227

ABOUT THE AUTHOR

Jacob Copeman is a research fellow in social anthropology at Jesus College, Cambridge University, England.